ACCLAIM FOR QUANTITATIVE MEDICINE

Quantitative Medicine Is a Complete Healthcare System__

Quantitative Medicine is a step-by-step guide to peak health. Degenerative diseases such as cancer, heart disease, adult onset diabetes, osteoporosis, and even aging can be held at bay or even reversed. This guide shows you how to assess your own health using simple blood tests and, more importantly, how to change your lifestyle to attain optimum health. This methodology has been used successfully by several thousand people over the last twenty years. Every single person has gotten better—many markedly so.

People Who Have Used Quantitative Medicine Say_____

Over the past ten years I have rigorously adopted the lifestyle and approach to diet and exercise outlined in *Quantitative Medicine*. My appearance and overall health are better than 25 years ago. At times I feel I have found "the fountain of youth" in Dr. Mike Nichols's scientific approach to not only improving but, in my case, totally eliminating lifestyle diseases. Thank God I found QM before it was too late!

——R Michael Miller, Insurance Executive

Dr. Mike's *Quantitative Medicine* really has changed my life. After my first heart attack I followed the broadly recommended "standard" medical advice, only to have a second heart attack within two years. A good friend recommended Dr. Mike and his Quantitative Medicine approach. Diet change + effective physical and spiritual exercise = new healthy life. Side benefits are: feeling years younger, stronger and happier (even lost 25 lbs, though that was not a specific objective).

——Dave Saxby, Silicon Valley Entrepreneur

This book connects the dots between lifestyle choices and health at the cellular level and makes it crystal clear why we should care. In the process it delivers terrific motivation to put that newly found knowledge to work.

——Ken Goldman. Silicon Valley Venture Capitalist

A Doctor's View of Dr. Nichols_____

Dr. Mike Nichols, a true medical visionary, was at the forefront of advocating lifestyle changes for the treatment and prevention of diseases since the 1990s. His brilliant and pioneering work in combining healthy nutrition, regular exercise, meditation, and adequate rest was years ahead of the mainstream thinking of practicing physicians and even of widely acclaimed national specialty organizations. He has seen significant improvement in clinical outcomes of his patients: in improved exercise tolerance, hypertension control, weight loss, diabetes control, lipid management, and general well-being.

I met Dr. Nichols in the 1990s. He was a mentor to me, and I incorporated much of his teachings in my own practice of Preventive Cardiology.

Dr. Nichols is that rare physician who combines in-depth scientific knowledge with a caring commitment and connection to his patients, thus bringing about extraordinary positive changes both physically and emotionally. He is a true "healer."

——Michael R. Nagel, MD, MPA, FACC
  Board Certified Cardiologist

Patients Views of Dr. Nichols_____

Mike is an incredible physician. He understands in great detail how the body works. He implements a medical practice based on the fact that the body can heal itself through proper diet, exercise and relaxation. This frequently means that drugs are replaced by exercise and dietary recommendations to deal with degenerative diseases. Best of all this treatment makes you feel young and vigorous again, much more so than you can imagine. It is amazing.

——Louise Wholey, Adventurer

Dr. Mike was 20 years ahead of his time 10 years ago. If you are interested in recruiting your body's natural potential to be and stay healthy *without* pills, let him be your guide.

——Ken Okin, Consulting Architect

QUANTITATIVE MEDICINE

A COMPLETE GUIDE TO
GETTING WELL
STAYING WELL
AVOIDING DISEASE
SLOWING AGING

Mike Nichols, MD
Charles Davis, PhD

GOLDEN LOTUS PUBLISHING   PALO ALTO, CALIFORNIA

QUANTITATIVE MEDICINE
Copyright © 2016 by
Mike Nichols and Charles Davis.

For information contact:
qm-info@goldenlotuspublishing.com

ISBN: 978-0-9862520-0-6

First Edition: February 2016

10 9 8 7 6 5 4 3 2 1

ACKNOWLEDGMENTS BY MIKE NICHOLS

I live in an amazing place and have amazing patients. Well, that is two uses of the word "amazing," and I've barely scratched the surface of amazement and gratitude I feel for getting to do the work I do.

All doctors see sorrow and suffering in the lives of their patients, and all of us were trained to see our role as dispensers of drugs. For some reason I felt this was not the best medicine.

My patients—thank you patients!—smart and hardworking to a fault, wanted more and expected me to deliver.

This book is the first step in delivering what they expected: a clear path to health.

Mike Nichols, 2016

DEDICATION

Dedicated to Jim and Anne Sorden AMDG

ACKNOWLEDGMENTS BY CHARLES DAVIS

Two years ago, I embarked on a project of recording and explaining the amazing and powerful methods of Dr. Mike Nichols: those of Quantitative Medicine. My sole objective was to spread the word, to make this knowledge accessible to all. I have been very fortunate in my 70 years, but ultimately, nothing matters more than health. Mine is excellent, and likely to remain so. For this I thank Dr. Mike, for without his guidance, this would not be the case. But he did not heal me. He empowered me. He taught me how to harness the healing resources of my own body. Resources that were already there, waiting. My hope is that Quantitative Medicine will make this priceless information available to everyone. No one needs to get sick.

Quantitative Medicine, though, would not have become a reality without the help of many, and I apologize for omissions I have surely made. Thanks first go to my wife, Liên Nguyen, for patience, advice, and very thorough editing. To Camille Davis of CamilleMaiIllustration.com for her wonderful illustrations. To Tahlia Day for excellent, precise, and thorough proofreading. To John Houchin, Mack Diltz, and Bernard Yosten for their early reviews and critiques of the book. To Dollie Davis, Sue Davis, Mélodie Davis, and Joan Murray for their assistance and encouragement.

Charles Davis 2016.

CONTENTS

PART I - CONTROLLING YOUR HEALTH

HOW YOUR BODY CAN PREVENT DISEASE AND AGING

1 - DEGENERATIVE DISEASE

There is no need to die from age-related diseases, yet 70% of us do. Included here are cancer, adult onset diabetes, heart disease, dementia, and several others. Sometimes these are called degenerative diseases, sometimes chronic diseases.

We can completely prevent all of these. We can reverse most of them. The tools are all there, inside each of us. Evolution gathered them for us. Evolution is continually at work, remodeling all of life, discarding items that proved useless, retaining those that aided survival. At this point we have amassed an enormous collection of healing and repair processes. Those that repair DNA date all the way back to bacteria. Processes fighting cancer are found in the earliest animals. The ones cleaning arteries emerged with the appearance of the vertebrates, a relatively recent development. In the countless eons of our past, this diverse and complex collection of repair and replacement processes has accumulated—layer upon layer. But what to call it? It's no single system, but an evolutionary parade of healing mechanisms and processes that began with the inception of life itself.

This collection is far more powerful than any drugs or surgeries conjured up by our wizards of medicine. For those whose habits or actions engage these processes, age-related diseases rarely occur, and aging itself is slow. These people don't get sick. They stay energetic and healthy, with fewer aches and pains and more exuberance. But they are the minority. For most of us it isn't working. All these disease prevention mechanisms and processes are failing. They are not preventing degenerative disease.

What went wrong?

Any living thing is the accumulation of that which went before, and we are, of course, strongly adapted to the human condition, or rather, what it had been for the last few million years. Evolution, however sure, creeps forward with a glacial step. It deals poorly with abrupt change, which is unfortunate, because the agricultural revolution, which began only 10,000 years ago, so thoroughly upended our lifestyle that we have only begun to catch up.

What began then, eventually spreading worldwide, was an abrupt shift from a million-year history of an irregular protein and fat diet, a lifestyle involving fierce bursts of activity, to a new type of starch-based diet, and a sedentary, though arduous, sort of life. In the preceding million years, we had successfully endured a huge confusion of ordeals and misfortunes, and were well adapted to deal with any of them, but the changes that arrived with the agricultural revolution were new, never seen before, and our wonderfully evolved health management systems and processes didn't know what to do with them—*and they still don't.*

This should be an era of ease and plenty. And in many ways it is that, but a strange paradox intervenes, casting an unexpected gloom: *all this abundance and ease convinces our body that it should prepare for a famine.* We will shortly explain the survival logic at work here, but as part of this famine preparation, all "unnecessary" processes are shut down, including much of the degenerative disease prevention. This has the unintended consequence of opening the gates and giving these diseases free rein.

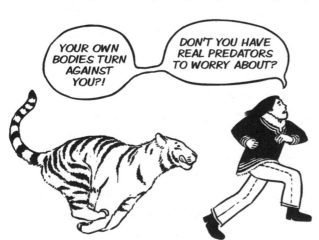

This is certainly an odd and unfortunate conclusion for our body to reach. How could unprecedented wealth and ease take such a sinister turn?

In all of us, there is a survival point of view operating behind the scenes, forcing a life script we cannot escape. It holds us to its ancient logic, a logic driven by survival, and despite the obsolescence of such primordial concerns, the unseen parts of us that manage energy and healing still heed the rules and remnants of those times long past.

Simply put, our body thinks we're starving, or about to. And its logic? We aren't doing the right things: we aren't hunting or gathering. Worse, we are eating food that normally would become available only before the cold, lean winter. The agricultural revolution immersed us quite suddenly into this new mode of life, and our body—the unseen part that manages energy and healing—is only just beginning, after all this time, to sort it all out.

Impressed firmly in our inner clockworks are certain constant rules, etched there by millions of years of life experience:

- To get food, you must hunt or gather. If you aren't doing this, the logical reason is that there is no food available.
- If you are getting anything sweet or starchy, it is late summer and a cold and hard winter lies ahead.

With food running out and winter approaching, perhaps an ice age one, survival is key. Best to store the immediate food supply as fat. Reduce energy levels. Put off anything that can wait for a time of plenty. Put off repair, healing, and replacement. Save these for another day.

The agricultural revolution has become the agricultural institution and we can never return to the old ways, nor would most of us want to. But can we construct a link back to the prior health? Can we convince our archaic inner processes to use the energy we consume to heal, and not store it as fat? Convince it to enable again all these powerful repair mechanisms? The answer is yes, and Quantitative Medicine will show how.

THE NATURE OF DEGENERATIVE DISEASE

Infectious disease involves an invader—a virus or bacteria perhaps. It invaded via a cut or by eating bad food and then spread. The immune system fights back, usually successfully. Once the disease is fought off, the invader is gone, having been fully annihilated.

Degenerative diseases are different. They are occurring continuously, starting from birth. The immune system fights them as well, but it's not always clear who has the upper hand. These diseases have a tipping point nature. Cancer is a good example. We have an astronomical number of cells—something like 50 followed by twelve 0's—not a number we can easily contemplate. At any given time, some millions of these cells are defective in some way. This is a lot of cells, but it is a very small percentage of the grand total. The immune system monitors for this, and will kill off these errant cells. However, some may malfunction in a cancerous sort of way. They may start aggressively dividing and growing, and if the immune system doesn't catch it, a new tumor has begun. Even so, the immune system will usually get on the job and kill the newly-formed tumor. But if it doesn't, the tumor will keep growing and a cancer can result.

Here we have bad cells pushing against the immune system. Who will win? On one side, we have the number of errant cells. If the number is low, problems are less likely. This can vary a lot. Smokers will have 20 times as many damaged cells in their lungs as nonsmokers. We also accumulate more defective cells as we age. On the other side, how active is the immune system? If the body is healthy and energetic, the immune system will likely be in a similar condition. A weakened immune system, however, might not be able to prevent a budding cancer from taking hold.

This same sort of tension seems to be typical of all degenerative diseases. Something is promoting them within the body, and some other process is trying to prevent them or repair the damage. The progression of the disease depends on the balance between the intensity of the assault and the body's ability to push it back. These two are locked into a sort of death spiral. If the assault succeeds, the body's ability to push back is diminished. Things then spin quickly out of control. They can spin the other way as well; anything that reduces the level of assault will increase the body's ability to fight back. So, being partly sick isn't a very stable situation. It will likely get worse or better—a tipping point situation.

Throughout the book, we tend to lump heart disease, cancer, and adult onset diabetes together; yet these seem like very different diseases. They are, of course, in their final manifestations, but their origins share a common ground. Something is amiss and off balance. At the microscopic level, various sorts of normal cellular trash—free radicals, products of oxidation, and other potentially damaging things—are allowed to accumulate, cause problems, and instigate inflammation. At this level, all degenerative disease is interrelated. One disease or another is taking hold because the usual processes—processes that are otherwise more than capable of rolling it back—are inhibited. Some of us are more prone to cancer, or heart disease, or some other diseases, but none of these need happen if the body's defenses are fully engaged.

WHO GETS SICK? WHO IS SPARED?

How can we know for certain that degenerative disease can be avoided? There are at least some identifiable groups that get almost none of these diseases. They are known as hunter-gatherers. You may be surprised to hear that there are any still around, but perhaps as many as 200 tribes are scattered here and there, in various isolated places. One island group off the coast of India is a complete unknown. Potential visitors, helicopters, and passing ships are all met with volleys of arrows.

Research into more accommodating tribes has been going on for at least a century, and a common thread runs through it all: members of hunter-gatherer societies rarely get cancer, heart disease, or other degenerative diseases. This contrasts sharply with our world, where 70% of us now die from one of these. This almost total absence among the hunter-gatherers strongly suggests that degenerative disease is not inevitable.

A hundred years ago, there were far more hunter-gatherer tribes, and much more isolation. There are numerous reports from various explorers and missionary doctors. From Albert Schweitzer, *"On my arrival in Gabon [1910], I was astonished to encounter no cases of cancer. I cannot, of course, say positively that there was no cancer at all, but, like other frontier doctors, I can only say that if any cases existed they must have been quite rare."* These sorts of medical surprises seem to have been the rule. Cancer, diabetes, and other diseases were nowhere to be found in the hunter-gatherer populations. There are a variety of references to hunter-gatherer health in the annotated bibliography.

Suppose we were to dive in and join a hunter-gatherer tribe today. Would that reverse degenerative disease? Apparently, the answer is yes! It is reported that various members of Australian Aboriginal tribes moved to the cities, and soon became afflicted with the various "modern" diseases. Some of these people saw the light and moved back to the bush, and within a short period of time, their newly acquired diseases disappeared.

Ideally, we'd like to achieve a healthy state that will reduce disease risk without becoming a hunter-gatherer, and that is what Quantitative Medicine is all about. But how far do we have to go? The French, for instance, have a much lower rate of heart disease—the lowest in the world actually (not counting the hunter-gatherers). Eating like the French wouldn't necessarily be such an ordeal.

What's underlying all of this? The body tightly regulates and controls internal processes like heart rate and hormone levels, or at least it tries to. Body temperature is a good example, but just about everything else is controlled as well. Testosterone, glucose, cholesterol, cortisol, insulin, and fat are other examples. All of these highly-regulated circulating hormones, biochemicals, particles, and molecules largely define your health. If your body is able to regulate these into their proper ranges, you will be healthy. If they are out of whack, your health may be compromised; degenerative disease can, and probably will, occur. This should seem odd. If these things are controlled, wouldn't they be controlled for our benefit, and so wouldn't degenerative diseases somehow be eliminated?

The short answer is: it's trying, but we have pulled things so far away from their natural primordial ranges, that it can't. The body is trying to get these levels under control, but it is simply overwhelmed by a diet that it has never learned to deal with. Almost all adult onset diabetics have dangerous blood sugar and insulin levels. This is primarily due to diet. Similar lifestyle attributes are strongly associated with the other degenerative diseases. The body can maintain a very healthy state and prevent these diseases, but, in a variety of ways, our modern lifestyle prevents it from doing so.

This is by no means a new notion. It occasionally shows up in the medical literature as the "discordance hypothesis," but so far this idea hasn't gotten much traction in the popular press.

But what about genetics? One would suppose that genetics must play a large role. Consider the Japanese. Their rates of both heart disease and cancer are much lower than those of Americans. It would be quite reasonable here to assume genetics was somehow protecting the Japanese, but this view fails to hold up: Japanese-Hawaiians generally follow the American diet and get disease at the American rate. So, looking at large groups, genetics seems to be less important. However, at the individual level, genetics clearly does make a difference. So, as is usual with nature versus nurture arguments, the conclusion is both.

For our purposes, lifestyle would seem to be by far the more important. First, genetics obviously can't be changed. Second, when whole groups of people are considered, the statistics are pretty overwhelming. Hunter-gatherers get almost no degenerative diseases, but for the rest of the planet, 70% die from these. 0% versus 70%. This is a huge difference, and points very strongly to lifestyle. Hunter-gatherers are not genetically different. In fact, when these "immune" hunter-gatherers are assimilated into our world, they rapidly begin to develop all our degenerative diseases as well.

Other than some specific situations, like celiac disease, you should view genetics, especially your own, as a predisposition, and no more than that. We may indeed be taller, shorter, skinnier, fatter, blonder, or whatever, but degenerative disease is different. We are NOT destined to get these diseases because of genetics. If we were, hunter-gatherers would get them too, but they don't. Since we have the same genetic mix, we don't have to get these diseases either. Let degenerative disease in, and some will get heart disease, others cancer. That's the role of genetics. If degenerative disease gets no foothold, genetics has little role to play.

QUANTITATIVE MEDICINE

Our ancient ancestors had an unbroken continuity of knowledge of the Earth: their Earth, their world, and their relationship with it. Sometimes this would mean difficult times, but not always. Often life was leisurely. They had evolved with what their world offered; they survived and thrived. Robust health was part of that life. Civilization dissolved the connection, and in a health sense, we are now cut loose and adrift.

Quantitative Medicine bridges that gap, which, by this point, has evolved into more of a chasm. Most of us don't want to return to a hunter-gatherer way of life, but there are other routes to the ideal healthy state—peak health. This is a goal well worth the pursuit. In this ideal state of health, degenerative disease is pushed back, held at bay, and aging is slow. This is the good life.

All those enjoying peak health have certain attributes in common with each other. These attributes are evident in biological markers, many of which will be familiar: blood pressure, glucose, triglycerides, etc. For these healthy people, all such measurements are in the same desirable ranges.

This is quite surprising if you think about it. It means a healthy Inuit and a healthy Australian bush man, people from opposite corners of the world, with vastly different diets, will have similar numbers. Odd indeed, but true.

Even more amazing is that it works both ways. If you can somehow push your own numbers to these healthy zones—push them there without the help of drugs—you will be healthy too, and degenerative disease will retreat. So besides being a universal measure of health—well worldwide anyway—these numbers are also the *levers* of health. Push or pull them all to their ideal zones and good health is yours. If some areas aren't right though, degenerative disease has a route in. The changes needed vary considerably from person to person, but the ideal numbers are the same for everybody. Knowing quite precisely which numbers are the key ones, what they should be for peak health, and how to drive them there is the essence of Quantitative Medicine.

Here is the simple premise Quantitative Medicine offers: if a person's numbers are in these ideal ranges, they won't get degenerative disease and they will age slowly. Further, no matter what condition someone is in now, or in what state of disease, if their numbers are driven to their ideal ranges, disease will stop occurring, and in many cases, existing disease will reverse.

So by measuring, you can determine your health, and also see how far it is from ideal. Quantitative Medicine explains exactly how to do this. Once you measure, you will know all your numbers, and you can then devise a lifestyle strategy to push those measurements into the ideal ranges. Quantitative Medicine is able to tell you how to do this too.

Quantitative Medicine is a complete health management system. Follow its suggestions and protocols and the risk for degenerative disease is very low. As far as degenerative disease prevention goes, it is complete. It alone is all you need. It has little use for supplements, vitamins, antioxidants, whole grain, high colonics, vegan diets, lotions, magic crystals, or the like. The tools to prevent disease lie entirely within oneself, but since everyone is different, the "best" lifestyle choices are unique to each of us.

Everyone is quite capable of maintaining pristine health into very old age. The body knows how to handle a wide variety of environments and lifestyles. Unfortunately, our "civilized" lifestyle appears to be a major exception, at least for many. We are still largely a product of what went on a million years earlier.

What Exactly Is Lifestyle

Clearly we're not talking about Versace versus Armani, or urban versus rural living. We mean the way you "style" your life from a health perspective. This may include many things, but the four to be explored in detail are:

- **Nutrition**. Which parts of your diet are improving your specific health, and which are damaging it.
- **Exercise**. Which types are best, what they help, why they help, and which should be avoided.
- **Spiritual Discipline or Meditation**. Reducing stress. High stress has huge negative health implications.
- **Sleep**. The ideal amount and its importance.

If all four of these lifestyle elements are right—right for you, that is—the risk of degenerative disease will be low, and you can look forward to a long healthy life. However, what is right varies from person to person, and determining this and acting on it through lifestyle change are the main purposes of Quantitative Medicine.

How Can We Know Our Own Health?

This mismatch between the ideal and the actual affects different people in different ways. For instance, can you eat grain? Or does it cause problems? Measure. If your numbers are OK, then eating grain is OK. Enjoy your grain. If the numbers are not OK, we can usually predict the dietary changes needed to correct them. This may mean cutting down on grain or eating more protein or different fats. So, try it and see. "Quantify" yourself.

Quantitative Medicine works, and works well. This methodology has been refined and used on some 2,000 patients in Dr. Nichols's practice over the last 20 years. The results have been dramatic, and the method can be used by almost anyone. It is straightforward, and it will be explained step-by-step in PART II of this book.

All degenerative diseases are interrelated. They are all manifestations of basically the same problem: our civilization has evolved in a way that damages our health. In this sense, our civilization itself is the disease. It creates an imbalance that allows these various degenerative diseases to advance, each in their own insidious way. Restore the balance, and they all retreat.

If we could know exactly what we should eat and how we should exercise, there would be little need for Quantitative Medicine. Many people *think* they are healthy, but this is usually self-deception. The abundant diet and physically undemanding life that our modern civilization has blessed us with *causes* 70% of us to die from degenerative disease. Yet, we don't see this connection until it is pointed out to us. These diseases are preventable, avoidable, but no fixed regime, no standard diet will work, at least not for everybody. There is an imperative need to quantify—to measure exact levels first—and then design a lifestyle that will optimize them.

The earlier that health is quantified, the better. The information needed is available via blood tests and scans. You may already have some such results. You will find out how to interpret these various numbers in PART II, and, more importantly, how to modify them. By doing so, you can, and will, improve your health. This is Quantitative Medicine in action. If your numbers are put right, the prevention and repair processes will be engaged, you will be energetic, disease will be pushed back, and aging will be slow. This is the good life! All factors that may be inhibiting the body's disease-fighting ability can be fixed with lifestyle changes.

How Did We Drift So Far Off Track?

Beliefs attempt to impose understanding and order on our chaotic world, a world largely beyond our control. Without some system of beliefs, we would be largely adrift, undirected, unfocused. Governments, schools, religions, and business interests constantly exploit this by supplying us with their preferred versions. This works. We adopt many of these beliefs, though this is not always in our best interest (to put it mildly). These beliefs may have a presumed basis in fact, or possibly not; they are at least thought to be true. The quality of the facts underpinning these beliefs varies enormously.

The biology of even the simplest creature still guards far more secrets than it has divulged. Scale this up to the level of a human being, and the problem compounds almost without measure. Though airs of deep knowledge and comprehension are cultivated by the learned classes, the true understanding of human biology is so shallow that beliefs overwhelmingly dominate (though often given the credence of established scientific fact). Much current medical wisdom is just belief. But good or bad, these beliefs tend to persist, often long after it is clear that people are being harmed.

You may already be managing your health according to a set of beliefs and you might do well to analyze them. For each of the things you are or aren't currently doing, things that could affect your health, ask yourself, "Why do I believe this is good for me?"

Some of the things you believe will be true, but others not. Some may apply to the general public, but not to you. Some may reflect older medical thinking that has since been revised. And of course—we are all human—some of our beliefs are there because we earnestly wish them to be.

There is absolutely no need to have a set of beliefs regarding your own health that is anything other than fact based. Health is entirely quantifiable. Though complex, health is not a "chaotic world largely beyond our control." Whatever the source of these beliefs, with measurement they can be tested, and then corrected, improved, or tossed out as necessary.

Health beliefs frequently come from government, business, or our own wishful thinking.

Here is a U.S. government-generated belief: "The food pyramid is how you should eat." The reality is this. The food pyramid is a high-starch diet. For 30-50% of the population, this is going to cause obesity and increase the risk of adult onset diabetes and heart disease. In fact, it already has.

An industry-generated belief: "Eat whole grain." This is an attempt to save high-profit grain-based products like cereal. While whole grain

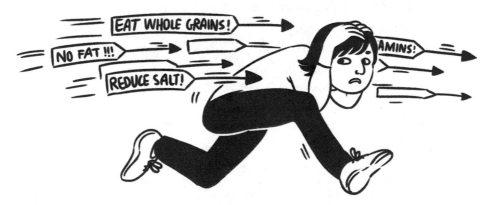

is slightly better than refined grain, the real question is, "Should you be eating grain at all?"

Wishful thinking belief: "Jeanne Calment lived to 122 and was a smoker. (True!) Therefore smoking couldn't be bad for you."

So as a preliminary step, try to put all your medical opinions and beliefs on hold, at least for now. After you have finished the book, or PART II at least, you can reassess. At that point, you will be far better informed, both about health in general and about your own specifically.

Quite a lot of the medical wisdom that has been drummed into our heads for the last 50 years is either useless or patently false. Here is a list of false medical folklore we plan to lay asunder:

- Saturated fat is bad for you.
- Foods with cholesterol should be avoided.
- Overweight is unhealthy.
- Skinny is healthy.
- High cholesterol is very risky.
- Low-fat diets are healthy.
- Whole grains are good for you.
- Red meat is bad for you.
- An hour of mild aerobic exercise daily is good for you.
- Statins should be prescribed for those with even a slight risk of heart disease.

Every single one of these is provably false. Many of these "beliefs" were generated to serve some agenda—typically not our own. You may have believed in at least a couple of these. No one can wholly escape the media barrage.

A few things that are true:

- Trans fats are bad (except those naturally occurring).
- Smoking is bad.
- Alcohol in excess of one or two drinks a day is bad.
- Rapidly changing weight, up or down, is bad.
- Not exercising is bad.
- Grass-fed meat and organic food are a lot better for you.
- Poor sleep is very unhealthy.
- Chronic stress is very unhealthy.
- Fat does not make you fat.

Key Points
1 - Degenerative Disease
- Currently 70% die from degenerative disease, cancer, heart disease, etc.
- The body can prevent all of this, leading to a long disease-free life.
- Modern lifestyle thwarts this repair and renewal process.
- The status of our own repair and renewal processes can be measured.
- This status can be changed through lifestyle modification.
- This book gives you all the tools you need to do this.

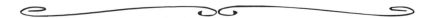

2 - HEALTH IS CONTROLLED

Why are we the way we are? We are the accumulation of what worked in the past. Things that didn't work, and the creatures that embodied them, were left behind. Natural selection is not sentimental. We descend from an unbroken line of vertebrates that successfully reproduced: perhaps 100 million consecutive generations. Quite a run! According to Richard Dawkins' fascinating book, *The Ancestor's Tale,* we are 22 species removed from the earliest vertebrate, a primitive and especially ugly eel-like thing called a hagfish.

This slimy creature oozed onto the scene around 500 million years ago, and 22 species later, here we are. That's about 25 million years per species. We parted company with the chimpanzee *only* seven million years ago. Evolution is in no hurry. We have little in common with the hagfish, but a lot in common with the chimp. However, one interesting brain organ shared by all three is the hypothalamus, which is the master regulator, and seems largely driven by survival. It is the hypothalamus that is controlling and regulating all those healing processes mentioned earlier. For the hagfish, and quite a few species that followed, this was about all the brain there

15

was. It is still the command center, and it has been on the job for 500 million years, so it's had quite a while to hone its skills.

Survival depends on many things. There are the obvious, like predator avoidance, as well as a large number of internal items, such as managing metabolism, sleep, cell repair, and renewal. These are all very complex and interconnected processes, even in the lowly hagfish. Given our impressively long record of reproductive success, we may reasonably assume that we have a very well developed and sophisticated hypothalamus. Natural selection effectively guarantees this for us.

EVERYTHING HAS A REASON

Living things, especially humans, are incredibly complex, and from an evolutionary point of view, little has been left to chance. Whatever features improved survival were nurtured, managed, and optimized. Unnecessary abilities were usually jettisoned as excess baggage because they used precious energy (food). Maybe it would be better to say that everything at least *had* a reason, as some things, such as the appendix, linger on with no apparent one. But to understand most bodily processes, the key is survival. Whatever is happening is happening because at some point in the past, it made a positive difference to our survival chances.

Survival usually implies economy. New features often cost energy, and for most of our 500 million years, energy—meaning food—has not been plentiful. For any new feature to make sense, it had to improve overall survival. Any additional cost had to be more than offset by the additional advantage the new feature conveyed.

We used to be able to make our own vitamins. But since we were getting them from food anyway, why waste energy making them on our own? Thus, this ability was lost. Though it might have come in handy to hang on to our vitamin-making skills, apparently it wasn't "cost effective."

Our big brains use a lot of energy. Are they worth it? Apparently, by

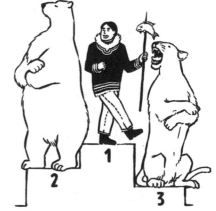

TOP LAND PREDATORS

using them, we could figure out ways to get enough additional food to power them. In fact, primarily because of our big brains, we became the most successful predator in history. We left Africa and thrived everywhere we went. No animal, small or large, slow or fast, was safe from us. And if today's hunter-gatherers are any indication, we were so efficient at it that it was practically a part-time activity. As we were becoming the apex predator, our primate cousins were, and still are, swinging from the trees, hoping to hold on to their unique habitats. So, the investment in brains definitely paid off. (Curiously, Neanderthals had slightly bigger brains.)

Energy management remains the big story, though. To conserve energy, our body will actually tear down bone and muscle if there is a food shortage. It will even do so if it *thinks* a shortage is coming.

EVERYTHING IS CONTROLLED AND REGULATED

By regulated, we mean something is set to a certain level. Body temperature is regulated to 98.6 °F. For this to occur, three items must be present:

1. Something called the "regulator" has to "know" that 98.6 °F is the "right" temperature (called the set-point).
2. This regulator has to be able to measure the body's temperature (called the monitor or sensor).
3. Finally the regulator has to be able to appropriately push the temperature up or down in order to drive it to the 98.6 °F set-point (has to be able to control).

Almost every key bodily function, hormone, cycle, response, and so on, is regulated, much of it tightly. Body temperature is highly regulated in birds and mammals. This has a huge energy cost, and both have evolved some form of insulation to help deal with it. Cholesterol is also tightly regulated, as are glucose, insulin, thyroxin, triglycerides, fat storage, sleep cycles, onset of puberty, rate of aging, and literally hundreds more. And regulated to a single end: to maximize the chances of survival. So summarizing:

- Everything has a survival-oriented reason.
- Everything is controlled and regulated.

It is the hypothalamus that is managing these two items. It is a little brain with a big agenda. Most of the controlling processes are located there, and its main concern is survival.

Soon, we will explain how the various aspects of modern civilization challenge the regulatory ability of our body, and force it into a state where it cannot maintain optimum health and energy levels. The net result is an imbalanced low-energy situation, which vastly increases risk of heart disease, cancer, adult onset diabetes, Alzheimer's, arthritis, osteoporosis, fat accumulation, and accelerated aging. Perhaps imbalanced isn't the right word. Overloaded might be a better choice. In either case, the body is attempting to react to the situation it finds itself in. The problem is that it is reacting in a way that doesn't make sense, given our modern conditions, but that indeed did make sense for the millions of years that came before. We can't change how the body reacts, but we can certainly change *what* it reacts to. By choosing this properly, we can restore the body's ability to maintain health and energy. Degenerative disease doesn't have to be the inevitable outcome.

We could add the obvious: all this survival optimization is glacially slow. It isn't really clear why that is best, as sometimes things change rapidly. Plants and animals that can't adapt become extinct, and 99.99% of the living things that evolution has hatched so far have indeed done so. Of course, extinction of one (dinosaurs) creates opportunities for others (us). Maybe it is survival in a larger sense. Life itself goes on.

THE HYPOTHALAMUS

The hypothalamus arrived with the vertebrates. A huge variety of regulation and control functions seem to have been gathered together and installed in it. It can't directly cause you to flex a muscle, but, interestingly, it knows if you do. It also continuously measures all the circulating biochemicals and hormones, and is constantly making adjustments. It has outbound nerves going to several other organs, and completely controls a tiny hormone factory called the pituitary gland, which is located directly beneath it.

We would probably benefit if we had a greater awareness of its ideas and actions. What would it have to tell us . . .

INTERVIEWER: What are you called?

HYPOTHALAMUS: I don't have a name. I live under the Thalamus so they named me Under Thalamus, but they changed it to Greek so it would sound fancier.

INTERVIEWER: So what is it you do, exactly?

HYPOTHALAMUS: Ask me instead what I don't do. I regulate and control metabolism, digestion, fat storage, energy level, sleep, puberty, fight-or-flight. I maintain your health. I control renewal and repair. I can order up a fix for almost anything. I can slow aging to a crawl. I can ...

INTERVIEWER: And you have no name? Incredible. Sounds like you're the Big Cheese.

HYPOTHALAMUS: I like it. Big Cheese. Call me that. Actually, let's translate it into Greek. Sounds more impressive. From now on call me Megalotyri. And tell that lumbering neocortex to show more respect. How am I supposed to keep things in order with all the messes it makes. . .

INTERVIEWER: OK, OK, thanks. Now, for the weather. . .

Would we really want conscious awareness of that little scold? Maybe, maybe not, but we'd best keep it happy. Though our "Megalotyri" is a bit of a stuffed shirt, it is only exaggerating slightly. It is definitely in charge of metabolism and energy management. It very directly decides what to do with the food you eat: whether to burn it or store it as fat. It decides whether or not to burn the fat you already have. It controls your sleep, overall energy, whether cells repair or degrade, whether muscle or bone is built or torn down, and so on. It decides the levels for many of the hormones and other circulating biochemicals, and tightly regulates several of them. It has numerous timers: some daily ones that manage sleep cycles, one for the menstrual cycle. It even decides when to start puberty.

The hypothalamus does not control your conscious self, though it can certainly affect your mood, alertness, pep, etc., but these are consequences of its actions, not an attempted takeover. You do have free will. You can do that which pleases the hypothalamus, or that which thwarts it. In this way, you affect some control over it. The hypothalamus is strong-willed, but pretty predictable.

Dr. Mike's Philosophical Sidebar
Paleo This, Cro-Magnon That

Many of you will have heard one version or another of "mankind is old and our diet is new and it is killing us." And, basically, it is true. Virtually all the world was colonized by our genetic ancestors over 20,000 years ago, and they survived until the end of the last Great Ice Age, about 10,000 years ago. Then "they" became "us." Out of deserts mountains, out of ice and snow and struggle, emerged a fast, strong, intelligent, highly athletic King of All Jungles, King of All Mountains, the mankind we know today. Out of such places and times emerged pretty much our entire genome and our entire metabolic heritage.

There are numerous theories of genetic change and drift, but no version gives a plausible account of why we should eat sugar or starch—frankly, because almost none of those things existed in the 50,000-year history of our ancestors.

So what? Well, the body always makes sense, and so it makes sense that eating these things might not be good for us. Thus the rise of agriculture, and I mean sufficient agriculture for grains to become a large part of our caloric base, is clearly associated with diabetes, coronary artery disease, and the like. As primitive cultures rise out of the dietary level of subsistence, they start developing degenerative diseases like diabetes. It seems fashionable to blame the Western Diet for the rise of diabetes in India, China, and elsewhere; it is not the Western Diet, but the inevitable consequence of getting enough to eat of what everyone wants: in China enough rice, in India enough wheat, and in Central America enough tortillas and cornmeal. It's the grains, the starch, in sufficient amounts that kills.

Still, "the body always makes sense," and our ancestors could not have evolved to tolerate such foods. Our modern (less than 5,000 years old) sensibilities may not like it, but we are genetic omnivores: hunters and gatherers of what the harsh landscape of the last Great Ice Age afforded. OK, you've have heard it before and it makes sense to you.

Well, this same line of thought will help you understand why endurance exercise, especially long distance running, or staying on the treadmill at the gym for prolonged periods, is so harmful. And be clear, it is harmful. Well done studies tracking the rate of the progression of coronary artery disease have shown that the only way to age your arteries FASTER than long distance running is not to exercise at all.

Our body evolved to cope with a wide range of conditions: times of plenty, times of scarcity, times of terror, and times of joy suffused with hope, gratitude, and peace. Our body can swing from making lots of new stuff, like muscle and bone and babies, to tearing down our very bone and hearts and brains to generate fuel to survive until the next time of plenty.

Times of SCARCITY meant running or walking, often great distances, to find new prey or new leaves and roots and nuts; to find new hunting and grazing grounds. It makes sense that this demanded a low-energy transportation method, which we call walking or jogging. The mechanism that turns down our metabolism, so we don't run out of fuel before those fields of plenty are found, is stress and eccentric exercise. Eccentric exercise is that use of muscles whereby they resist getting longer rather than forcefully getting shorter. Jogging increases the metabolic effects of stress so that we will burn fewer calories for work done. But lest you be misled, sprinting does just the opposite.

You will always need your ability to hunt, to gather, to fish. Exercise that increases strength, foot speed, hand/eye coordination, flexibility, agility, multi-planar capacity, and power is a positive adaptive capacity for the good times, not for famine. This kind of exercise increases your metabolism, your immunity, your intellect, your memory—your fun!

But we live in the modern world and eat food from a depleted food chain, and most of us would wind up dead if we depended on bow hunting and the outcome of wrestling crocodiles. So we need a method to approximate the benefits of such a life without the risks. This is an attainable goal.

The hypothalamus thinks we are still hunter-gatherers, at least as far as food and exercise are concerned. That is so central to health that it bears repeating: The hypothalamus manages virtually all of our bodily functions, but does so as though we were still hunter-gatherers. Of course, 10,000 years ago, we all were, and this is an eye-blink in the grand scheme of things. Evolution simply doesn't move that fast. There are some changes, but basically, the hypothalamus is managing us now like it managed us in ancient times.

Our own hypothalamus has broad abilities to effectively metabolize food and can adapt to just about any combination: mostly fat, mostly protein, or in some cases, mostly carbs. This, in turn, gives us great adaptability, and no need for any particular "habitat."

The Grand Hypothalamic Gotcha

We changed from hunting and gathering to the agricultural lifestyle way too fast. The hypothalamus will eventually catch up, but this may take tens of thousands of years. In the meantime it continues to manage us as it always has, and therein lies the grand hypothalamic gotcha: for most of us, scarcity is a thing of the past, but in our millennia of evolution, an ample food supply was fleeting at best. So long protracted periods of prosperity appear to be something the hypothalamus simply can't grasp.

Almost anything out of the ordinary tends to set into motion the well-oiled famine management machine. If we aren't hunting (the hypothalamus monitors your exercise), it most likely means there is nothing to hunt, and that means a famine. If you get a lot of sugar and starches (the hypothalamus monitors sugar levels), it must mean it's late summer and thus winter is coming, yet another famine, and on and on. The hypothalamus seems ever ready to go into famine mode, store everything it can as fat, cut

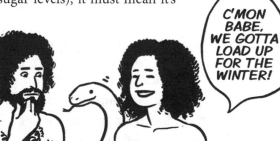

C'MON BABE, WE GOTTA LOAD UP FOR THE WINTER!

the energy level, shut down renewal and repair, and alter and adjust a variety of other bodily functions. All this made all sorts of survival sense 10,000 years ago, but many of these actions have now become obsolete, if not downright detrimental.

So, keep your hypothalamus happy. Convince it that famine preparation isn't the appropriate response, and the good life is yours. You will be well, or will become well. You will live a long, happy life. If you are doing something the hypothalamus interprets as hunting or gathering, and eating stuff that would be plausible bounty from those activities, it will turn on all the astounding prevention, repair, and renewal processes.

So how do we do that? What will convince the hypothalamus that we are not in any danger of starvation, and that it needn't toss us into some unhealthy low-energy conservation mode? Generally the right combination of diet, exercise, sleep, and low stress will do the trick. It takes all four, and determining how to optimize each of these is a major part of Quantitative Medicine. We will take a look at the same circulating biochemicals (glucose, cholesterol, etc.) that the hypothalamus is monitoring and then undertake to adjust them to known healthy levels. Interestingly, even though people vary enormously in their body chemistry and response to lifestyle changes, the ideal levels of the various blood markers are the same for everyone. This is quite fortunate, because it gives the entire human race a common health target. If this weren't the case, this book wouldn't exist.

To summarize: We know where we want the levels to be. Quantitative Medicine is then used to figure out where the levels actually are and how to send them in the right direction.

WHAT EXACTLY IS REGULATION?

To most people, regulation means rules or guidelines. However, in our context, it means forcing something to a precise value, and we will use terminology like "body temperature is regulated to 98.6°." In spite of a huge variety of foods and metabolic demands that would especially be part and parcel of the hunter-gatherer lifestyle, the body attempts to create a "standard" and optimal internal environment by doing exactly this sort of regulation.

Feedback Control Theory

It sounds like an exotic engineering discipline, and indeed it is, but you are already an expert at feedback control theory. Let's suppose you are on a road trip. Speed limit 65 mph, light traffic, on a particularly boring but speed-trap-infested Interstate. Your wife's second cousin, the highway patrolman, has told you they only ticket 10 miles over the speed limit, so you decide you are going to go 74 mph. If you go over this, you risk a ticket: if under, you waste your precious time.

So how do you do this? You know how, of course (no fair using cruise control), but let's walk through the steps. Do you keep the gas pedal at a certain spot, say depressed one inch? Of course not. You don't even think about that. Besides, to maintain 74 mph, you'll need to give it gas to get up hills and let off or maybe even brake going down. How do you know you are going 74? You watch your very accurate speedometer like a hawk. You step on the gas till you are close to 74, then ease off. If the speed starts to pick up, perhaps due to a tailwind, you ease off some more. The gas pedal is getting adjusted all the time, depending on various external conditions, so that the speed is maintained at exactly 74 mph.

In control theory parlance, 74 mph is your *reference* or *set-point*. Your actual speed is your *output* and ideally is the same as your *reference*. You *monitor* this output by looking at the speedometer, the *input* is the gas pedal and sometimes the brake, and the *controller* is you. In this situation, other things besides the gas pedal input are affecting the output speed: uphill, downhill, headwind, tailwind, and so on.

So, you are riding along at 74, over hill and dale. You are in homeostasis. You are able to control the speed to exactly 74.

However, if you come to a hill that is steep enough, you won't be able to climb it at 74 mph, even with the gas pedal all the way to the floor. Your speed will fall off. You have exceeded the capability of your system to regulate. At this point, you are no longer in homeostasis.

Now, the purpose of this book is not to teach you how to evade speed traps, but rather to gain an understanding of the things that the body regulates, and if necessary, means by which to alter them. For most people, the desired set-point or reference for blood sugar (glucose) is around 74 mg/dl. This translates to about one teaspoon of sugar in your five quarts of blood. This is not a lot of sugar, but if it goes too low, below 40 mg/dl, say, a coma can result, so this one is critical. Less critical, but far more common, is that it goes too high. The hypothalamus is in charge of all of this, and has a variety of ways to control the blood sugar level (output) to match its 74 mg/dl reference.

Suppose you eat some sugar or starch. This gets quickly into the bloodstream as glucose. One teaspoon of sugar would bump the glucose to maybe 110 mg/dl. Or at least it would try, but such an increase wouldn't happen. The glucose level is monitored by the hypothalamus, which has a vast spy network of neurons located in every nook and cranny. As soon as the sugar level starts up, the hypothalamus orders insulin to be secreted. This is our *input*. Insulin will clear out that excess sugar, driving it into muscle, fat, or storing it in the liver. How much insulin? This is hard to say. The hypothalamus will dump as much as it needs to bring the level back to 74 mg/dl. As soon as 74 mg/dl is reached, the insulin dumping is curtailed. If the level goes below 74, the hypothalamus can boost it back up by causing another hormone to be secreted. As long as the hypothalamus can adjust the glucose level to the 74 mg/dl *reference* or *set-point*, your bodily system is in homeostasis, at least, as far as blood glucose is concerned.

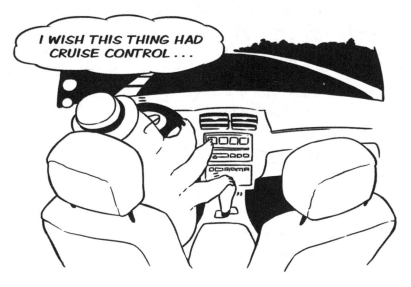

If too much sugar or starch is consumed (all starches are converted straight to glucose as soon as they arrive in the intestines), the hypothalamus will continue to boost the insulin level in an attempt to bring it down. Eventually, the insulin pedal is to the floor. The insulin level reaches a maximum and can no longer clear out the excess. The glucose level then goes up, up, and up. Sustained high levels of either glucose or insulin are bad for you. How much sugar/starch will trigger this overload situation? This varies from person to person, but a couple of bagels and a glass of orange juice would run the sugar up for several hours for a lot of people. During this period of time, they would no longer be in homeostasis. Many people eat a high-carb diet, and their sugar level is out of homeostasis much of the time. The hypothalamus is still trying to control things, but its ability to do so has been swamped by the excess sugar. The sugar hill is too steep. Glucose is too high, and insulin is kept high to try to deal with it. With adult onset diabetics, both these levels are too high 24/7.

We will be referring to input, output, controller, reference or set-point, and monitor later. Here's a little review in chart form:

Activity	On the road	Eating bagels
What is to be controlled	Speed	Blood glucose level
Reference or set-point	74 mph*	74 mg/dl
Output	Speed of car	Glucose level
To be overcome	Hill	Excess dietary glucose
Input	Gas pedal	Insulin secretion
Monitor	Speedometer	Glucose-sensing nerves
Controller	Driver	Hypothalamus

*The authors have no idea how much tolerance is given and decline all responsibility for any tickets.

Your body has hundreds of such systems, if not thousands. The key ones are controlled and regulated by the hypothalamus. If homeostasis is attainable—the hill's not too steep—the hypothalamus will regulate the key hormones to optimal levels. There is no need to eat or exercise in some precise way. You only need to manage yourself in such a way that the hypothalamus can "lock-in." This varies from person to person, but can be determined by measurement. One person might be able to eat a lot of starch and still maintain a glucose level of 74 mg/dl. Another person might have to give up starches entirely to achieve this.

The typical modern lifestyle tends to push us into regions where homeostasis cannot be achieved. This allows degenerative disease to gain a foothold. With proper lifestyle choices, this trap can be avoided.

So, in the end, health is managed and controlled to a certain degree of perfection by a neural system we are largely unaware of, with a complexity beyond all description, perhaps forever beyond human comprehension. Whether this came to be by the blind guidance of evolution or was the work of a Divine Hand may be equally unknowable, but whatever the cause, there is something of truly remarkable beauty and awe residing in each of us: as close to a miracle as one can likely get. If there is a corporal soul, it surely resides therein.

Dr. Mike's Philosophical Sidebar
Belly Be Gone!

There are different kinds of fat. The first kind is fat under the skin; the second is inside the muscle layer, and is also know as "mesenteric," "visceral," or "organ" fat.

The inside fat is toxic and both related to and causative of many kinds of metabolic diseases like diabetes, high blood pressure, osteoporosis and stroke: bad stuff. It makes us look funny in a Speedo too.

Now, surprisingly, even skinny people can have a lot of this "beer belly fat." I used to call such people "skinny fat people." Some better diplomat than I dubbed them TOFI: thin outside, fat inside. Same thing. Still bad.

Genetics is always at play, but this is mostly a behavioral problem. The sad part is that conventional exercise can actually make the problem worse. You can grind away on the treadmill and get fatter. Really? Really!

This is where the old confusion about "calories in, calories out" comes into the picture. There are two elements to this:

1. What the calories do to your own hormones is much more important than the calorie count and it is the hormones that determine if the calories are stored or burned. Eat the right calories and they are literally metabolized away. Eat the wrong calories and they wind up as seat pads.
2. The second element is the exercise aspect. Simply burning calories in the wrong way can actually increase the body's tendency to store them. Conventional aerobics does this neat storage trick very nicely.

I remember many years ago, in my own endurance aerobics phase, being amazed at the number of beer-belly-bearing pretty good runners I would see at various 10K and marathon venues. It was years before I finally understood.

It doesn't much matter about your family history or your personal fat history; what matters is it is all largely under your control.

PREVENTION AND REPAIR PROCESSES

Many prevention and repair processes are distributed throughout the body, while others are centrally controlled. Almost all the centrally controlled ones are managed by the hypothalamus. If this little computer-like brain is allowed to function properly, it will set up the conditions that prevent almost all degenerative disease.

The 70% that are suffering and dying from these diseases are, in various ways, confounding the operation of their hypothalamus. If we change our ways so that the hypothalamus deals with a situation it is familiar with, one it has seen before in its millennia of evolution, these diseases won't occur, or, if they are already occurring, they will be halted or even reversed.

Since we cannot know our ancient ancestry, we cannot know in advance which lifestyle choices will work, but this can be determined from measurement, and that is the topic of PART II. The measurements are blood tests and scans. Far more information is gathered than in a typical annual physical. This is the Quantitative part. This greater amount of information very exactly describes your current state of health, and quite accurately predicts where you are headed. The majority of us are headed in an unhealthy direction. Quantitative Medicine suggests changes to rectify this.

Quantitative Medicine is unique in having no standard advice. People are too different for that to ever work. Quantitative Medicine differs from other medical philosophies or disciplines in two important ways:

1. **We know how measurements relate to health.** This is the result of Dr. Nichols's 20-year practice of Quantitative Medicine. Using these measurements, one can develop a personal health strategy and, in some cases, embark on a cure to existing disease.

2. **It actually works.** The methodology has been applied by Dr. Nichols over the last 20 years and has altered the lives of several thousand people—dramatically for many. Not a single person got worse.

This book is intended to complement standard Western medicine, not replace it. Indeed, if a degenerative disease has already struck, a heart attack or cancer, for instance, Western medicine is by far your best chance of recovery and survival. These sorts of interventions are where it shines.

This book aims largely at preventing such maladies in the first place, and its methodologies have already proven very effective for the people who have practiced them. We suggest you fully consult with your doctor should you decide to try the recommendations and methods in this book. However, don't let your doctor malign the methodology without good reason. Other things being equal, this book can save your life.

Much medical research today addresses these "modern" diseases. The maladies that were killing us 100 years ago have largely been slain, mainly through medical breakthroughs, but also through improved sanitation and food standards. Cholera, for instance, is caused by contaminated water, and is really a civil engineering problem. Deaths associated with childbirth, once common, have been greatly reduced. Life-threatening childhood diseases are all but gone. People now live longer. Long enough to get the diseases of our age: heart disease, cancer, adult onset diabetes, Alzheimer's, and the rest. Medical research has been on the attack on many fronts. The War on Cancer, declared by Nixon in the '70s, is one such example. (Not a war we're winning, by the way.)

A fundamental difference with these new diseases is the absence of pathogens: bacteria, viruses, and other invaders. We are inflicting these diseases upon ourselves, starting in childhood. In this book, we are going to explore how we are doing this, and what can be done about it. Everything will turn out to have a reason, almost always rooted in survival.

Key Points
2 - Health Is Controlled
- Every attribute we possess is there because it improved our survival chances.
- Anything "new" had to pay for itself: it had to provide a greater benefit in terms of survival than it cost in terms of energy (food).
- The hypothalamus controls most essential repair and renewal processes. It controls major organs. It is survival oriented.
- The hypothalamus maintains a precise list of ideal key hormonal levels.
- The hypothalamus will tightly regulate these.
- The hypothalamus still thinks we are hunter-gatherers and that food will frequently be in short supply.
- If the hypothalamus decides to economize, repair and renewal are shut down to save energy, and degenerative disease progresses. The hypothalamus frequently reaches this conclusion.
- If the hypothalamus thinks you are successfully hunting and gathering, it turns on repair, renewal, creativity, disease prevention and so on. We want this.

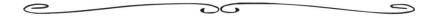

3 - ATTAINING PEAK HEALTH

Peak health, the condition where degenerative disease is halted, even reversed, has two components, ideal homeostasis and anabolism. To achieve peak health, these two need to occur frequently. Ideal homeostasis means the body is in a healthy enough state to be capable of performing repairs and fighting disease. Anabolism means that it is actually doing so.

IDEAL HOMEOSTASIS

Your hypothalamus will attempt to regulate numerous circulating hormones and biochemicals. Regulate means driving the levels to specific targets or set-points. Regulation of glucose was discussed extensively in the last chapter. The targets or set-points that the hypothalamus uses are tucked away internally. We are born with these numbers already set, though many of them slowly vary over the course of our lives. If the hypothalamus is able to do its job, all the regulated biochemicals and hormones will be at the same level as their targets. But what are these target levels exactly?

If we knew that someone was in homeostasis, we would only need results from blood tests. But unfortunately, we don't know when someone is in homeostasis. There is no little green light that comes on and tells us.

The way out of this conundrum stems from this observation: for almost all people, the ideal homeostatic set-point or targets are very nearly the same. Using the data from several thousand patients, Dr. Nichols was able to determine the ideal ranges. He observed that if someone was sick, did the Quantitative Medicine protocols, and got well, their blood measurements almost always ended up in certain narrow ranges. So we call these the ideal ranges. There is strong confirmation for this: the hormonal numbers we have from hunter-gatherers, be they Inuit or desert bushmen, fall into these same ranges. So at this point, there seems to be a very strong case that these ranges are the ideal ranges, and that they apply to all of humanity.

The ideal range for fasting glucose is between 60 and 80 mg/dl. Since we don't specifically know the level of your own target numbers, we make an assumption, a strongly justified one, that the target number is in the ideal range and the hypothalamus will adjust to this *if it can*.

A given individual's set-point might differ, and his hypothalamus could be targeting some number outside the ideal range. This happens, and has turned up in Dr. Nichols's data, but it is fairly rare. We really don't know if this oddball number is, for some reason, ideal for that particular person. We think that it is not, and that the hypothalamus has goofed, or has gotten pulled off track by a long period of bad lifestyle choice, but we don't know that for sure. The following section has a couple of examples.

The Quest for Ideal Homeostasis

Suppose that for some period of time, a person had a lifestyle where regulation was impossible: perhaps a period of high stress, or of no exercise, or a diet which caused a slow but steady weight gain or blood pressure increase. Measurements can be made. Some of these measurements will probably be out of the ideal homeostatic range. Let's suppose fasting glucose is measured and is high: 110, say. Likely cause: too much sugar or starch. We already know that we want it at 74 mg/dl. Actually, anything from 60 to 80, the ideal fasting range for glucose, would be fine. The reason our "patient" has a glucose level of 110 is because she has made the "glucose hill" too steep. Try as it might, the hypothalamus cannot reduce that glucose into the ideal range. So what should she do to help the hypothalamus out? There could be many strategies, but cutting out starch and sugar for three months would be fast and effective. She can then re-measure, and perhaps she will find that her fasting blood glucose is down at 77 mg/dl. That is a big win. She can infer, with considerable confidence, that her particular homeostatic reference point for fasting glucose is around 77, which is in the ideal range. She is now able to regulate properly, and is achieving ideal homeostasis, at least as far as fasting glucose is concerned. She has quantified her personal glucose level, along with its ideal set-point, and has gained knowledge on how to attain the ideal. She could experiment at this juncture and see if she could get away with a bit of sugar or starch. Possibly, she could, and still have her glucose regulate at 77.

This is the whole idea. The hypothalamus will be able to lock-in and regulate over a fairly broad span of nutrients and physical activities. Just get into the "ballpark" and the hypothalamus will do the rest. There is no need to hit some precise sort of target. The big problem for many of us is that we are outside the zone where the hypothalamus can lock-in. However, for most people, getting into a region where the hypothalamus can regulate properly is quite possible.

Sometimes, the picture isn't quite that tidy.

Possible problem #1: Tiny homeostatic range. Here, the person can drive himself to the ideal range, but it doesn't hold very well. A modest bit of backsliding and the numbers immediately start to go askew. This could happen with age. Cells are not as vigorous and supple as they once were. Self-discipline will be needed to keep the numbers in the right range. There is a bright side. Making all of those changes will greatly improve cellular health, which will, in turn, help regain some of that lost flexibility.

Possible problem #2: A number goes partway toward the ideal and then sticks. It may be the case that some kind of set-point was reached, but one not in the ideal range. Maybe cutting out starch and sugar moved fasting glucose from 140 mg/dl (a dangerous level) to 110. If that 110 persisted for years, it probably means that it is a homeostatic set-point, though clearly not an ideal one. This is unusual, but not unknown. The set-point may stay there forever. Or it may, over time, creep toward the ideal range. In either case, the "treatment" for both of these problems is the same: Cut the glucose (sugar and starch). Keep pushing it toward the ideal.

ANABOLISM

Achieving ideal homeostasis is only half of the story. To get well and stay well, we need to get our body into an anabolic mode. Anabolism is the building, repair, and renewal of the body. The opposite of anabolism is catabolism, which is the tearing down and disposal of the old and worn. Normally they work in turns: catabolism clears the terrain and anabolism builds anew.

But anabolism doesn't just automatically occur. Even though the body is in a state of ideal homeostasis, and is ready to renew, repair, and repel disease, nothing will happen unless the hypothalamus also declares, in effect, that the body is *allowed* to proceed and do all this. It is that direct. Cells needing repair will sit and wait for a hormonal signal from the hypothalamus to go ahead. We obviously want all those healthy renewal processes occurring. Why would the hypothalamus curtail them?

The hypothalamus puts a high priority on conserving energy for possible lean times. Unless you are actively hunting and gathering, it will conclude that food is going to be scarce and will start economizing. All those desirable healthy processes use energy, and the hypothalamus is still managing our energy expenditures by the same stingy rules worked out over the last several hundred thousand years. Economy is always its reaction to uncertainty. It has barely begun to adapt to our modern lifestyle.

So how can we get the hypothalamus to stop this scarce-food nonsense and enable the healthy restorative processes? You would think that getting regular meals would convince it. This helps, but it's not quite enough. You also have to prove that you were doing something to *deserve* those meals. The hypothalamus requires, in effect, that you were hunting and gathering. Otherwise, it thinks the food was just some temporary store and will soon run out.

Of course one method of jump-starting the desired repair processes would be to simply become a hunter-gatherer. However, some of us may feel we don't have the requisite skill set, and have perhaps become very fond of our modern creature comforts. Is there any hope for us then?

As it turns out, it's enough to do physical activities that resemble hunting and gathering. The hypothalamus will enable the renewal and repair if it detects this. We are saved!

A nice place to perform this pseudo hunting and gathering is at a nearby gym. Such activities could be done at home, or even in the great outdoors (if you want to get closer to the real thing). But whatever the locale, convincing the hypothalamus that you are hunting and gathering is a little tricky. The type of exercise is very important. Exercises that look like *migration* will cause the hypothalamus to again conserve and curtail repair and renewal activities. Why? Because migration usually means that the current location has no more food available, so the hypothalamus is again confronted with a scarcity situation. And what might the hypothalamus interpret as migration? Aerobic exercise fits the bill to a tee. And it is easy to see why: it's a long, moderate, and sustained activity. Ditto brisk walking and golf.

Medical Drill-Down Sidebar
How Does the Hypothalamus Know What We Are Doing?

The hypothalamus make some major decisions based on its perception of near-term food availability. Specifically, if you are hunting, it expends energy (a situation we want). If you are migrating, it conserves, and turn off the repair and renewal processes. But how does it know this? The answer is amazing.

The hypothalamus has a huge network of specialized nerves that detect this and that. Some detect glucose level, some body temperature, and there are some that can detect types of muscle movement. The hypothalamus knows if you are using your muscles, and also knows how you are using them: is it concentric or eccentric movement?

In concentric movement, the muscle is working while shortening. In eccentric movement, the muscle is working while lengthening. Most exercise involves both in turns, but one type usually predominates. If you are about to spring on an unsuspecting gazelle, you crouch very slowly (lightly eccentric) then spring with all your might (explosively concentric).

Walking, though, is largely eccentric. For each step, you effectively fall forward and catch yourself. The catch is the main energy expenditure and is primarily eccentric. Walking is very efficient. We are "designed" to migrate without expending much energy. Good thing, no doubt.

So concentric means hunting. Food supply assured. OK to expend energy. Eccentric means migration, searching. Food is not assured. Conserve. Shut down processes that can wait.

Does this mean that aerobics, the doctor-recommended, ideal-in-every-way exercise, the one peddled and pushed for three decades, actually thwarts the body's inherent repair and renewal system? Sorry folks, but that does seem to be the case. That sort of exercise will cause the hypothalamus to turn down the desirable repair processes in order to save energy. Aerobics are far better than sitting on a couch, to be sure, but fall far short of initiating the processes we need to effectively combat degenerative disease.

The type of activity that causes the hypothalamus to turn on anabolism and launch the various repair and renewal processes is exercise of an intense explosive nature. Brief and intense. Exactly the sorts of activity that go on in ancient hunting. Hunting with spears, clubs, stones, and the like.

This is not speculation on our part. Tests after tests have proven that high-intensity interval exercise, as it is now known, will provide far more health benefits than aerobic, and in far less time.

There is still plenty of aerobic exercise going on at most gyms. We find it tedious and would far prefer something strenuous that lasted only a minute or so. But we are getting ahead of ourselves here.

Metabolism = Anabolism + Catabolism

Medical Drill-Down Sidebar
Is Glucose Always Bad? Isn't Glucose Necessary?

Some people can deal with glucose without any problems. However, this ability diminishes with age. The principal sources of glucose are sugar and starch. Many, perhaps over half, of those over 50 have some degree of difficulty metabolizing the sugar and starch they are currently consuming. Recall that our hunter-gatherer ancestors got very little of either. In our long pre-agricultural history, we had correspondingly little opportunity to evolve or adapt any effective strategies for dealing with them. On the grand evolutionary scale, 10,000 years simply isn't long enough to make that leap. Further, sugar is strongly implicated in the big four degenerative diseases: heart disease, cancer, adult onset diabetes, and Alzheimer's. It plays different roles, but it is always found lurking at the scene of the crime. Dietary fat isn't implicated in any of these diseases, and that includes saturated fat (but trans fat is indeed bad news—avoid). The body is all set up to deal with fat. Protein is innocent as well.

Unregulated glucose levels invariably have long-term consequences, especially if coupled with high insulin, and unfortunately, this is a pretty easy situation to slip into.

A certain level of glucose is necessary, and you may wonder where that necessary glucose is going to come from if a person eats no sugar or starch. Actually, there will be plenty of glucose available in non-starchy vegetables, and we recommend eating a fair amount of those. The glucose from these is digested slowly, and usually does not cause an overload.

The body even has a system for dealing with a complete absence of carbohydrates. If a person, an Atkins dieter for instance, eats no vegetables at all, their body will make glucose from protein and fat. This likely won't be enough, but the body has yet another trick up its sleeve. It has a substitute for glucose called ketones. The liver makes up ketones from fat, and any organs that need glucose, especially the brain, will do just fine with this ketone substitute.

WHY AREN'T WE NATURALLY IN IDEAL HOMEOSTASIS AND ANABOLISM?

We "naturally" are. We are quite well equipped to deal with all that life threw our way when we were "at one" with nature. In fact, we are well equipped for many different sorts of natures, from the arctic to the desert to the jungle. And this was everyone's lot until very recently. Very recently in evolutionary terms, anyway.

And we didn't just survive, we thrived. The capabilities of our direct ancestors tell us that we are easily able to deal with all this variety and difficulty. We have a proven hypothalamic versatility, if you will, and in those vastly different environments, we were in ideal homeostasis, were often anabolic, and, importantly, we didn't get degenerative disease.

An entirely different situation arises if the hypothalamus is strained or pushed so that most of the time it cannot regulate to the ideal range. It can then no longer control and regulate the various hormones and other critical levels. Things stop working. Biological infrastructure is broken down: Health deteriorates. Renewal and repair are curtailed, and degenerative disease is not pushed back. Worse still, the hypothalamus usually interprets all the confusion as a cause for conservation, and further pushes the body into an energy-saving catabolic state: just what we do not want.

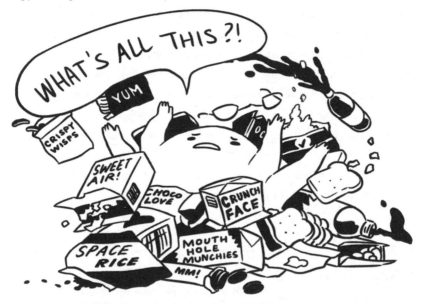

Starting 10,000 years ago, we began making a series of changes that would bring all those undesirable changes crashing down upon us. The agricultural revolution had the net effect of pushing our hypothalamus out of its normal equilibrium, and into a place where it could no longer regulate and operate properly. And worse, it pushed it into an energy conservation state as well. The early agriculturists (the elite excepted) lived almost solely on grains and other low-quality, mass-producible foods. And seldom enough of even that.

This was a health disaster without precedent. There have been archaeological digs where skeletons were found from both early agriculturists and nearby hunter-gatherers, and the difference is dramatic. The hunter-gatherers were several inches taller, more robust, non-arthritic, had better teeth, and were generally a lot better off. They likely worked less, too. At least today, hunter-gatherer societies typically spend only three to five hours daily obtaining their immediate needs and use the rest of the time, well, playing. We don't know what the ancient farmers' schedules were, but doubt they were leisurely. The health and durability advantages the hunter-gatherers had over the have-nots of the agricultural society (almost everybody) would persist until the 19th century. On the basis of degenerative disease, you could argue that it persists still.

The agricultural revolution didn't happen overnight. It spread slowly, and many of us remained hunter-gatherers for several thousand years. Perhaps as recently as 1,000 years ago, half of us still were. All of the Americas were. At the dawn of the 21st century, a few tribes still remain. They may be the last.

Given the huge variation in hunter-gatherer cultures, it should come as no surprise that humans have a wide genetic diversity, especially metabolically. This has both benefits and drawbacks. One major benefit is that we can thrive on a huge variety of diets, with the significant exception being our Western one. The disadvantage of all of this diversity is that we are all quite, one could say, diverse. This isn't bad in and of itself, it simply means that we cannot know in advance how we will respond to changes in diets or exercise patterns. Determining this is where Quantitative Medicine comes into the picture.

Ask Dr. Mike
The Value of Fasting

Q: As the hunter-gatherers seemed to have either "feast or famine" and you claim that this is our evolutionary and genetic legacy, why don't you include fasting in your dietary advice?

A: The answer to this has more to do with clinical experience than the evolutionary anthropology underlying most other advice. It has been my experience that most people engage in compensatory eating behavior when they attempt a fasting regimen: they wind up eating more and worse food than when they eat on a regular basis. Besides eating poorly or too much, eating all of the time is another way to fail and thus "grazing" suppresses some of the advantages of the intermittent eating of regular meals and snacks. Eat every three hours but do not graze.

THE KEY TO A LONG, DISEASE-FREE LIFE

Achieve ideal homeostasis and anabolism, at least some of the time, and the good life is your. You will look healthy, feel healthy, and be healthy. The risk of degenerative disease will be low and aging will be slow. The rest of the book is about why this is, and how to meet the requirements without joining a hunter-gatherer band. Quantitative Medicine will lead you to this ideal state. Though the degenerative diseases are different, they share a common cause. And a common cure. In these senses, they are all interrelated.

Difficulties Meeting the Ideal Homeostasis Requirement

Here is a list of lifestyle attributes that tend to push the hypothalamus out of ideal homeostasis:

- Chronic consumption of sugar and starch
- Lack of sleep
- Chronic stress
- Chronic overeating
- Irregular sleep, irregular circadian rhythms, artificial light
- Sedentary lifestyle

These are all prominently featured in our modern civilization, but mostly absent in the hunter-gatherer's world.

Stress could be a frequent component of the hunter-gatherer lifestyle. Of course, if there is a saber-toothed tiger lurking in the cave, the stress response is appropriate, but one way or the other, that situation is transitory. But chronic stress? We really don't know.

Chronic stress is very unhealthy. The immune system is suppressed, repair put on hold, inflammation increased, mental acuity decreased, and excess food stored as fat. All in all, very undesirable.

Nowadays, for many, the day-to-day coping seems to be a cause of chronic stress.

Difficulties Meeting the Anabolic Requirement

There are two lifestyle features that cause the hypothalamus to enter and remain in a catabolic state, thus suppressing renewal and repair:

- Sedentary lifestyle
- Chronic stress

Sedentary lifestyle has already been discussed. The hypothalamus thinks you are unable to hunt, so it conserves. No energy-consuming anabolism is permitted.

Less clear is the reason for the anabolic shutdown in the presence of chronic stress. The stress response, again managed by the hypothalamus, consists of shutting down processes that can wait, and that would include energy-consuming anabolism.

We now know where we want to be. We know also how to determine where we are. The step-by-step procedures that will be developed in PART II explain how to make the transition. It's a question of willpower, coupled with an awareness of what is going on. We'll supply the latter; the former is up to you.

Key Points
3 - Attaining Peak Health

- If the hypothalamus cannot maintain the regulation of the key levels, the body may be in a perpetual catabolic state. Renewal does not occur; aging is rapid. Degenerative disease advances.
- Various lifestyle choices can get the body into the range where the hypothalamus can achieve ideal homeostasis.
- The agricultural revolution presented a nutritional and physical situation that thoroughly confounded the hypothalamus. The net result was a huge deterioration in health of the agricultural populations.
- The key to a long disease-free life is to present the hypothalamus with a lifestyle that causes it to engage its vast repair and renewal capability.

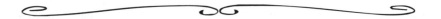

4 - QUANTITATIVE MEDICINE: MEASUREMENT AND MODIFICATION

You cannot know whether you are experiencing the benefits of ideal homeostasis and frequent anabolism without measurement. You may think you know, which could add to the problem. You may feel fine, but if your hypothalamus is out of balance or overloaded, there will be underlying processes heading in undesirable directions. Since this cannot be known directly, it is determined and quantified by testing. This step is necessary and the results are frequently surprising. Some things needn't be worried about, but others should be dealt with.

Your hypothalamus knows exactly what is going on. It gets continuous measurements from many places in the body, which is far better information than the occasional fasting blood draw. It is too bad we have so little awareness of all this information. It would be very convenient if we could tap into this hypothalamic information center with some yet to be imagined medical gadget: perhaps a nifty hypothalamic wristwatch. There could be a little dial that indicated anabolic (green) and catabolic (red). It would go well into the green when you exercised. Another dial would indicate homeostasis. It would go into the red if you ate a cheesecake or got stressed out.

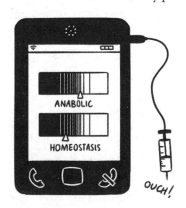

ILLUSTRATOR'S NOTE: THE HOMEOSTATIC WATCH HAS BEEN REPLACED WITH AN APP FOR ACCURACY.

39

Such a gadget could have quite a beneficial effect on our behavior, as we would be getting immediate feedback on our actions (or inactions).

Back here on terra firma, we have no such gadget (yet), but we can measure and quantify these things, it's just not as convenient and is somewhat indirect. However, it is absolutely necessary to do this if you want to develop the healthy habits and practices that will reap the innumerable benefits of ideal homeostasis and anabolism.

Ideal homeostasis means the hypothalamus is able to keep the various hormones, nutrients, and biochemicals regulated in their proper zones. Since these biochemicals circulate in the blood, they are readily measured with a blood test. Anabolism can also be measured this way.

If you are over 40 or have a family or personal history of heart problems, you should also get a scan to measure heart calcium and bone density.

Blood tests and scans will define your health just as well as our hypothetical hypothalamic wristwatch. If you change your lifestyle, you will change these measurements, and that will mean your health has changed as well. This is the fundamental reason Quantitative Medicine works so well.

MODIFYING YOUR HEALTH TRAJECTORY

Although it is difficult and perhaps dangerous to meddle directly with the functions of the hypothalamus, it is fair game to push it in a desired direction by consciously controlling the energy supplies and demands. The hypothalamus looks directly at these to reach its energy management conclusions. To modify our health trajectory, we need to get our hypothalamus into ideal homeostatic and anabolic modes. This is both a communication problem (what does it want us to do?) and a problem of execution (are we willing to do it?).

The hypothalamus is a very old system. It evolved well before much was going on in the way of brains, and there isn't a lot of mental connection with our neocortex, at least not the conscious part. Watching sports on TV isn't going to convince it of anything. However, any sort of physical motion that might actually be involved in hunting or gathering would be a valid signal.

Imagine what our hunter-gatherer ancestors were doing to try to get food. They could be shoving boulders onto an unsuspecting mammoth or charging a buffalo. These animals might equally be chasing them. This is explosive stuff: stalking, stalking, and then in for the finish. Further, that meat's got to be dragged back to the cave or igloo. More work. On the way back, the local wolf pack might take some interest in the spoils. More activity, likely vigorous.

Can this be done at the gym? Fortunately for us, the hypothalamus really can't tell the difference. Cook up some explosive and strenuous, but brief, exercises, and the hypothalamus is likely to conclude hunting season is on and there is no need to conserve. Typically, a couple of vigorous 45-minute sessions a week will accomplish this and set the hypothalamus into the highly desirable anabolic mode. Two short, intense sessions represent a huge time saving over the typical five-hour-per-week aerobic sessions often recommended., but they do need to be as intense as you can manage. Intensity is far more important than duration. Will this work for you and do you even need to do it? It definitely works, and you probably need it, but measurement is the only way to tell for sure.

Exercise is the "energy-out" piece of the equation, but what about "energy-in?" Again, everyone is different. A safe bet is to avoid eating anything hunter-gatherers couldn't get their hands on. Still, this varies from person to person. Some people do fine with starches (rare in the hunter-gatherers' world), while others cannot metabolize them well, which causes their glucose and insulin levels to soar, leading to disease vulnerability and unhealthy weight gain. The measurements reveal this too.

HONEY

FRUIT & VEG

MEAT, BUGS & GRUBS

ORGANS AND BLUBBER

HEART HEALTHY FOR 100,000 YEARS!

The hunter-gatherer diet is not necessarily a healthy one. Intestines (full of parasites) or scavenged meat (don't even know where to begin) are obviously quite dangerous. However, bad meat or starvation is a choice most of us don't have to make.

It turns out that today most hunter-gatherer societies are consuming 60-90% animal product. This is probably what we are "designed" to do. This doesn't mean some can't do well on a vegetarian diet that includes eggs and dairy products, but they are possibly bucking the system. Vegan is another story. A lot of supplementation will typically be needed to avoid serious health issues.

Eat things that the body, in its evolutionary past, has seen before. Pastured animals are healthier than feedlot animals. Organic vegetables are better. Sugars, starches, cereals, breads, and so on were not even on the Paleolithic menu. Again, some people do fine with these and for others they are practically toxic. This can be quantified by measuring.

The meats (here including fish, fowl, dairy, and eggs) and vegetables also have essential micronutrients. You have already heard of these as minerals, vitamins, and the like. You need to get a reasonable amount of these micronutrients, and just about any sensible mix of meats and vegetables will do. Starches and sugar come up quite short in this area. Sugar has none. Starches have little to none. You can survive on sugar and starches, but cannot thrive. This was probably abundantly clear any time a hunter-gatherer troop opted (or was forced) to join the grand agricultural revolution, but in the ensuing years this has been largely forgotten.

STACKING THE ODDS IN YOUR FAVOR

Risk is chance, not certainty. However, the tendencies are there, and if the numbers are not in the right ranges the diseases are pretty likely to be advancing, particularly heart disease. That said, we want to go:

- From destruction to renewal
- From catabolism to anabolism
- From accelerated aging to slow aging
- From disease to health

These are all really the same thing, and everything is regulated and centrally controlled by the survival-oriented hypothalamus. If ideal homeostasis can be achieved and anabolism started, these fall into place.

Anyone with the will to do so can accomplish this. The hypothalamus isn't really in charge, it's just running things in your absence. Armed with the knowledge of how it reacts, and the will to change what it reacts to, you can take over. It's entirely up to you. However, to effectively exercise this will, you need to know your genetic and biologic predispositions. Otherwise you will likely fail. Cutting this metabolic Gordian Knot is what Quantitative Medicine is all about. It supplies the focus and specificity necessary to pull it off.

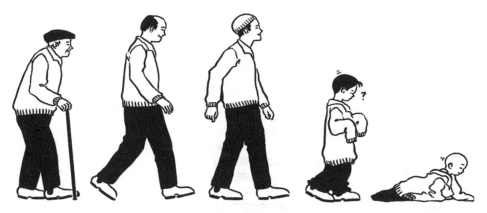

⚠ *WARNING: DO NOT REVERSE THE CLOCK TOO FAR!* ⚠

Health as a Business Proposition

Are you an investor? Or a gambler? Both? (For many they are the same thing.) If so, consider this investment proposition: undertaking this program can reasonably add 10 good years to your life. Maybe more. Consider it 33% from diet, 33% from exercise, and 33% from de-stressing. Just guesses here. Which component is more important depends on the individual. For our hypothetical "Judy," it's 33-33-33%. She started optimizing all these at age 55 and added nine healthy years to her life, cashing in at 95. Let's compute some returns on investment.

Judy has to eat, so a diet that is optimal for her specific metabolism gets her three years right off. That was practically free.

For exercise, we typically recommend two strenuous 45-minute sessions a week. Judy starts doing this at 55. Forty years later she will have exercised 3,100 hours. That's a lot of sweat, but timewise, it's slightly over four months. What did she get for that? Three more years. That's a pretty good payback. That works out to about 7 hours of additional healthy life for every 45 minutes of exercise, a 9:1 payout. So even if you hate exercise, this is a really good investment.

Stress is a huge part of modern civilization, and entering the program, Judy was a bit of a stress-ball. She got this under control and added another three years. For Judy, this required a daily 10-minute meditation like activity. Thus Judy got around 12 more hours of additional life for the 70 minutes of weekly stress reduction activity. The payout here, an impressive 11:1, even beats exercise.

There is a catch: You can't just do one thing. The body is too interconnected. All three are necessary.

Here are six-month results from 25 Judies and Joes:

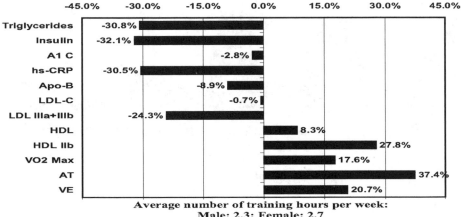

Average number of training hours per week:
Male: 2.3; Female: 2.7

These are the first 25 people who began a program Dr. Nichols launched in 2001. These are stunning results. These people's health has dramatically improved in a very short time. There were no drugs used to achieve these results. In fact, any drug that could achieve anything remotely similar would be the blockbuster of all blockbusters.

Do you want to go ahead and do all this? If so, there's PART II, which spells it all out, step by step, and PART III, which explores the underlying science. If you've had enough, here are four pieces of advice that should make a difference. You may or may not need to do any of these things, so this is not "standard advice." Measurement is the only way to be sure; this is the essence of Quantitative Medicine. However, these items may help and will definitely do no harm:

1. If you seem to be gaining a pound or two a year, cut down on sugar and starch. Or cut them out entirely. They are the most likely cause of that weight gain. Most of us are not well designed to deal with sugar or starch. Don't worry about meat, fat, or high-cholesterol foods. Try to eat two to three times as much vegetables as protein (meat, eggs, cheese). Eat snacks between meals. Eat

colored vegetables and vary your meats. For fruit, eat berries, or better still, nothing: fruits are loaded with sugar. Eat nuts. Buy organic when you can.

2. You *should* exercise. You already know that. However, quality trumps quantity. Do explosive stuff. Run your heart up and down. (See a doc first if you have *any* reason to suspect heart problems.) What's explosive? Instead of swimming for an hour, swim like mad for 30 seconds, rest 2 minutes, repeat 5 times. Jogger? Change to the same sort of pattern: 30-second sprint, 1 minute walking. Don't do the one-hour swim or 5-mile jog. Do some resistance exercise too. If you are over 50, be sure to include squats and deadlifts. This and only this prevents and reverses osteoporosis. Two hard 45-minute sessions per week will reap huge rewards.

3. Reduce your stress level. This may be the most important point, and it is certainly the one most frequently ignored—a huge mistake. Chronic stress is very unhealthy, far more so than is generally recognized. Chronic stress contributes more directly to a degenerative disease state than either poor diet or lack of exercise and further, is often the cause of both of these. Do what you can to minimize the stress of your day-to-day life, but take it a step further. Give your inner voice a chance to be heard. What inner voice? Well, maybe your hypothalamus, or some other inner consciousness. Your soul perhaps. Here is how: Stop the constant thinking and chattering of your conscious brain. Simply think of nothing at all. This is a lot easier said than done. Once you begin this, your conscious brain will soon restart the chatter, rudely taking over. The trick is to start with short targets. See if you can shut the brain-computer-chatterbox up for 30 seconds. Or 15. Try to work your way up to 10 minutes a day. This activity could be called meditation, but no need to label it. Don't put on saffron robes or bother with the lotus position. Just get comfortable and shut the chatter down. This will accomplish a lot. Meditative activity is known to reduce stress, cortisol, and inflammation. This boosts the immune system, which helps push back cancer, but the effects seem to go much further. Things change for the

better in numerous other subtle ways. Try it. Above all, do what it takes to get your stress level down.

4.   Tune in to your circadian rhythms. Our Paleolithic ancestors were locked into the hours, lengths, and colors of the days. This foretold the coming seasons and initiated the substantial metabolic changes needed to survive them. Did we know how to hibernate back then? Not exactly, but we certainly have many of the requisite abilities. A long and severe ice-age winter requires an ability to quickly store a lot of fat and to down-regulate energy expenditures. Does this ring any bells? It likely still rings a few in our hypothalamus, which has these expectations hard-wired in. If we violate them, are there consequences? The is surely the case. Seasonal Affective Disorder is connected to this, and shift workers have significantly higher rates of cancer. In any case, sleep well. Quality sleep is best. Seven *solid* hours is probably enough. Nine is even better. Be sure to make it dark and quiet. Tape over all those red lights from your electronic gadgetry. Perhaps your sleep patterns do need to vary with the seasons. Pay attention to sleep. A lot of repair and renewal goes on during sleep. Make it count.

Do you need to do these things? We don't know and neither does anyone else. We suggest them because first, they are common problems, and second, they won't hurt you. No one needs sugars and starches. Exercise is universally beneficial, and quieting your mind is always healthy. If you want to refine this, you can get a lot more benefit, but you will have to measure and go from there. That is the topic of PART II and PART III.

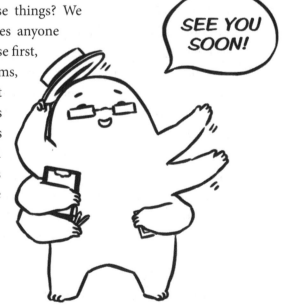

GUIDE TO THE BOOK

Hopefully, PART I answers the "what" of Quantitative Medicine.

There are two more principal parts:

PART II - USING QUANTITATIVE MEDICINE (the "how")

PART III -THE SCIENCE OF QUANTITATIVE MEDICINE (the "why")

You can stop after PART II. Should you go on? Read this paragraph:

Life span amongst mammals is generally proportional to weight. Mice live about 2 years and elephants as much as 70. We are exceptions, as are our primate cousins, living longer still. However, there is a very small mammal with a very revved up metabolism that represents a far greater exception. This animal is lighter than a mouse but consumes several times as much food daily. Whereas a mouse may live 2 years, this animal—the common bat if you haven't already guessed—lives 25. What is the bat's special trick? Well it's not the 100% bug diet, it's flying. Flying means being able to summon up a huge burst of energy. This means a very modified metabolism, and this modification also gives the bat (birds too) an extraordinarily long life for its weight. The modification lies in tiny sub-cellular organelles called mitochondria. These organelles were once free bacteria and were enslaved by our single-celled ancestors perhaps a billion years ago. Mitochondria still have their own DNA. They create energy from glucose and fat. The more mitochondria you have, the more energy you can conjure up, and the slower you wear out. We all have some mitochondria, but bats have a lot more. This has serious implication for us. If we can improve our mitochondrial function, it can have a profound effect on....[and so on]...

Now take this "quiz": Did this interest you? Could you follow it? Then read PART II and then go on to PART III. No advanced degree required. B's or better in high school science and an inquisitive mind are useful, especially the latter.

Did this seem like a needless digression? Would you rather get straight to the point? Do you have better things to do? Then just read PART II, which won't be diving as much into technical detail. This is not to say it is in some way easier or dumbed down, just less technical.

There are also various appendices, including an annotated bibliography of medical research papers.

Quantitative Medicine is a complete medical system for preventing degenerative disease. It began 20 years ago, largely as an investigation into the various reasons standard medicine wasn't making people well. (In fact, in a lot of cases, it was making people worse.) It became a synthesis of what is known about the cause and prevention of degenerative disease.

Some of the material is common knowledge, some has been known and ignored for decades, and some is new. Its effectiveness has already been proven on a diverse cohort of over 2,000 patients. Effectiveness is largely a matter of compliance, which is to say application of willpower, self-discipline, or just plain old-fashioned gumption.

If you are stopping at PART I, thanks for dropping in, and come back if you need to go further. Good luck.

Key Points
4 - Measurement and Modification
- We are too genetically diverse to know our own health.
- A blood draw and full-body scan will elicit considerable information.
- The hypothalamus doesn't know if you are actually hunting, or emulating something like that at the gym.
- If you eat mostly what you, in principle, could have hunted or gathered, the hypothalamus will make good use of it.
- Starches and sugars have little nutritional value and we are ill equipped to deal with them. They weren't in the Paleolithic diet.
- In any case, your health will not deteriorate, and will likely improve, if you 1) cut down on sugar and starches, 2) turn up the intensity of your exercise, 3) undertake a meditative activity, and 4) get quality sleep.

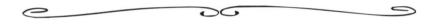

PART II - USING QUANTITATIVE MEDICINE

QUANTIFYING THE HEALING AND REPAIR PROCESSES

5 - PREPARATIONS

Welcome to PART II, which guides you through the whole process of self-quantification and determination of your optimum healthy lifestyle. Included are how and what to measure, how to interpret the results, and if needed, which modifications are most likely to improve them. Do it and you are on the path to a long, disease-free life. Heart disease, cancer, adult onset diabetes, Alzheimer's, osteoporosis, and other degenerative diseases can largely be avoided.

PART II stands alone. It is a complete guide to degenerative disease prevention and recovery. It is the "how to" of the Quantitative Medicine method. "Why" it works is found in PART III.

THE QUANTITATIVE MEDICINE PROCESS

Normally a doctor will order blood tests and scans of various sorts, often as part of an annual physical. Interpretations of the results vary widely. Many simply check that the numbers are within some acceptable range. In fact, often the "normal" ranges that are shown on the blood work results are literally that: the range of the numbers the blood analysis lab typically sees, and not a medically relevant OK/not OK classification at all.

Many doctors are unaware of ideal homeostatic set-points, the body's feedback mechanisms, anabolism indicators, and their importance to health. This information can be pieced together from the medical literature, but it is rarely taught specifically in medical school. When it is, it is usually called

"Lifestyle Medicine," but even there, the Quantitative Medicine "measure and modify" feedback methodology is missing.

Though possible, it is not advised or even desirable to pursue the Quantitative Medicine lifestyle changes without your doctor. But even with your doctor on board, you are, in a sense, taking matters into your own hands. The day you turn up at your doctor's office asking for a requisition for the 16 or so blood tests we recommend, you will likely find you have a confused physician on your hands. Hypochondriacs excepted, having the patient wanting to order additional tests is a bit off the standard medical track.

Dealing with Confused Physician Syndrome (CPS)

Explain exactly what you are doing and why. Other than paying for them, there is no potential harm in getting all these tests, and of course, there are many substantial benefits. Indeed, the measurements could indicate a serious problem. You will want to work with your doctor for any such thing as that. Second, your doctor knows you and can facilitate your proposed transformation, or should anyway.

Chapter 7 lists the tests, along with strategies for dealing with potential costs. So get the blood draw and scan prescriptions and so on, but analyze the results with the doctor, using this book. Discuss what you intend to change and why. There is no logical reason any doctor should have major objections to all this. Actually, they ought to be very interested. They can do better doctoring by adopting these techniques. They too can (and should) practice Quantitative Medicine. CPS is usually curable.

Logical or not, it goes without saying that many doctors won't see things quite this way. They may have the attitude that they and they alone are the keepers of your health. They may discourage the whole approach. A very typical response might be to disregard any numbers that aren't notably problematic and recommend more exercise and less saturated fat. They may try to put you on statins. This response corresponds to an internal doctor thought process that goes something like this: "This patient is not in serious trouble now, maybe the statins will slow the inevitable, maybe he will follow the exercise and dietary advice. Unlikely. Little else to be done. We'll wait for something more serious and hope for the best."

This could be called "standard practice," and if you accept as a given that people won't change, it may indeed be the best advice. However, if you are reading this book, then clearly this is not the kind of medical advice you are seeking When you elect to use Quantitative Medicine, you are taking personal control of your health, and you can bring about substantial improvement by doing so. The method is familiar. It is about health measurement and lifestyle modification.

DOCTOR SHOPPING

Perhaps you do not have a doctor who knows you and whom you regularly see. Or you may have been using a walk-in clinic, or could have relocated. Or perhaps you do have a doctor, but he or she rejects or denigrates the Quantitative Medicine principles. If you feel a change would be appropriate, here are some search tips.

First and foremost, choose a doctor with whom you can communicate, with whom you feel comfortable. If you feel the doctor is not engaged in your issues and concerns, or has an overloaded schedule, you may need to move on.

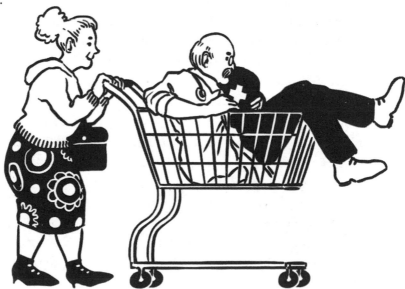

Bear in mind that a doctor may have over a thousand patients, most of whom are seen once or twice a year. It is not necessarily reasonable to expect genuine engagement with every patient, but if the doc shows interest in your proposed program, he will probably become quite involved in your own quest.

But try to push beyond "curious medical observer" and find one that will embrace the principles of Quantitative Medicine, at least provisionally. It is always a good sign if the doctor participates in your investigation of possible measurement-driven lifestyle changes. Will he or she be a detached observer or a co-conspirator? Seek the latter.

Ask the doctor his or her ideas on heart disease prevention, cancer prevention, diet, and the like. Get an idea how they tick. Are they mired in the past or open to new ideas? Probe around.

STANDARD PREVENTIVE MEDICINE ADVICE

Normally it's these four words: "Eat right and exercise." This advice is slung around so casually that it has lost any meaning it may have had. But the four words beg the questions: what should I eat and what sort of exercise must I do? And here is where the troubles really begin. High up on the list of recommendations will likely be found the words "whole grain" and "aerobic." Any advice advocating either of these in any form is a sure sign of belief-based BAD MEDICAL ADVICE. Fact-based reasoning is rare enough in many medical realms, but almost wholly absent in nutritional and exercise recommendations. Neither are taught in medical school, and both are subject to huge cultural and business influences.

Here's a good place to raise your hand and ask a few hard questions. If your glucose is too high, and your doc says eat whole grain and take 45-minute brisk walks daily, you may want her to explain exactly why that is going to help, because as you will soon learn, grain (whole or not) is a likely *cause* of high glucose, and brisk walks aren't going to have any effect on it.

There is no universal best diet. There is a diet that is best for you, but unless you match diet, exercise, and other changes to your specific needs and deficiencies, there will be little improvement. Things may even get worse. The big surprise is that if you do match them, you can make enormous improvement, enough to make an immediate difference, as well as a substantial long-term benefit. Enough to prevent and even reverse degenerative disease. Enough to extend a healthy life. These are the astounding benefits of Quantitative Medicine.

This slowing of aging and blocking of degenerative disease is achieved by giving your hypothalamus free rein to achieve ideal homeostasis and to put you in an anabolic state. These catalyze renewal. Homeostatic misalignment is the root cause of all degenerative disease. In this sense these diseases are all the same.

You, the conscious you, will need to provide an environment that will facilitate this, but to get started, you must resolve four unknowns:

- First, how do you know which parts of you need fixing? Which are in homeostatic alignment and in an anabolic state, and which are not?
- Second, if you need to change something, what, precisely, do you change?
- Third, what will be easy and what will be hard?
- Fourth, how will you know when you've gotten there?

Quantitative Medicine will provide the missing links, or rather show you how to provide them for yourself. To determine which changes might be needed, you have to measure hormones, biochemicals, and the like with blood tests, and take a look inside with a scan. There are known ideal levels, and if these aren't met, they will indicate a direction to take. At this point, you can choose to accept this. It's not an impossible mission, and further, you can make a change, get another blood test in three months, and see if it worked.

To quantify homeostatic alignment and anabolism, we will focus on these five groups of numbers. Get these right, and your rate of aging will be slow and your risk of degenerative disease low.

- Sugar/Starch Management - how well do you metabolize these two?
- Lipid Management - your risk of heart disease. How is your hypothalamus managing fat?
- Stress Management - are you under physiological or psychological stress? Is this impairing your health?
- Anabolism - is your body spending time in anabolic mode, renewing and repairing at the cellular level?

- Organs, Iron, and Bones - are your liver and kidneys working right? How is your iron storage? What is your risk of osteoporosis?

For some of the population, all of these are OK. These lucky people needn't change their lifestyles. For most people, several of these areas will be OK, which then suggests a focus on just the one or two that aren't. For some people, there will be broader problems, which will call for broader solutions.

Depending on your specific results, various changes will be proposed. These will include diet suggestions, exercise suggestions, and stress reduction methods. After all is said and done, you should be eating a delicious diet, but possibly with some of your old favorites gone, exercising vigorously a couple of hours a week in a very specific way, and doing some sort of stress reduction. This would be a typical program. The specifics would be determined from your actual test results.

Summoning up the willpower, drive, gumption, self-discipline, resolve, or whatever you wish to call it, is entirely your affair. You will have your style. You can tiptoe in or take the plunge. If you do *some* of it, you will get *some* of the results, which is always better than none. Plus, this isn't some sort of makeover or rehab. If you have to make changes, you probably have to make them for the rest of your life. So you need to have the wisdom to make changes you can actually stick with; that you are willing to tolerate long-term.

Along the way, you are going to learn a lot about how the body works and a lot about degenerative diseases, both its causes and cures.

Key Points
5 - Preparations
- You may encounter skepticism on the part of the health care providers. Persevere.
- Measurements will indicate how close you are to ideal homeostasis and how anabolic you are.
- Measurements has been divided into four groups—glucose management, lipid management, stress and inflammation management, and anabolism—with a fifth group for several other individual measurements.

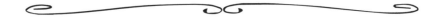

6 - WHAT YOU ALREADY KNOW AND ITS IMPORTANCE

Y ou are already partly "Quantified." You know certain things: your weight, blood pressure perhaps, cholesterol, possibly more. This is a start, but unfortunately these common numbers are, in most cases, badly misinterpreted, as you will soon see.

YOUR "WATE" AND FATE

These machines were once ubiquitous, costing only a penny, but offering mostly non-medical fates. However, attempts to predict health from body weight go back at least 150 years to the Body Mass Index or BMI. There are innumerable (and identical) BMI calculators found on the Internet. By entering your height, weight and sometimes your sex and age, your BMI will be computed, and you will often be sorted into a thin, normal, overweight, obese, or *really* obese category. Normal is 18-25, overweight is 25-30, and so on. Now as measures go, BMI is a really lousy one. What is a lot more important is the percentage of that weight that is muscle, and (not unrelated) 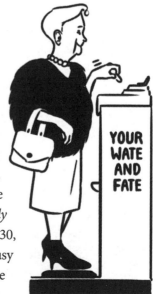 your waist measurement. But lousy or not, a large amount of medical advice is dispensed based on BMI, and a surprisingly large amount of medical research has been conducted connecting it with expected mortality.

Now here's where it gets really interesting, or maybe odd is the right word. Virtually all the medical *authorities* say that the ideal, healthiest BMI is the "normal" range, 18-25. However, virtually all the medical *research* says the healthiest BMI is "overweight." Really! For men the best BMI number is around 27 and for women around 30. This is well into the "overweight" range. There is a 15 to 40 pound difference between "normal" and the ideal "overweight." How can overweight be best? Well, again we have (another) case of doctors appearing to ignore their own research. What is going on here? The doctors are advising a BMI 15 to 40 pounds lower than their own researched optimum. That many pounds is quite a lot to lose, as most of us can attest. Why the disconnect? Here are some possible reasons:

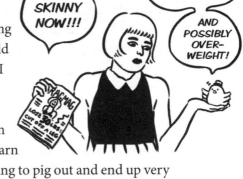

- Doctors watch too much TV. We learn from TV that one notch up from emaciated is ideal.
- The published advice is lagging behind the research. Could be, but some of this BMI research is 15 years old.
- Moral hazard. A medical profession favorite. As soon as we, the general public, learn overweight is best, we are going to pig out and end up very obese. Possibly, but after all, are we really that stupid...?

Does this mean you should plump up? Not really. The overweight health advantage, though real, is quite slight. We will be exploring many other factors that make huge health differences. The real message is that quite a broad range of weights are healthy. For a 5' 10" male 130 to 210 pounds is likely OK; for a 5' 6" woman, a weight of 115 to 185 is in the "don't worry about it" zone. If your weight is changing for no reason, up or down, worry about that.

So what is important weight-wise? It's simple enough. Belly fat is bad. Other fat is not bad. Muscle is good. Don't worry about fat for now. If you are in some sort of dangerous area, too fat or too skinny (which can be dangerous too) the numbers will show what is amiss and will also indicate the best lifestyle changes. Starvation dieting and marathon brisk walks are not going to be among them.

THE GRAND UNIFIED THEORY OF FAT

You have heard by now that fat doesn't make you fat, carbs make you fat, which seems confusing. Why wouldn't fat also make you fat? Rarely is a cogent answer supplied for that one. Here's the answer.

The amount of fat you have is regulated to an ideal homeostatic set-point by our dear friend and master controller, the hypothalamus. If you have more fat than it thinks appropriate, it will burn it. If you have less, it will add fat. If the hypothalamus thinks you need more fat, it will convert everything you eat to fat: carbs, fat, and even protein. It will regulate you to a level it thinks is appropriate—not fat, not skinny.

Fine, you think, so if fat is regulated, why does anyone ever get fat?

Well, there's a catch, and it's a big one. If insulin is high, this hypothalamic fat regulation apparatus is shut down, and fat is stored, not burned. This includes both the carbs you just ate and any fat or protein you consumed as well. It's all converted to fat and stored. Circulating fat in the form of triglycerides will also pile up in your blood.

But fat and protein by themselves don't raise insulin. Glucose—meaning carbs—is the only food that does. So this is why carbs, especially sugar and starch, make you fat. They increase your insulin, block the fat regulation, and basically put you in a fat storage mode.

If you are a kid and can metabolize all those carbs without running up your insulin, then these sorts of dietary habits won't make you fat. That's why kids can get away with that sort of thing, but if those kids eat enough carbs, you get the childhood obesity epidemic.

This hypothalamic regulation is why the Atkins diet works well at first and also explains why there is no more weight loss after a few months. Atkins is a very low-carb diet. This causes the insulin to drop, which allows the hypothalamus to regulate the fat to its desired level. If there is excess fat, it will burn it off quite quickly. It actually burns it. An Atkins dieter will feel hot and sweaty. This burning of fat yields the rapid weight loss this diet is famous for. As soon as the fat has burned down to the ideal hypothalamic reference level, fat is regulated. No more weight loss or gain.

With today's social pressure to be forever skinny, many will not be pleased with the fat level their hypothalamus has chosen for them. Eating less will not work well. Your hypothalamus will fight it tooth and nail. It will lower your energy level, your mental acuity, your creativity, your immune system, your cellular repair level, anything to hang on to that precious fat. You will be irritable, anxious, and depressed. If you starve yourself enough, you can lose more weight, but you will effectively become a zombie.

Why is the hypothalamus so enamored with fat? And why does it shut down the fat burn when we eat a bunch of carbs?

Fat is your reserve fuel. As far as the hypothalamus is concerned, we are all still hunter-gatherers. If we run out of food, that stored fat is our lifeline. So it will let other stuff slide in order to hold on to it. But why does it let the carbs derail the regulation process? Recall that hunter-gatherers ate little or no starch, maybe some honey when they lucked into it, and fruit in season.

This meant carbs were a summertime thing. Since a long ice age winter was soon to follow, it made sense to store up all that sugar as fat. So that's what it does. The hypothalamic set-point for the fat storage is largely genetic. The northern hunter-gatherer populations needed better fat preservation skills. Though of little benefit now, many of us wouldn't be here if our ancestors hadn't had this ability.

BLOOD PRESSURE

This also hasn't a lot of diagnostic value, though high blood pressure is a risk factor for heart disease and should be dealt with.

The conventional medical wisdom among many doctors (sometimes more weightily called "standard practice") has been that anyone with a blood pressure over 140 should be on statins. Some say anyone over 50 years old should be on statins, and some have even proposed them for children. Finally, there is one doctor who has advocated adding statins to the drinking water. (His actual name: Dr. Reckless.)

Other drugs are usually prescribed with the statins, the most common being beta-blockers and ezetimibe.

Here is what the Mayo Clinic has to say:

- If your blood pressure is below 120/80, fine.
- If above 120/80, but below 140/90, it's "Pre-hypertension," and drugs are not recommended.
- Above that, but below 160/100, it's "Stage 1 Hypertension." Try to reduce it with a lifestyle change and failing that, consider drugs.
- Above that, do a lifestyle change and "discuss" taking medication with your doctor.

As far as drugs go, the Mayo Clinic doesn't seem to be in any hurry to pull the trigger. Why then are so many doctors writing endless prescriptions for hypertension? Here, Mayo is perhaps reflecting more recent research, which appears to rather sharply limit the groups of people that benefit from these drugs. Normally, these drugs are specifically targeted at some cardiac risk factor. They may well reduce that risk, but apparently this comes at the expense of other problems. In particular, most of the drugs, singly or in combination, do not appear to lower all-cause mortality for most groups, and for some combinations, there is an increase in death rate.

High Blood Pressure Is Not the Disease

The additional drugs frequently tossed into the mix usually do no good and some harm. The general reason for this is simple: high blood pressure isn't the disease, it is a symptom. The body is raising blood pressure for a reason, such as ensuring that blood gets where it is needed. In most cases, high blood pressure is due to clogged arteries, and the right "medicine" is to unclog them. Unfortunately, neither statins, nor ezetimibe, nor beta-blockers, nor any of the other commonly prescribed meds, reduce the clogging—arterial plaque. The cure is diet and exercise of the right sort, and stress reduction.

However, there are categories of people with dangerously high blood pressure, say 180/110 or higher, that need immediate treatment. Levels this high need to be brought down, but this should be looked upon as an interim measure: something to bridge the gap till lifestyle change can solve the underlying problem.

Here is a list of typical drugs that may be prescribed, in varying combinations, for hypertension.

Statins. These drugs reduce LDL cholesterol, but show no benefit overall. Heart attacks are reduced, but risks of other mortal illnesses are commensurately increased. As mentioned, statins are widely prescribed.

Ezetimibe. This drug is frequently prescribed with a statin. It further lowers cholesterol, but does not appear to lower heart events, and increases cancer.

Beta-blockers. These inhibit adrenalin production and slow the heart down. This lowers blood pressure, though it means less blood to critical areas such as the brain and muscles. Beta-blockers are commonly prescribed for hypertension, but have never been proven to be of benefit to any cohort. They increase mortality.

Calcium channel blockers. Blood pressure is controlled by the tension of the muscles surrounding the walls. Calcium channel blockers relax these (and all other) muscles. Calcium channel blockers are frequently prescribed for hypertension. They have been found to also increase mortality and breast cancer risk.

ACE inhibitors. These also relax the muscles surrounding the vessels. For people with high blood pressure, these drugs show a slight decrease in all-cause mortality (~7%). This appears to be the only drug in the lot that actually shows any benefit (albeit a slight one).

Thiazide is a diuretic and causes the body to dump fluid. It also reduces blood pressure, though the reason for this isn't known (after 60 years on the market). One serious side effect is adult onset diabetes.

It goes without saying that most of these drugs are doing little if any good. None of them reduce atherosclerotic load, the usual cause of high blood pressure, whereas proper diet and exercise will.

If blood pressure is not dangerously elevated, we support the Mayo recommendations: fix it with lifestyle change. This works well and improves every other aspect of your life as well.

Even people with normal blood pressure sometimes have heart disease. Ten percent of all fatal heart attacks involve people with blood pressure below 120/80 - the "ideal" range. However, the higher the blood pressure, the greater the risk. If your blood pressure is over 120/80, you already have some heart disease. It is reversible without drugs. The only way to really determine existing heart disease is a scan for heart calcium. We will be recommending that you get an initial full-body scan and virtual colonoscopy regardless of your age. If you are over 50, have a blood pressure over 120/80, or have any reason to think you may be a cardio risk, we strongly recommend it. Blood test measurements will also provide additional information. You may not be at risk at all, or you may need to make immediate changes. Heart disease is preventable, even reversible.

CHOLESTEROL

Many people will know their total cholesterol number, and perhaps their "good" and "bad" cholesterol levels as well. These numbers haven't a lot of value really. The medically useful information is much more nuanced. Lumped in with "bad" cholesterol we find "really bad" cholesterol and "not bad at all" cholesterol. Similarly, within "good," there is "really good" cholesterol and "more or less neutral" cholesterol. The "really bad" and the "really good" are the important ones. If you don't have much of the "really bad" cholesterol, you may not need to worry about cholesterol—period. And what's more, you are at quite low risk for heart disease. If you do have the "really bad," then you would be advised to make serious efforts to keep it on a short leash. There are several ways to lower the amount of "really bad."

The cholesterol molecule is a major cell wall building block. Without it you would probably melt. It's so important, cells make their own. The cholesterol floating around in the blood is a backup supply manufactured by the liver. The liver packs fat molecules along with cholesterol into little balls called Very Low Density Lipoprotein, or VLDL, and sends them off into the bloodstream. As the VLDL particles circulate about in the blood, hungry cells pick at them and tear off the fat molecules for fuel and structural needs. As the VLDL particles continue their journey, they shrink. As they get smaller, they are renamed LDL (Low Density Lipoprotein), though they are really still the same particle—minus much of its original fat. At this point there is a possible problem. LDL particles, especially the smaller ones (the "really bad ones"), can get stuck behind the artery wall. This causes atherosclerosis (hardening of the arteries). For this reason, LDL is called the "bad" cholesterol.

Your body has developed an interesting way of dealing with these stuck LDL particles. The liver manufactures an even tinier particle, which also circulates in the blood, yanks bits of the stuck LDL particles out of the arteries, and hauls them back to the liver for disposal. These wondrous little particles are called HDL or High Density Lipoprotein, and are known as the "good" cholesterol. As the tiny HDL particles vacuum up the stuck LDL mess, they grow in size. If you have a lot of the "fully grown" HDL particles, your body is doing a splendid job of managing stuck LDL problems and is thereby reducing and reversing atherosclerosis. These fully grown particles are the "really good" cholesterol we mentioned earlier, and are also known as HDL2b, mature cholesterol, or very large HDL particles.

Medical History Sidebar
The Lipid Hypothesis

The lipid hypothesis is that LDL cholesterol causes heart disease. Cholesterol became implicated as a possible culprit in the early 50's when it was found that cholesterol, along with various fats, were principal components of arterial plaque. Therefore get rid of cholesterol and fat. This led to the banishment of eggs, meat, and so on. Well, not entirely banished, but relegated to the tiny top of the food pyramid.

Sounds good, but cholesterol isn't some toxin. It is an essential body building block. Cells make their own, but it is so critical that the body has a backup supply, manufactured by the liver and distributed in the blood.

Furthermore, and here's the key point, the body will keep a certain fixed amount of cholesterol circulating no matter what you eat. If you eat no cholesterol, the liver will manufacture the full amount. If you eat food containing cholesterol, the liver will use that, and make up the difference. Eating has almost no relationship to circulating cholesterol. This has been a cornerstone of Quantitative Medicine dietary advice since inception.

Saturated fat too is innocent. Test after test has shown that saturated fat either has no effect on your health or is good for you.

Then what does cause heart disease? It is LDL cholesterol, all right, but a very specific type. LDL cholesterol particles come in varying sizes. The tiniest sizes do most of the damage. If you don't have those tiny sizes, you probably won't get heart disease no matter what your cholesterol level is.

The cause of these tiny LDL particles is high triglycerides. High triglycerides and tiny particle size are in lockstep. This is solidly established.

Now here's the grand irony of the lipid hypothesis. High triglycerides are not caused by dietary cholesterol, nor are they caused by dietary saturated fat. They are caused by excess carbohydrates. So the "cure" to the heart disease problem—the high-carb food pyramid—actually made things worse. It greatly increased incidence of heart disease.

Later, with measurement, you will learn how much of the troublesome sort of LDL you have and how well the HDL garbage collection fleet is working. If these need fixing, there are ways.

One very important thing. Unless some drug interferes (statins, for instance), the liver, under the direction of the hypothalamus, determines your cholesterol level. It will regulate the level quite *precisely* regardless of what you eat. This means that if you eat cholesterol-rich food, it will make less, and vice versa. The internal level will be kept the same. And this in turn means you can eat any high-cholesterol food you want, with no risk whatsoever. This includes eggs, meat, butter, etc. Don't worry about the cholesterol in what you eat; your body's way ahead of you on this one.

YOUR FAMILY GENETICS

Most health questionnaires ask about your parents, grandparents, and other close blood relatives, and for good reason: you're cooked up out of the same stuff.

You should use this information to jump-start the process. If heart disease is rare in your family, but cancer is not, paying special attention to any lifestyle modifications that fight cancer is clearly in your best interest.

Still there are definite limits as to how much your ancestors can be held accountable. Some problems are recessive and could show up in the child but not the parents. Other problems are simply not genetic.

The several conditions that are genetic in origin merit special attention. There are generally preventive steps that can be taken. For the following, additional information can be found elsewhere in the book:

- **Lp(a).** People with high concentrations of Lp(a), an LDL variant, are at increased risk of heart problem and should focus on heart-healthy practices (exercise, low carbs).
- **APO-E4.** Apolipoproteins are a family of proteins that coat LDL, HDL, and chylomicron particles in order to make them water soluble. The APO-E4 subtype is a strong risk factor for Alzheimer's and heart disease. Again, the best way to fight it, indeed, the only way, is through heart-healthy practices.
- **Celiac Disease.** This is caused by a reaction to gluten, which is found primarily in wheat. It can be quite serious if undiagnosed. Some cannot digest wheat. The solution is simple, though: no wheat or other glutens.

- **LDL particle size.** A predominance of small LDL particles causes heart disease. The size is determined by diet and exercise, but also genetically. Again heart-healthy practices can counteract this.
- **Homeostatic weight.** If you are on a low-carb diet and exercise, your body will regulate to the weight that your hypothalamus thinks is your healthiest. Further weight loss is difficult. The specific level is largely genetic.
- **MTHFR.** A deficiency of this could result in high homocysteine. Homocysteine is a toxic breakdown product of the essential amino acid methionine. Stress and poor diet also raise homocysteine.

See the specific sections or the index for details on these conditions.

Needless to say, there can be numerous other situations affecting overall health that are genetic in origin. Genetic information should be used to advantage, and not as an excuse. For instance, a tendency to store starch and sugar as fat is common and is an adaption to the realities of northern seasons. This doesn't mean that starches must be avoided, or that such weight gain is inevitable. It means only that the levels of the hormones that control all this must be frequently measured and tightly managed. If this is done, the problem can be controlled. Of course, more discipline will be needed.

Genetics can work in you favor as well. Things may turn up indicating that there are certain problems you will never have to worry about. So don't shun genetic information, but use it wisely and sensibly.

Key Points
6 - What You Already Know and Its Importance
- Weight in general and Body Mass Index (BMI) in particular are poor predictors of health.
- "Overweight" is the healthiest weight, though its advantage over "Normal" and "Obese" are slight.
- Normally a weight 20-40 lbs. lighter is recommended by the medical profession.
- Hypertension (high blood pressure) below 140 does not need to be treated with drugs, including statins.
- Total cholesterol is a practically useless measure. More important are certain types of LDL cholesterol and certain types of HDL cholesterol.
- If you have very few of the small LDL particles, your heart disease risk will be low regardless of your overall cholesterol.

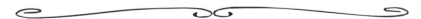

7 - STEP I - TESTING

QUANTIFYING YOUR HEALTH

Health is measured with scans and blood tests. Unless there is a problem, scans would be done infrequently: every couple of years. Blood tests, though, should be done more frequently, some quarterly. There are five categories of blood tests to be considered:

- Tests done only once.
- Tests done in response to a specific symptom.
- Tests done annually.
- Test done twice a year.
- Tests done quarterly.

This may mean, initially, that quite a few tests should be done. There may be some expense involved depending on a variety of factors. Quantitative Medicine is not completely covered by most insurance. More on that later. The test list will evolve. Before diving in, consult QuantitativeMedicine.net for the latest list (and pricing). Enter "Blood Test Panels" in the search box. The availability and usefulness of the various tests are moving targets. Several important tests are no longer available. The reasons for this are unknown, but almost surely financial. We hope they return, along with some useful new ones. Good health depends on good testing.

I'M CRAMMING FOR THE BLOOD TEST!

Tests Done Only Once

These tests tend to indicate things you either do or do not have, but if you have them, you are basically stuck with them. So why bother? These particular tests mean certain risks. For instance, high Lp(a), a cholesterol variant, significantly increases the risk of heart disease. It's genetic and around 10% of the population has it. There is currently no cure, but having it doesn't mean you are condemned to get heart disease, You are predisposed to it though. By adopting lifestyle practices that reduce heart disease risk, you can effectively counteract high Lp(a).

You might already have had these tests. If so, there is no need to repeat them. Here is the list of do-once tests:

- **Lp(a).** Already mentioned, Lp(a) is a lipoprotein (cholesterol) variant that increases heart risk. About 10% of the population is at risk. See the "Is Your Lp(a) High?" section in chapter 9 for details.

- **APO-E4.** Apolipoproteins are a family of proteins that coat LDL, HDL, and chylomicron particles in order to make them water soluble. The APO-E4 subtype is a strong risk factor for Alzheimer's. See "Do You Have the APO-E4 Variant?" in chapter 9 for details. Again, the best way to fight it, indeed, the only way, is through heart-healthy practices, and knowledge of its presence provides strong motivation. Normally this test is ordered after it is too late. Caught early, the risk can be substantially reduced.

- **TTG and Gliadin Antibodies - Gluten Intolerance.** Gluten intolerance is a severe reaction to gluten, found primarily in wheat. In the extreme, it is called celiac disease. Some cannot digest wheat at all. The solution is simple though: cut out wheat and other glutens. See "Are You Gluten Intolerant?" in chapter 9 for details.

Though pricey (~$200 for the lot), these tests need not be repeated.

If either APO-E4 is present or Lp(a) is high, a serious lifelong discipline will be needed comprising a strict diet and strenuous exercise program. It's bad luck to have these, but by acting now, the consequences can be avoided. A strict diet and strenuous exercise program, if begun early, will prevent just about every other degenerative disease too.

Tests Done Once and in Response to a Specific Symptom

Some tests should be done once and also if a problem is suspected:

- **MTHFR.** A persistently high level of homocysteine, a frequently measured blood marker, could indicate an MTHFR deficiency. See "Do You Have MTHFR Deficiency?" in chapter 8 for details.

- **H. pylori** is a stomach bacteria and a nasty one. It causes stomach cancer, ulcers, and other serious problems. It is fairly common in the west, but endemic in much of the developing world. It should be treated with antibiotics. It is a tough bacteria, and several courses of antibiotics could be needed. Normal practice is to treat it when a symptom develops. It's better to be preemptive. H. pylori should be tested once, and retested again after any trips to countries having a strong prevalence. Re-test for this if living in Asia, visiting, or experiencing chronic stomach distress.

We are about to dive into the tests that should be done on a periodic basis. There is one test that should be done annually, and a couple of tests to be done bi-annually, and then a panel of quarterly tests. It is these quarterly numbers that run the show.

Tests Done Annually

Thyroid. Test Thyroid Stimulating Hormone annually. The test is called TSH and could indicate thyroid problems if too high. In such cases, energy levels will be low, and exercise will have less benefit. The standard "too high" level is 4 uiu/ml (or miu/L), but the warning bells should chime at anything above 2.5. For men, a doctor should be seen if this is the case and total testosterone is below 350/dl. For women, T3 and T4 should measured, and a doctor seen if they are low. We cannot give a precise number here, because different labs use different tests for this one. So here "low" should be taken to mean low according to the lab report. The cure for a weak thyroid is levothyroxine, a very inexpensive prescription medicine.

Test Tumor Markers Twice a Year

There are many tests available that could indicate cancer, and indicate it at a stage early enough for effective treatment. These are PSA, for the prostate, and

CA-125 for ovarian cancer. If CA-125 is above 20 u/ml, see your gynecologist. For PSA, trend is important, meaning more than one measurement is needed. If PSA rises more than 0.6 ng/ml in a 12 month period or less, see a urologist. If PSA is over 3, a urologist should also be consulted.

By the time you read this book, these tumor markers may be out of date. There is an enormous amount of work going on in this area. A fair amount of it is trying to come up with a machine that can match a dog's cancer sniffing ability. (Some trained dogs can reliably detect several cancers better than any machine and with an astonishing degree of accuracy.) In just a few years, it may be possible to detect most cancers at early, curable stages. Be sure to keep an eye out for these. Caught early, most cancers are curable, but caught late can be an entirely different story.

GET SNIFFED TWICE A YEAR!

The All Important Quarterly Tests

There are about a dozen or so key blood markers that strongly determine your health, and if not in the ideal range, strongly indicate which areas need to be changed. All these markers should, ideally, be measured quarterly. This is not that expensive, probably under $250, and certainly worth the money. The sicker you are, the more insurance will pay, but it's hard to get a dime out of them for prevention, but prevention is the cornerstone of Quantitative Medicine. There is detail on how to get these tests, how to figure out which ones insurance will pay for, how to avoid overcharging, and how the insurance companies dictate medical care in the "GETTING THE TESTS AT A REASONABLE PRICE" section, later in this chapter.

Sixteen or so tests is a lot to become expert on, so we have sorted them into five groups that specifically relate to degenerative diseases.

- Sugar/Starch Management Group—how well you can metabolize sugar?
- Lipid Management Group—HDL and triglycerides.
- Stress Management Group—is external or internal stress affecting your health?

- Anabolic Management Group—is your exercise level getting you into a healthy anabolic state?
- Organs, Iron, and Bones.

Each group has two or three measurement numbers in it, which often tend to move in concert.

If you "fix" all these numbers, your risk of degenerative disease will decline. If you *really* fix them, substitute "plummet" for "decline." Here is an example where one size really does fit all. The various diseases may look different, but their root causes are all the same.

However, beware: "fixing" the numbers with supplements, as opposed to lifestyle changes, WILL NOT WORK, and usually backfires. Niacin is a perfect example. It raises HDL, the "good" cholesterol, but shortens lives, not the direction we want to head. However, HDL when raised by lifestyle change, increases longevity, and reduces both heart disease and cancer.

Many people are taking all sorts of supplements, and there are innumerable books on the topic. Over-the-counter supplements are

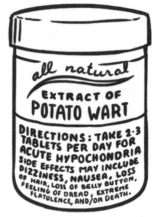

basically drugs, and ought to be viewed that way. We would suggest you stop taking them all if embarking on the Quantitative Medicine program. Other than vitamin D, and in some cases B-12, we know of no case where supplements are beneficial, and frequently, they are harmful.

Your numbers may not need fixing. They may all be OK. You would then already be at low risk and could count yourself very lucky indeed, or maybe you have been taking very good care of yourself or maybe you are a hunter-gatherer. Otherwise, with just reasonable luck, you may have a single main issue. It could be sugar or stress management or something else. When you focus on this issue, you are performing this experiment: Will making this lifestyle change fix that number? Suppose you succeed. You have "proved" the lifestyle change did what you hypothesized. Doesn't mean it will work for anybody else, but that doesn't matter. The experiment you are performing is all about you.

Results vary. People vary. To our knowledge, no one has ever gotten worse using the Quantitative Medicine methodologies contained in this book. Without exception, everyone has gotten better and many considerably so. We are talking about a couple of thousand people here. Many reversed degenerative diseases, and will keep them reversed. No other medical interventions have anything like this level of success.

Avoid the trap of deciding that you will simply do every lifestyle change suggested, so no need to bother with the tests. Be honest. Without that gun at your head, you won't keep it up long term. Take the tests, see specifically what is going on, and determine the lifestyle modifications that will tend to drive the numbers to their ideal zones. You can win. It just takes work. We won't belabor this point, but bear in mind that in things related to health, it is invariably better to ask the hard questions up front, by actual testing, than to make assumptions based on gut feel, or worse, wishful thinking. The reality always contains surprises, both positive and negative.

Here is a summary. This test lists may change. For the most up-to-date ones, and other info, go to the website, QuantitativeMedicine.net, and search for "Blood Test Panels." There may be new, improved tests, or price breakthroughs.

Medical Testing
Blood tests

It is said that it is best not to know how laws and sausages are made. This might well apply to blood tests. In most cases, it is a multi-step process, and they measuring something that is related to something else, that is related to something else, etc., and that is finally related to the item of interest. For example, total cholesterol is extracted form the blood using one chemical which produces two forms of cholesterol which are then combined using a second chemical, and that reacted with a third chemical, which produces a purple colored result, the shade of which is interpreted as the total cholesterol. At least this is one way to do it. The various commercial labs *do not say* how they make the measurement. Seems odd, but it's true.

LDL cholesterol and VLDL aren't measured at all. They assume that 20% of circulating triglycerides are tied up in VLDL, and then manufacture the VLDL number by multiplying triglycerides by 0.2. LDL is computed by subtracting VLDL and HDL total cholesterol.

Several of the tests are standardized and verified by the FDA to match across different labs. This would include HDL, total cholesterol, glucose, triglycerides, TSH, cortisol, ALT, bilirubin, AST, and creatinine. This is a nice start. Other tests might vary from lab to lab. With the exception of Lp(a), they do not seem to vary much. Even so, it is a good idea to stick with the same lab, as a trend in results is likely to be more reliably.

The most inaccurate test is Lp(a). Lp(a) is a risk factor for heart disease. It is an LDL particle with an additional protein string attached. The cholesterol content of Lp(a) is included in the LDL measurement. Lp(a) should therefore never be higher that LDL, but in reality, the measurements often indicate that it is, a logically impossible situation.

We hope that the future brings better, cheaper, and more accurate measurement. We follow this very closely. Before a blood test, it would be good idea to consult the QuantitativeMedicine.net web site for the latest information. Search for "blood test panel."

Test Once:

- Lp(a) - an LDL variant that greatly increases cardio risk
- APO-E4 - a risk factor for Alzheimer's
- TTG and Gliadin antibodies - gluten intolerance

Test Once and When Necessary

- MTHFR - possible cause of elevated homocysteine
- H. pylori - presence of a dangerous stomach bacteria

Test Annually

- TSH - indicator of thyroid function

Test Every Six Months

- PSA (men) - indicator for prostate cancer
- CA-125 (women) - indicator for ovarian cancer

Test Quarterly

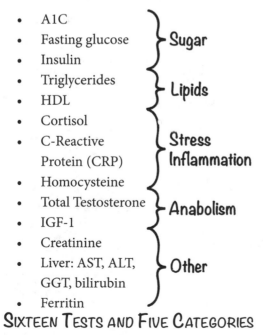

- A1C
- Fasting glucose — **Sugar**
- Insulin
- Triglycerides — **Lipids**
- HDL
- Cortisol
- C-Reactive Protein (CRP) — **Stress Inflammation**
- Homocysteine
- Total Testosterone — **Anabolism**
- IGF-1
- Creatinine
- Liver: AST, ALT, GGT, bilirubin — **Other**
- Ferritin

SIXTEEN TESTS AND FIVE CATEGORIES

UNDERSTANDING THE FIVE CATEGORIES

The five categories, built around 16 different quarterly test numbers, are shown above. These drive your health and are the numbers we are going to work with. Changing these numbers will change your health. You will soon be an expert, but before we dive into their meanings, and how they affect health, we should offer a couple of caveats. First, everyone is different. Basing health improvement decisions on these numbers works well for 80% to 90% of us. For some, it may not work. It won't be dangerous, but the desired result may simply not occur, or may occur very slowly. Second, other things have to be in a functioning state. For example, if your liver is not working well, the Quantitative Medicine program will be less effective. This applies equally to other organ functions. However, waiting for a thyroid, liver, or kidney to come into line is no reason to delay the process. The Quantitative Medicine lifestyle and protocols will speed up those recoveries as well.

The Sugar Management Group

This includes fasting glucose, A1C (average glucose), and insulin. These should be measured quarterly. Why insulin? The body secretes insulin in order to clear out excess blood glucose. Although triglycerides officially belong to the lipid group, we will have them make a guest appearance. Triglycerides tend to be created out of excess sugar in general, and excess fructose in particular. Read all about sugar in the STEP 2 - PUTTING IT TOGETHER chapter coming up.

How serious is the need to manage sugar? In most of our ancient past we only got sugar from fruit and occasionally honey, and those only a few months of the year. Only in the 20th century did sugar become something that could be separately manufactured and added to other food. And added it is! The health impact of this is hard to overstate. Suffice to say that if sugar had been discovered in the last 20 years or so, it would almost certainly be a banned

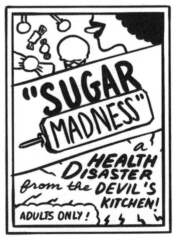

substance along with heroin, cocaine, crack, and the like. It is implicated in many of the degenerative diseases, particularly heart disease, cancer, adult onset diabetes, and Alzheimer's. Without sugar and starch, these diseases probably wouldn't be occurring, or would at least be far less pervasive.

The Lipid Management Group

Lipids (fats) of interest here are HDL, triglycerides, and Lp(a). Lp(a) need be measured only once. HDL and triglycerides are measured quarterly.

Usually, it is cheaper to get a lipid panel, which will also include total cholesterol, LDL cholesterol and VLDL. The drug tests usually just "compute" VLDL (20% of triglycerides) and LDL (total-HDL-VLDL).

Dr. Mike's Cohort Data

Triglycerides

Someone with high triglycerides, say over 200, is already insulin resistant and in the early stages of adult onset diabetes. The pharmaceutical industry has thrown considerable resources into finding a nice, profitable drug they can sell to this group. Some drugs have been shown to reduce triglycerides 20% over a period of several years. This isn't much of a cure. Ideally, triglycerides should be below 100.

In Dr. Mikes cohort, 292 of around 450 patients had two or more triglyceride measurements. Of those, 43 had triglycerides over 200 and were therefore at risk.

In just three months, this group managed to reduce their triglycerides 45%. This is a huge improvement. Of the 43, 29 got their triglycerides below 150. This is about 3/4 of the "at-risk" group, and they are now turned sharply away from adult onset diabetes.

Twenty percent of the group reduced their triglycerides below 100, a very healthy level. Nine people were over 300, and they managed to reduce their triglycerides 50%. Only three people in the entire "at-risk" group had an increase.

There were 46 people between 150 and 200. They reduced their triglycerides 30% in this three-month period. Of the 46, 25% managed to pull their triglycerides below 100. Only one person in the 150-200 group had an increase.

Getting triglycerides below 100 sharply reduces the proportion of "really bad cholesterol," and has many health benefits. Most of the people in the cohort have altered their health trajectory and many have achieved healthy levels, all in a very short period of time.

LDL particle size varies. A predominance of larger ones is called Pattern A, and is a major key to heart health. Pattern B means that primarily smaller LDL particles are present, and this is undesirable.

The principle cause of atherosclerosis is the leakage of circulating junk that occurs during arterial cell wall replacement. The larger LDL sizes tend not to leak through, while the smaller ones definitely do. For this reason, the larger Pattern A sizes mean a much lower risk of heart disease.

We would propose to have the pattern or the size measured, but at this time, the test isn't standardized, and different methods yield different results, though they are similar.

We can estimate pattern type using the triglyceride measurement. Low triglycerides = large particle size = Pattern A. High triglycerides = small particle size = Pattern B. At some triglyceride threshold, people will flip from Pattern B to Pattern A and will stay there as long as they stay below this threshold. Unfortunately, this threshold varies from person to person. Almost everyone will flip to Pattern A if they can reduce and maintain their triglycerides to a level lower than 100 mg/dl. Many will achieve Pattern A with triglyceride levels as high as 150, but reducing triglycerides isn't difficult, so there is no reason not to aim for a lower number, 100 say, or even 75.

Dr. Mike's Cohort Data
LDL Particle Size, LDL Pattern

LDL particles come in different sizes, and there is typically a spread. A blood test that measures sizes reports the most predominant one. The sizes are tiny. A predominance of smaller sizes is dangerous for two reasons. First, there are more of them, and second, the principal route to the atherosclerosis region behind the arteries are dead or dying endothelial (artery wall) cells. These cells are in the process of being replaced. Considerably more of the smaller particles are able to penetrate these "under construction" sites. Based on the sizes, patterns are defined: Pattern A is the larger size, and, Pattern B, the smaller.

The relation between particle size and heart disease is profound. Pattern A is where you want to be. B is high risk, A is low. Those with Pattern B tend to be insulin resistant, have high triglycerides, high glucose, high blood pressure, and low HDL; all risk factors for heart disease.

Pattern A people are at low risk, needn't worry particularly about their cholesterol, and certainly do not need statin drugs. This has been known 20 years, but oddly, has not found much traction in standard medical practice.

Other things being equal, particle size is genetic. About 50% of the population have Pattern A and their inherent risk for heart disease is low. But other things don't stay equal very long—lifestyle soon makes its mark. High triglycerides will lower particle size as will smoking and trans fats. Exercising and reducing triglycerides will increase the particle size.

In Dr. Mike's cohort, about 400 people had their particle size measured using the GGE test (a test no longer available), and 210 had a second measurement, which allows us to look at the change. (Most of those that only did a single measurement had Pattern A already.)

Of the 210, 140 had "A," 27 were intermediate, and 43 were Bs. After 3 months, 13 of the Bs were still Bs. Eight of the Bs had improved to intermediate, and 22 of the 43 Bs, a full 50%, had improved to "A." All but 4 of the 27 intermediates had become As, and those 4 eventually would as well.

Now these results are something truly astounding. Half of the people at high risk for heart disease went from high to low risk in just three months. Over 80% of these initial B people eventually got to the A pattern. This saves lives. Heart attack for those at risk has been reduced by 65%. This was achieved by proper lifestyle change. There is no pill that does this, or even comes remotely close.

As pills go, statins are the most commonly prescribed. They lower risk of heart disease only modestly. They are prescribed equally to Pattern A and B people, which makes no sense whatsoever. Statins actually decrease particle size, which may explain why they are not very effective and why LDL pattern information has not found its way into standard practice.

Smoking and trans fats cause particle sizes to shrink. Fortunately trans fats have largely disappeared from the Western diet. (Naturally occurring trans fats—palm oil for instance—are no problem.) Exercise will cause an increase in particle size. This is likely to be one of its more important benefits. Diet has a greater affect, with excess sugar or starch being strongly implicated. High triglycerides cause small particle size.

You can, if you wish, get a test for LDL pattern type. The Gold Standard for this test was a method called Gradient Gel Electrophoresis (GGE). The company that developed and performed this test was acquired by Quest, and the test has disappeared. Three other tests are out there which will perform a Pattern A/Pattern B analysis: Ion Mobility, NMR, and VAP. We prefer them in that order. If your triglycerides are below 100 mg/dl, you are highly likely to be Pattern A, and it is a near certainty if triglycerides are below 75.

High Lipoprotein(a), also designated Lp(a), is a special condition that significantly increases the risk of heart disease. This can be ameliorated by a serious lifetime discipline. See the "Is Your Lp(a)High" section in chapter 9.

The Stress Group

Stress may have many causes. There could be internal physiological stress. If ideal homeostatic reference points are not being met, this will typically happen. The damage that results will produce inflammation, which indicates that the body, more specifically the immune system, is battling something.

To most people, though, stress means the psychological sort. Our modern civilization itself seems, for many, to be a direct cause. In any case, chronic stress, psychological or physiological, is a formula for cancer and other diseases. Dealing with the stress is every bit as important as exercise or optimizing a diet.

The body reacts in surprisingly similar ways to these two sorts of stress. One common denominator is inflammation and you will often hear

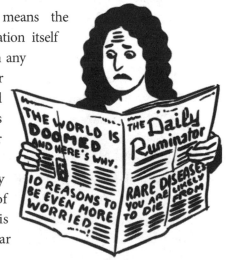

that inflammation is bad. Actually, it is the cause of the inflammation that is bad. Inflammation, though damaging in and of itself, is the lesser of two evils. The cause would do more damage if the body did not combat it. Atherosclerosis is a good example. Inflammation is the body's attempt to stabilize stuck oxidized rancid LDL particles. The immune system will try to remove them in various ways, and failing that, will attempt to wall them off. If it didn't do this, the oxidized material would be likely to eat through the arteries or poison us in some way.

Continuous stressful situations lead to elevation of several blood markers. In particular, we look at, cortisol, homocysteine, and C-Reactive Protein (CRP). These should be measured quarterly.

The Anabolic Group

IGF-1 stands for Insulin-like Growth Factor-1. It got this odd name because it resembles the insulin molecule, and not because it behaves like insulin. It's produced by a different organ (the liver) and has different functions. Specifically, it accelerates cell turnover and growth. Its normal level in childhood is around 100 ng/ml. With the onset of puberty it soars to 1000 or more, attesting to its potency. Most readers will have had some experience with this. IGF-1 then drops to around 200 in adulthood, gradually declining to maybe 100 in old age. If you are exercising, your body will raise your IGF-1 level. This signals cells to repair, grow, and divide. This is anabolism, the building of new body parts.

Testosterone has a life track similar to IGF-1 and has anabolic properties in both men and women. Testosterone levels increase with exercise, but whereas IGF-1 turns on repair and building in specific areas that need it, testosterone is more broad brush, up-regulating anabolism and muscle building throughout. Women produce less testosterone than men, but use it far more wisely. You probably knew that.

IGF-1 and testosterone should be measured quarterly.

Kidneys and Microvascular Health

Microvascular health is just what it sounds like: the health of your tiniest blood vessels. These are the capillaries, of course, and eventually all the arteries branch down to them. They are hardly larger than the various blood cells and biochemicals flowing through them, but they are very numerous. Most of your 50 trillion cells must reside close to a capillary to get their necessary nourishment. Unravel the capillaries and lay them end-to-end, and they go twice around the earth. That's quite a lot of capillary.

Capillaries clog easily. This does not carry the life-threatening specter of a major clogged heart artery (heart attack) or brain artery (stroke), and indeed, if a few capillaries clog, usually no big deal. But what if a lot of them clog in a specific region? That would cause that region to start to die. Where would this be likely to occur? Generally the extremities: the toes, the fingers, the eyes, the brain, and the kidneys. In the worst cases, this means amputations, blindness, loss of cerebral function, and so on. Not a pleasant picture.

Even though microvascular health issues may lack the drama of heart attacks or strokes, they are perhaps just as important, and unsurprisingly, they respond to the same lifestyle modifications as the big arteries: Anaerobic exercise will significantly improve microvascular function.

We would like to measure this. Microvascular health would not show up on a scan, but there is an interesting blood number we can use: creatinine. Creatinine is naturally produced bodily junk and one of the kidney's tasks is to get rid of it. Now the kidneys are very complicated, but one major part is an elaborate strainer, constructed by a huge network of tiny blood vessels. This is a handy microvascular proving ground. If the tiny blood vessels are clear, the kidneys will work well, and creatinine will be removed. If the microvascular health of the kidneys is poor, creatinine levels will rise.

Now the microvascular health of the kidneys is going to be pretty much like the microvascular health everywhere else. So this one measurement is going to give us the big picture—microvascularly speaking. A creatinine level at or above about 1.2 mg/dl is bad. This indicates serious microvascular disease. Often the lab reports will indicate a normal range of 0.7 to 1.2. Ignore that. Anything over 1.0 is a red flag. However, high creatinine levels are reversible. With appropriate exercise, the level can be moved from the danger zone, 1.2, to a very healthy level, 0.9 or even lower. Measure creatinine quarterly.

The kidneys also have several hormonal functions. They additionally regulate several key circulating electrolyte levels. Kidney function is very key to overall good health.

The Liver - the Body's Swiss Army Knife

While the kidney or pancreas may have half a dozen functions in their repertoire, the liver has at least 500. Besides having first dibs on just about everything you eat or drink, it is responsible for all production of VLDL and HDL. It manages an intermediate storage facility for glucose and runs an alchemy operation on the side where it can perform the following transformations: sugar into fat; protein into sugar; even fat into sugar.

Not surprisingly, the liver is an organ you cannot do without: it is just too complicated. If there are any disruptions to the liver, numbers throughout the body tend to go haywire. (If your liver numbers are bad, you should ignore other numbers, fix the liver problem, and retest.)

The liver numbers are AST, ALT, bilirubin, and GGT. They should be within the normal ranges, which will be indicated on the test results. The three main things that affect liver function are hepatitis, fatty liver disease, and excess alcohol. Acetaminophen can damage the liver too. The liver is otherwise a very robust organ, constantly regenerating itself. Make sure your liver numbers are in their normal ranges. Liver health is crucial. Measure quarterly.

GETTING THE TESTS AT A REASONABLE PRICE

If you are starting our program in conjunction with an annual physical, begin with the "test once" type tests, and all appropriate "test if" types, plus the six month tests and the quarterly group. The most up-to-date list, along with the best cash prices we have been able to find, are on the QuantitativeMedicine.net website; search for "Blood Test Panels. The tests are listed above and described below. We have made every effort to streamline this process and get the desired results with as few tests as possible. Still, all this will seem like a huge amount of testing to many doctors (and even more so to most insurance companies).

It's not. Prevention is always cheaper than the disease, cheaper than the surgeries, cheaper than the intrusive procedures, cheaper than a lifetime of pills. However, it is necessary to quantify yourself and measure frequently in order to obtain long lasting energetic health. Here the issue of costs does rear its ugly head, but we have quite a lot of advice on that front, most of it very promising.

Expect to Pay Some of it, But Expect Prices to Drop A Lot

It is just plain STUPID that insurance doesn't pay for preventive medicine, but that is how it is. They have apparently concluded that it is not cost effective (for them). Blood testing, if it weren't so outrageously overpriced, would cost around $150/quarter. Or less. But a nice standard garden variety heart bypass procedure, a procedure that Quantitative Medicine will almost surely help you avoid, goes for $75,000. That's about 120 years worth of blood tests. This is the American price. Divide by around (at least) five for the rest of the planet. But then divide the blood work cost down too.

However, these dark financial clouds have some silver linings: prices are falling rapidly, and insurance will often pay a portion of the bill. Since we advocate thorough and frequent testing, this is good news. To make wise decisions, you need to know how the insurance, doctors, and test labs play together. It is far from harmonious.

You, Your Doctor, Your Insurance: Who is making the calls?

It should be you, in conjunction with your doctor, that determine your medical trajectory, but the way medicine is currently set up, at least in the United States, it's your insurance company, or possibly Uncle Sam, in the case of Medicare.

Now the insurers best interests may not be our own. The less spent on us, the better for them, at least in the short-term. The insurance companies are for-profit, so their interests and objectives should be perfectly clear, and clearly not the same as ours. Plus if they can stall you long enough, you will become Medicare's problem.

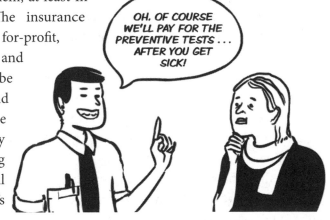

Medicare is worried about running out of money, but at least they have to deal with the long term picture. Whether they do so or not is debatable, but in any case, they are stuck with us to the end.

Though hardly our goal, we also save the insurance industry and Medicare a lot of money. Those that follow Quantitative Medicine are much less likely to need expensive surgeries and other such procedures, and this is where most of the money is going.

However, we are advocating spending money now, on blood testing and scans, in order to eliminate these down the line problems.

That insurance won't pay for prevention is, well— STUPID doesn't really come close, but even though we think it's a no-brainer, preventive medicine is not "standard practice." At least not yet. Other than annual physicals, insurance won't pay an iota for prevention. They were forced into paying for physicals by Obamacare. Still, you have had some blood tests before, and your insurance has probably paid for some of it. So what's the deal on that? There are things going on you don't know about . . .

Every Test Must Have An Appropriate Symptom

Every single test a doctor prescribes has to be triggered by a symptom. And the doctor has to justify it. After he packs you off to the blood draw center, he gets a notice either from the insurance company or sometimes by the blood draw center itself asking him why the test was prescribed. What was the symptom? Now "just making sure the guy isn't sick" or "looking for early warning signs" are not any of the acceptable responses. But obviously, that is exactly what we are doing here. So this puts the doctor in the odd position of having to sort of fish for symptoms. Low-energy could justify a thyroid test. Weight gain could be used for glucose.

The current state of affairs is ugly. If anything, we have understated the insurance company's influence. In many cases, they are actually dictating treatment: "Explain why you are not prescribing statins to patient 4427." From the doc's side, the discomfort level is high. They maintain a general state of infuriation, worsening on occasion. The docs do not want some committee in a for-profit company or some government bureaucracy telling them how to do medicine on their own patients; patients they usually know quite well. And of course, neither do we. And the docs don't like to talk about how constrained they are these days. It's embarrassing. If you do get them talking, you'll probably get an earful.

We are all individuals, yet are subjected to this one-size-fits-all medicine dictated by people that we never see, people that have no idea who we are, and what we are trying to accomplish. It's ugly. Medicine is all set up to prolong all the illnesses it is failing to prevent, or in some cases actually causing.

What does this mean to someone wishing to follow the precepts of Quantitative Medicine? It means that for the time being, until the medical world comes to its senses, you should expect to pay some testing costs out of pocket. How much and for what? The lists of tests and the best cash prices we can find are found on QuantitativeMedicine.net (search "Blood Test Panels"). To keep it in context, expect a cost of between one and three tanks of gasoline quarterly.

These numbers are for America. Elsewhere, gasoline costs (at least) twice as much, and medical tests cost (at most) half as much. So half a tank? Or maybe your national health service will actually pay for preventive medicine.

This is a moving target; keep an eye on the website. We believe that a lot of testing is a key component of peak health, and we are making considerable efforts to find ways this can be made affordable.

Be Up Front With Your Doc

Don't get him in trouble. Show him the list and tell him why you want to do the tests. But, in the same breath, tell him that you are aware that some of the tests may not be covered, and that you want him to identify a safe set of tests that can be sent to the insurance, and another set that you would be willing to pay for. For the tests where you pay cash, he won't have to write justifications, and he can't get in trouble, so he really shouldn't have any objections other than a possible concern for your pocketbook (and we are about to get to that).

So what would be covered by insurance? This varies a lot. Annual physicals are covered at least, sort of, more or less. And some blood work may be covered as well. If you have a symptom, or known disease, this is ample justification for coverage. Your doctor will know all this. But, remember, it is important that your doctor understand that *you know* that some tests are likely not to be covered. Otherwise, he may say that it is not justified, or not cost effective, or something like that. He probably won't want to say that the insurance company won't let him order that test, thus acknowledging that the insurance industry is really, in a sense, running the show. Is this an exaggeration? Below is a letter to Dr. Mike from an insurance company telling him to put his patient on statins. A computer probably generated this. It's rather stronger than a "suggestion." Doctor's reactions vary. Many comply.

Tracking Number: PL 164001730
Date: April, 30, 2015   4858

▶ 1. REVIEW THIS CARE CONSIDERATION for Patient

Tracking Number: 164001730   Date: 10/01/2015   3869DB4C

<u>Care Consideration</u>: Diabetes - Consider Adding a Statin - #1312L
Your patient has evidence for diabetes and has no evidence for a statin. The 2013 ACC/AHA Guidelines on the Treatment of Blood Cholesterol to Reduce Atherosclerotic Cardiovascular Risk in Adults recommend statins to lower the risk for major vascular events in people aged 40 to 75 with type 1 or type 2 diabetes. If your patient fits this clinical profile, and if not already done or contraindicated, consider adding a statin to your patient's medical regimen.

Circulation 2013 ACC/AHA Guideline on the Treatment of Blood Cholesterol to Reduce Atherosclerotic Cardiovascular Risk in Adults: A Report of the American College of Cardiology/American Heart Association Task Force on Practice Guidelines 2013

Relevant Patient Data:

Code	Description	Starting	Ending
250.00	DIAB W/O COMP TYPE II/UNS NOT STATED UNCNTRL	02/26/2015	07/07/2015
00093104901	METFORMIN HCL	03/12/2015	09/02/2015

Controlling The Price of the Blood tests

The simplest method is to not live in America. Then you can just get the tests and be done with it. The cost will likely be under $100, and of course, they may be paid for by the national health coverage anyway.

However, things are not so sanguine in the United States of America. With one major exception the "list" price for blood tests is absurdly high. See the chart a few pages along for some example list pricing. Your doctor may be unaware that much lower pricing is available to you, and available via several different routes, and may be worried that things are going to spiral out of control, cost-wise. However, you are never going to have to pay those outrageous list prices. Below, we explain exactly how to avoid it.

In any case, you can always ask your insurance company what they will pay for directly. However, since our sort of testing is not something they are usually handling, this may be somewhat futile. Or unreliable.

For those tests that the doc thinks can't be justified, plan to pay cash. The doc can write a separate requisition for cash tests.

There are two effective ways to deal with the test-price issue, both reasonably economical, and a third way, just now becoming available, that is yet a further cost improvement.

Method 1: Explore your inner Persian carpet merchant. Walk in, say: "no insurance, what's the cash price." You don't need real cash, you can still pay with a credit card. They will probably quote you a pretty good price, but they may quote list price. Insist on the cash discount. They all have one, but some of them make you ask for it. However, you will have consulted the QuantitativeMedicine.net website in advance, and will know that the tests can be gotten for some certain price, so unless they quote lower, negotiate. Tell them to contact the mother ship and get a lower price, the Medicare price, or the Medicaid price. Some lower price. Wheedle and whine. This nearly always works. The staff in the draw center is usually sympathetic. Print the material from the website and show them lower prices. They are still making plenty of money, so have no mercy.

Method 2. Get your own tests. This is easy, legal (in most states), safe, and completely identical to the tests your doctor would request. If you have any misgivings, discuss them with your doctor. Listed on the web site are "retail outlets" for two major nationwide blood draw centers. There are dozens of such outfits. They will take your money on-line, email you a prescription signed by some mysterious doctor, and instruct you to proceed to the nearest Quest or LabCorp blood draw center. From that point on, it is no different from walking in with your doctor's prescription, except no more cash changes hands. They will take your blood, do the analysis, which will be exactly and completely the same as the one that would have been ordered by your doctor. In a couple of days, the results will be emailed back to you and only you. These can then be forwarded to your doctor.

Costs here vary, but as of this writing, one of these outfits has 13 of our 16 quarterly tests for a $141 grand total. The other two tests are available at their arch rival for $90, so the grand total here, if you paid 100% out of pocket, should never exceed $231.

I'M READY TO TAKE YOUR BLOOD NOW!

That's three tanks of gas. Now if you just waltz into the blood draw center and let them take some blood, a single test might cost more than that.

Method 3. Local Labs. While Quest and LabCorp are nation wide, there are numerous regional labs. Theranos, for instance, is a startup, and the grand plan is that they will offer blood draw and analysis services in 8,200 Walgreen's all across the U.S. Their prices are quite low, and it would be a great benefit for the Quantitative Medicine approach should they succeed. The Theranos requisition is interesting in that it lists the actual prices you will pay, an absolute first for the American blood testing industry. For our 16 quarterly tests, the Theranos cost is only $94.57.

There are other regional labs, and they might have competitive prices. Your doctor should be well aware of them.

There are also other start-ups with various proprietary technologies that may revolutionize test in other ways. Some are specializing in early detection of cancer.

The approval process for new test methods can be onerous, sometimes taking years, and we further expect the established providers to become very defensive.

In any case, both you and your doctor should go over the blood test results. Best if you review them together, but don't become overly concerned if some of them are not in their normal ranges. This usually isn't serious and can usually be fixed.

About Panels

The blood test companies love batch testing. Their machines are set up for it. For instance, the "comprehensive metabolic" panel, costing between $10 and $30, includes glucose, creatinine, AST, and ALT, four of our 16 tests. Likewise, a lipid panel, costing about the same, will provide triglycerides and HDL. Panels often represent a significant savings.

Insurance Co-Pay and Deductibles

Many types of insurance will have co-pays, where you pay part of the bill, and most policies have a deductible, where you pay 100% until the deductible is reached. Now the cost is relatively well contained here, because the insurance company has negotiated a low rate, and usually a good one.

But again—buyer beware. You may be better off paying cash. The price may be lower still. You can inquire on the spot at the blood draw center. Just tell them that you don't think you will hit your deductible, so could you instead have the cash price. That's usually lower. Of course, if you pay cash, you don't use up your deductible, so you will have to strategize as to which would be best for your case. Medicare has no co-pay or deductible, but there is another pitfall there: ABN.

Medicare Recipients: Beware of ABN

ABN stands for Advance Beneficiary Notice, and is intended to protect Medicare from unnecessary procedures, and the patient, you, from unpleasant surprise charges. However, the charges are still unpleasant, just not a surprise.

From the blood draw industry's point of view, ABN is a license to steal. It works like this. If the physician wants to order a test for you, but doesn't think Medicare will cover it, he is obliged to have you sign an ABN, which is supposed to include the price you will have to pay. Rules are changing, and there is a lot of confusion. However, if you sign an ABN, and if Medicare doesn't cover the procedure, you will be stuck with blood work charged at the hugely inflated "list price," not the nice low Medicare price.

There is no need to take this risk. Don't sign the ABN, but do get the test. Just tell your physician to remove the test from the requisition that would be submitted to Medicare, and write a separate one for the test(s) that Medicare may not cover. Then follow the procedures outlined in the preceding section.

As of late 2016, Walk In Labs is the lowest price "retail outlet" we have been able to find that sells blood draw requisitions for LabCorp. New Century Labs seems to be the lowest for Quest. We are not endorsing these companies. There are dozens of other "retail outlets," and there may be lower prices. Do your own shopping. These outfits even have sales and coupons!.

So just say NO to any ABN that your physician wants you to sign, get him to write a separate requisition, pay cash, and avoid the ABN price trap.

Ready for some shock therapy? Here are ABN prices from a lab that carelessly put their ABN procedures document on-line. This document has fallen into the wrong hands (ours). The name of the lab has been fictionalized. Excerpts:

Test	ABN Price at "Welcome To My Parlor" Labs	Theranos	Walk in Labs, LabCorp Retail	New Century Labs, Quest Retail
Fasting Glucose	$44	$2.70	$27	$10
PSA	$130	$12.65	$35	$17
Triglycerides	$77	$3.95	$27	$15
Hemoglobin A1C	$68	$6.67	$27	$14
HDL Cholesterol	$87	$5.63	Included with triglycerides	Included with triglycerides

SCANS

Blood tests, though valuable, have their limits. The other major technology available to take a non-invasive look inside is the full-body scan. The scan will measure several important things that blood tests cannot. We advise that one be done periodically, perhaps every five years if there are no problems. There are several sorts of scans, but the one of interest here is the CT (Computed Tomography) or "cat" scan. The CT with the lowest exposure is called EBT (Electron Beam Tomography). The exposure is very moderate and will not likely be a problem. All these machine work by rapidly spinning an x-ray around you. The EBT accomplishes this by moving the x-ray beam electronically, which is inherently much faster than moving it mechanically, as is done in a normal "cat" scan.

If the scanner is an EBT machine, they will say so. Otherwise it is the mechanical type, the "normal" cat or CT scan, and is designated by the number of "slices," the range being 4, 8, 16, 64, 256, and 320. This refers to the number of x-ray sensors the machine has. From the manufacturer's point of view, each sensor depicts a "slice" of you. More slices means it's over quicker and hence less exposure. The exposure from a 256 or 320 slice machine is on par with the EBT and is thus quite low.

We need to mention that both the CT and EBT machines are X-ray measurements and excess exposure to x-rays increases your risk of cancer.

However, the increase in cancer risk with the recommended machines is well under 1%, likely closer to a tenth of that. Such risks are hard to measure and are more than offset by the life saving information that you will be obtaining. Further, if you follow the protocols given in this book, you will be decreasing your cancer risk between 50% and 100%, which completely swamps any tenth percent increase.

Try to find an EBT machine or one of the newer 256 or 320 slice machines. If the scan center is offering any of these, they will usually advertise it. Otherwise, ask, or assume it's 64 slice or less. Since insurance doesn't typically pay, the scan industry tends to have reasonably competitive pricing. We know what you are thinking: reasonably competitive pricing couldn't exist in American medicine. But it does. They even have sales and specials. At least one outfit offers a couple's deal. How romantic.

We recommend a full-body scan with a virtual colonoscopy, even if you are under 50. If you have any reason to suspect you may have a heart problem, have ever smoked or been exposed to second-hand smoke, or are over 50, we strongly recommend it. This is the most complete scan, though lesser scans are also useful. A complete scan will reveal the presence or absence of several life-threatening problems, and most importantly, will provide enough advance notice about these potential problems to take an early and effective action.

The full-body scan will reveal these:

- Amount of heart calcium—the best non-invasive measurement of atherosclerosis.
- Bone density—how far are you from osteoporosis?
- Colon problems—any early signs of colon cancer.
- Thoracic or abdominal aneurisms—these can be fatal and ~4% of people over 65 have one.
- Cancers or pre-cancerous condition in various organs— includes lungs, liver, gall bladder, spleen, kidneys, adrenal glands, etc.

It is good to know precisely what is going on. This allows a more directed health strategy. Here is some detail about the items in the above list.

Heart Calcium. Calcification is one of the body's (many) defenses against arterial plaque. It is just what it sounds like. The plaque is turned into stone. As such, it is stable and won't break loose and cause a clot, heart attack, or a stroke. However, it can restrict blood flow and reduces the flexibility of the various arteries. Men over 50 and women over 60 usually have some heart calcium. It is not a threat.

However, the heart calcium will double every two to four years unless measures are taken. With the exercise and dietary program you will be developing, the increase can be vastly slowed down, even reversed. We will warn you that some very firmly entrenched medical dogma clearly states that this is impossible; that there is nothing you can do to even slow the heart calcium increase. You will be proving this wrong, as have several hundred other people that undertook the Quantitative Medicine approach.

Bone Density. The amount of calcium and other minerals in your bones. Calcium gives them strength. A typical 40-year-old will have a bone density of 175 mg/cc. These are strong bones, hard to break and quick to heal if they do. With age, there is about a 2% loss per year. This adds up. By seventy, other things being equal, the density will have sagged to around 105, with is the "fracture threshold." This is as serious as it sounds. The bones can no longer support the weight of their owner and start to crush in on themselves. This is osteoporosis. Calcium supplementation will slow it, but calcium supplementation significantly increases heart attack risk—not a good trade-off. Dynamic, load-bearing exercise, though, can actually reverse osteoporosis.

Medical Tests
Scans and Early Detection of Cancer

Early detection of cancer can save your life. Cancer has not shown the marked reduction in mortality that heart disease has. In some countries it is rising. The best defense by far is to catch it early, and except for a couple of specific cancers, the scan is the only tool we've got.

There are dozens of types of cancers, varying considerably in both lethality and speed. The full-body scan looks at every organ except the brain. It will detect tumors as small as ¼ inch. There are also frequent false detections. As is well known, early detection greatly improves survival prospects.

For lung cancer specifically, a scan will detect about 85% of the highly treatable Stage I cancers, and if treated, over 90% will survive beyond 10 years. Untreated, it is essentially fatal. Colon cancer is similar: largely curable if caught early, usually fatal if not.

Other cancers are not so easily defeated, even with early detection. Liver and pancreatic cancer are in this category with one-year survival rates around 30-40%.

If you have a significantly elevated cancer risk, you might want to discuss an annual scan with your doctor since many cancers develop too quickly to be caught by a five year scan.

Who are at risk? Anyone who ever smoked or lived with some who did. Those who have a close blood relative who died of cancer. Those who have had previous cancers.

Colon Cancer. The virtual colonoscopy will turn up possible cancerous or pre-cancerous conditions in the colon. Colon cancer is not rare and is the most common fatal cancer among non-smokers. Caught early, it's usually curable. Caught late, it's usually fatal. People under 50 seldom die from colon cancer, and because of this, many doctors will not advise a colonoscopy. However, a study has shown that 20% of people between 40 and 50 have some sort of abnormality in their colon. Now, these people probably won't develop cancer until they are over 50, and if they do, it will likely be caught by a colonoscopy then, or so the medical reasoning goes. We find this foolhardy. If you know there is something there (and if you are in your 40's, there's a 1 in 5 chance there is), you should keep a close eye on it. Lifestyle modifications may make it go away. If it doesn't and treatment is needed, it can be done early and safely. With better screening, deaths from colon cancer could be substantially reduced.

Thoracic or Abdominal Aneurism. An aneurism is a weak spot in an artery wall that then balloons out. This alone will cause a lot of damage if it happens in the brain. However, in the chest (thoracic) or gut (abdominal), it will probably go unnoticed. But if this "balloon" pops, it can be fatal. About 4% of people over 65 have an aneurism, and are therefore at risk. The scan will detect these. Aneurism should be treated. Treatment is usually surgical and very effective.

Cancers or pre-cancerous conditions in various organs. The "full-body scan" starts at your neck and stops at your nether regions. Though not literally "full-body," such a scan looks at every organ except your brain. It can reveal cancer or potentially cancerous areas as well as other items, such as gallstones or kidney stones, generalized infections, or inflammations. It gives you a very nice, thorough, and reassuring picture.

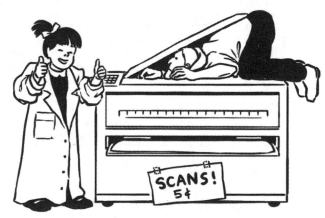

DON'T OVER-ECONOMIZE.

So to further answer the original question: "Should you get a scan?" we would respond: definitely. In the absence of problems, get another one every five years.

If there is any likelihood you are prone to cancer, consider getting a scan annually. If there are problems, the frequency of the scans will be driven by the doctors treating them. If there are one or two specific things of interest, it allows you to focus. For instance, to treat low bone density, dynamic, load-bearing exercise would be appropriate.

Dr. Mike's Philosophical Sidebar
Get Well With Aristotle!

Against the backdrop of genetics and environmental hazards like infections and toxins, we become ill as a function of our character.

Those familiar with my work know that I advocate changing nutritional and exercise patterns and adopting a spiritual discipline as the most effective medicines there are, and with which we can beat back the encroachment of aging and degeneration.

It is clear from this that I hold that changes in behavior going forward in time can alter the effects of already emergent disease caused by past behavior. Simple enough.

Unfortunately it is not as simple as that, and here is the instance where Aristotle becomes our physician.

I have a fascinating example to illustrate my general point. I have one member of a pair of identical/maternal twins in my practice. He came to me with out-of-control adult onset diabetes already, with a positive nuclear stress test, and he promptly accepted my direction and cured himself of diabetes and completely reversed his nuclear stress test evidence of severe coronary artery disease. "Promptly" was a few years but it was certainly more prompt and efficient than years of medications and a series of stents in his coronary arteries.

Well his identical twin has the same diseases and, by narrative from his brother, to the same degree. Yet he has not adopted any of the healthy lifestyle changes that my patient, his twin, has so successfully undertaken.

A quickly judgmental person (myself sometimes, I must admit) would say "what the heck is wrong with that guy?"

But that's the wrong question; the right one is: "what does it take?"

What it takes is what Aristotle has to offer: an understanding of what moves us to change our minds, to have us see ourselves in a new light.

It takes drama, it takes tragedy, it takes the narrative power of a well told story, a moving hero or flawed protagonist, it takes seeing our lives not as a completed story waiting for the last chapter to be read but one that is dynamic and fluid with the possible and with chapters yet unwritten by our authorship.

Stories have a beginning, a middle and an end; when understood we identify with the protagonist and are moved by his dilemma and long for a just or happy resolution to his story.

About Pills and Supplements

Now obviously if you have something a pill will usually cure, such as a bacterial infection, then it's clearly appropriate. A day seldom passes that Dr. Nichols doesn't write a prescription to someone. However, a pill that is to be taken every day for the rest of your life merits some deeper consideration, and in the absence of a clear, well-defined benefit, it's generally best to avoid such a commitment.

It should be abundantly clear that the most effective prescription is lifestyle change, and pills or supplements aren't generally recommended. This is not because of any notions of holistic medicine or other such principles. The reasoning is much simpler. For the most part, pills and supplements simply don't work. Not all, but most. Here is a short list of two pills and a supplement which may be indicated.

Thyroxin and Testosterone. With age, the thyroid gland reduces production below the hypothalamic set-point. Testosterone may be low as well. However, give Quantitative Medicine a real and determined try before considering supplementation. The thyroid can turn on under the influence of proper diet, exercise, and stress reduction. If you don't get the expected boost after at least six months of serious, compliant effort consider taking thyroid and/or testosterone replacement. Start with the thyroid supplement. Testosterone may improve with the thyroid. Of course, consult your doctor first.

Vitamin D. Vitamin D is not actually a vitamin, i.e. we can produce it ourselves. Vitamin D acts like a hormone, and properly should be considered to be one. There are several forms of vitamin D over-the-counter. Choose D3. Consider supplementing until your total vitamin D level is in the mid-range of what is reported as normal. Do not get caught up in the "high doses of vitamin D cure everything" craze. Keep you eye open. There is still a lot not known about vitamin D.

As to the drugstore aisles full of other supplements—leave them alone unless you have a specific solid reason. There are simply too many unintended consequences. Consider these four items before buying any supplement:

- Reliability of the manufacturers. There have been numerous scandals involving mislabeled ingredients.
- Overall effect on mortality - do you live longer or not?
- NNT - Number Needed to Treat. How many need to take the pill before one person benefits? This could be 1 in the case of an antibiotic—it works nearly 100% of the time—or could be as high as 300 to 1 for a statin, where it means that 300 must be treated for one of them to experience a benefit.
- NNH - Number Needed to Harm. How often do the side effects harm someone?

Thyroxin, testosterone, and vitamin D, used as we suggest, all decrease or have no effect on mortality, none cause any known harm.

Here is some information on some of the most widely used pills and supplements:

- Medications for mild hypertension (blood pressure<140): No one benefited, 1 in 12 were harmed.
- Statins for people with no known heart disease: No effect on mortality. Heart attack prevented in 1 in 60. Caused diabetes 1 in 50, caused muscle damage 1 in 10.
- The only vitamin supplement that doesn't appear to do any harm is vitamin D. A large study of older women (Iowa Women's Health Study) found the following alarming result: Daily multi-vitamin increased mortality 2.4%
- Vitamin B$_6$, folic acid, magnesium, and zinc increased mortality 3-6%
- Calcium supplementation also increased mortality 3% in one study at least.

Key Points

7 - STEP I - Testing

- We recommend you start with our standard lists.
- There are many measurements. We group them into sugar management, lipid management, stress management, anabolism, and other.
- Measurements that are out of the "normal" range should be addressed by your doctor. Most cases are no cause for concern.
- You will probably have to pay for some of your tests.
- There are many ways to avoid the overpricing endemic to the blood draw industry.
- A scan is recommended, but wait till you have access to a newer scan machine.

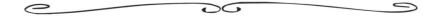

8 - STEP II - QUANTIFY YOURSELF

Wе'll suppose now that you got the tests mentioned in STEP I - TESTING or have decided to analyze some numbers obtained in the past. This section will show you how to interpret them. You may want to do this with your doctor.

Before we dive in, a couple of items need to be mentioned. First, the blood tests usually come back with "normal" ranges indicated on the test report. These ranges represent what the test labs usually see, and not necessarily some OK value. Second, different labs use different methods, and numbers can vary somewhat.

THE BIG HOMEOSTATIC-ANABOLIC PICTURE

In PART I, we hypothesized a gadget that would tell us how we were doing anabolically and homeostatically. We promised that this could be done with measurement. Here is how.

Your Anabolic Score

Score 2 points if your IGF-1 is in the range 130 to 170 ng/ml (higher is dangerous) or else score 1 if in the range 100 to 130. If your total testosterone in ng/dl is greater than 500 (men) or 20 (women), score a point. If your HDL is greater than 65 mg/dl for males, or 75 mg/dl for females, score 2 points, and score 1 point if HDL is below that, but above 55 mg/dl for males or 65 mg/dl for females. A total of 3 is good. 4 is superb, and 5 is Olympic material. These are exercise numbers. If you want to improve them, consider increasing the intensity of your exercise rather than the duration. Keeping the score high will promote cellular health, retard aging, and stave off degenerative disease.

Your Homeostatic Alignment Score

We have repeatedly spoken of ideal homeostasis or alignment. Here are the markers that matter the most, along with their ideal ranges:

- Fasting insulin between 3 and 6 μu/dl
- A1C less than 5%
- Triglycerides below 100 mg/dl
- HDL greater than 65 mg/dl (male) or 75 (female)
- Cortisol below 12 μg/dl

Score 1 for each one of these you meet. The top score, 5, is great, and 4 is good too. A score of 0, 1, or 2 indicates a need for improvement.

Add your two scores together. You could be a perfect 10—perfectly aligned and anabolic. For most people this is achievable, though it would take some dedication and discipline. The reward for doing so is a long disease-free life. Most sensible and active 25-year-olds and most hunter-gatherers of any age would score a 9 or a 10. Any combined score below 5 should sound an alarm. Above 6 is pretty good. An average 55-year-old American would probably come in between 4 and 6. Someone with adult onset diabetes would likely score below 3.

Suppose the homeostatic score is good, but the anabolic score is not, or vice versa. What would this mean? A good homeostatic score with a low anabolic score would be found in many thin people. An older person in this category might be considered frail. The good homeostatic numbers mean degenerative diseases are not developing, but the low anabolic numbers mean the resources needed to combat these diseases are limited. Basically the body is conserving. Energy levels will be low. Cell renewal is suppressed. Osteoporosis could be a significant problem.

High anabolism with low homeostatic alignment could describe the athlete who takes steroids, or any individual who exercises, but perhaps overindulges. Cancer would be the main risk for this group.

For most people, some of the numbers will be in the desired range, and one or two others will not. This indicates where the efforts need to be deployed. Below, the numbers are broken down into groups and may be analyzed more deeply. It is important to know exactly where the risks lie. Some of us are naturally prone to heart disease, others to cancer, and others to adult onset diabetes. All of these can be effectively combated.

Before we plunge into all this, we want to add this caveat—no cheating is allowed. By this we mean that pills, drugs, and supplements that might improve these various numbers won't improve your health prospects. It simply doesn't work that way. Niacin is a good example. Niacin raises HDL—the famous "good" cholesterol—and lowers triglycerides as well. However, niacin doesn't reduce all-cause mortality. In fact, it increases it. This is certainly an unwelcome surprise. Exercise will also raise HDL, but exercise increases life span. The moral: it's not the numbers *per se* that are causing the improvements; what counted is what you had to do to get those numbers. Unlike niacin, exercise improves HDL, but also improves a variety of other things. Niacin is not a substitute for exercise even though they both improve HDL. So far, no magic pill.

THE SUGAR MANAGEMENT GROUP

SUMMARY	SUGAR MANAGEMENT GROUP
MEASURES	Ability of body to metabolize sugars and starches
SCORING	Special Case 1 - Insulin less than 3 µu/dl - See "Hypoglycemia" Special Case 2 - Insulin less than 3 µu/dl- See "Are You Too Thin?" "A" - Fasting glucose below 80 mg/dl, A1C below 5%, Insulin between 3 and 6 µu/dl "B" - Fasting glucose below 90 mg/dl, A1C below 5.5%, insulin below 12 µu/dl "C" - Anything else
RISKS	"A" - Healthy "B" - Slight insulin resistance - early warning for adult onset diabetes "C" - Insulin resistant - significant risk of adult onset diabetes.
REMEDIES	"A" - No changes needed "B" - Cut some sugar and starch "C" - Cut all sugar and starch, or as much as you can tolerate.
TIMING	Results should be apparent in 3 months, retest at that time.

All About Sugar and Starch

Glucose seems to be a major player in most degenerative disease: The plaque that gums up arteries, causing atherosclerosis, typically has some glucose components in it. Excess sugar raises triglycerides, a major heart disease risk factor. Excess glucose leads directly to insulin resistance, weight gain, and if carried far enough, adult onset diabetes. The brain damage seen in Alzheimer's tends to have glucose products present. Finally, glucose is a cancer promoter. Cancer cells usually can only survive on glucose, and they need a lot of it.

Sugar usually consists of a 50–50 mix of glucose and fructose. This is true for table sugar and high fructose corn syrup and roughly true for most fruit. Starches, however, are converted to 100% glucose. Both fructose and glucose go first to the liver, but after that, their fates diverge markedly.

Most of the glucose you consume passes through the liver and then directly into the bloodstream. The body then generates insulin, which acts as a delivery service, carrying the glucose through the bloodstream and delivering it to waiting cells. The muscle, brain, and other cells have first shot at this, but if there is glucose left over, it's stored as fat in the fat cells. So excess glucose makes you fat!

Fructose doesn't make it out of the liver in one piece. The liver first uses it to replenish its glycogen, a high-density form of sugar the liver builds and stores for later use. Once this is topped up, the liver converts the remaining fructose to triglycerides, the basic molecule of fat. It then packs lots of these little fat molecules along with cholesterol into VLDL particles and sends them off into the bloodstream. VLDL stands for Very Low Density Lipoprotein, and is a fluffy wad of triglycerides and cholesterol. As the VLDL particle floats by, cells can snatch a triglyceride and use it for energy. Muscle cells, fat cells, and in some cases brain cells do this. As the triglycerides are stripped off, the VLDL particle shrinks, eventually becoming LDL, the infamous "bad" cholesterol. So excess fructose increases your triglycerides and LDL cholesterol!

For these reasons, there is currently a lot of press suggesting that fructose is worse than glucose. Excess amounts of either are quite dangerous over the long run, and excess amounts of both are a prominent feature of the Western diet.

Fructose isn't really needed at all. The ever versatile liver can replenish its glycogen storage from glucose alone if need be. Glycogen is a massive molecule made up of perhaps as many as 30,000 little glucose molecules rather elegantly tacked together. It looks like a dandelion about to be blown. If the liver is building glycogen by using fructose, it converts it to glucose before attachment. After a meal is digested and there is no blood glucose available from food, the liver will supply it by disassembling the glycogen-dandelion back into individual glucose molecules and letting them loose into the bloodstream. Quite versatile, the liver.

The muscles also store glycogen. (Actually, altogether the muscles store several times more than the liver.) They make the glycogen from the circulating blood glucose. The muscle glycogen is consumed first in exercise.

The amount of circulating glucose is tiny compared to the glycogen store: 5 grams circulating glucose versus 100 grams stored in the liver and 400 grams in the muscles. A fifth of an ounce of sugar in the blood, a pound of sugar in the muscles.

Young cells can metabolize glucose more efficiently than old cells. It is for this reason that children can get away with a sugar/starch intake that would rapidly get stored as fat in many adults. However, this obviously has its limits too, as we are reported to be in the midst of a childhood obesity epidemic. The obesity is the visible effect, but arterial plaque is developing, cellular stress is developing, along with insulin resistance, the hallmark of adult onset diabetes. If for some macabre reason you wanted to jump-start degenerative disease, excess sugar and starch in childhood would be very effective.

The Sugar/Starch Management Group Score

How is your sugar management? You get an "A" if fasting glucose is below 80 mg/dl, A1C is less than 5%, and insulin is between 3 and 6 μu/dl. Fasting means 12 to 14 hours after your last meal. Circulating sugar from that meal should be long gone and the hypothalamus should be regulating to your ideal reference point somewhere below 80. At this point, it's adding sugar to the blood by directing the liver to dump glucose from the glycogen that was stored earlier. There should be little need for the insulin escort, so its level should be below 6 μu/dl, effectively turned way down. A1C is an indirect measure of average sugar. The average includes the fasting levels as well as the higher levels that occur right after a meal. A score of 5% on A1C means an average level of 100 mg/dl. This in turn means either your body rapidly took up all the sugar and starch you ate, or you aren't eating much of it in the first place. If your A1C is less than 5.5%, fasting glucose less than 90 and the insulin less than 12, the score is a "B" for now, but if any of these three are near these limits, you are not on very solid ground and should make a dietary change, and cut sugar or starch somewhat. If you are over any of these limits, the score is a "C" and you are showing signs of insulin resistance. You definitely need to cut sugar and starch in this case. This will have to be a lifetime decision, so cut it in a way you can live with. This isn't always easy, especially at first. More on this in the LIFESTYLE CHANGES section.

THE LIPID MANAGEMENT GROUP

SUMMARY	LIPID MANAGEMENT GROUP
MEASURES	How the body is dealing with fat and cholesterol
SCORING	Special case - Lp(a) greater than 30 mg/dl - see "Is Your Lp(a) High?" "A" - Triglycerides below 100 mg/dl and HDL above 65 (men)/ 75(women) "B" - Triglycerides below 150 mg/dl and HDL above 55 (men)/ 65(women) "C" - Anything else
RISKS	"A" - Healthy "B" - Atherosclerosis is developing "C" - Significant heart disease risk. Rapid plaque development.
REMEDIES	"A" - No changes needed "B" or "C" - High triglycerides indicates a need to cut starches and sugars. HDL should respond to higher intensity exercise.
TIMING	Result should be apparent in 3 to 6 months, retest at those times.

All About Lipids

Lipids are fat. Fats are essential to life; carbohydrates are not. Fats are the preferred energy source for the body. Carbohydrates, though, especially starches, are a lot cheaper. This is how they got into our diet in the first place, as a cheap, low-grade food for farm laborers, who were largely enslaved or in some way indentured.

Hopefully, you read the earlier material on cholesterol and are no longer afraid of it. If not, here's a short summary. Your hypothalamus will regulate cholesterol to a specific ideal. If you eat food that contains it, less will be made, so as to keep the total at its ideal reference level. If you don't eat such foods, it will generate more cholesterol from scratch to make up the difference. It doesn't matter one way or the other how much you eat.

Statin drugs interfere with the cholesterol process and reduce the levels. It is far from clear that this is a good idea, and for many people, possibly most, it is a not a good idea at all. Statins also decrease the benefits of exercise. Given the endless inundation of statin advertising, being well informed is important.

A lipoprotein is a bunch of fat particles coated with a protein so that it can float around in the blood. This packaging is needed because blood is mostly water, and fat and water don't mix. Lipoproteins come in five species: VLDL, ILDL, LDL, HDL, and chylomicrons. The first four, from large to small, stand for Very Low, Intermediate, Low, and High Density Lipoprotein. All these originate in the liver.

The oddball, the chylomicron, is constructed by the intestines while digesting a meal, and released directly into the bloodstream. As blood tests are performed after a 12 to 14-hour fast, almost all the chylomicrons are gone. Its life story is much like VLDL, but without the cholesterol.

VLDL particles have a short but perilous journey. VLDL is manufactured in the liver. It is a small wad of triglycerides (fat) with a cholesterol core and a surface coating of protein. The VLDL is set loose in the bloodstream and circulates about, passing near cells. Any cell needing some energy can snatch a triglyceride molecule and use it for energy or other purposes. As the VLDL particle gets repeatedly plucked by the hungry cells, it shrinks, and at about half its original size, it is renamed IDL. When further stripped, it is renamed again, to LDL, though it is still the same original particle, minus most of its triglyceride (fat) content. It is well over half cholesterol at this point.

Cholesterol is so important that cells make their own. Circulating it via these LDL particles is a backup plan in case the cells can't make enough. If a cell needs cholesterol, it will actually engulf the entire remaining LDL particle and disassemble it internally.

Those circulating LDL particles that don't get engulfed continue to shrink and this is not good. Below a certain size, they are able to migrate behind the artery wall and get trapped. These stuck particles, now a mix of fat, glucose products, and cholesterol, don't keep well. In a short period of time they will get oxidized (made rancid) by the infamous free radicals. Once this happens, the immune system gets involved and a cascade of further problems can occur, leading to atherosclerosis—hardening of the arteries.

Some people inherently have the small LDL particles and others don't. The reasons aren't 100% clear, but genetics plays a role. We have the picture of the shrinking VLDL particle, with cells greedily plucking triglycerides until nothing much is left but an LDL particle full of cholesterol. This particle circulates until some needy cell engulfs it entirely. It does seem clear that the cells won't engulf the particle until most of the triglycerides are gone and mainly cholesterol is left. High levels of triglycerides cause the more dangerous, tinier final particles.

Finally there is High Density Lipoprotein or HDL. This is a completely different creature. It is also cooked up in the liver, but its mission is garbage collection, and what a superb job it does of it. HDL particles start out small and flat, like microscopic dishes. These are much smaller than LDL. They circulate around the body, pick up all sorts of junk, and swell up into "mature" HDL particles (also termed HDL2b), at which point the liver takes them out of service and recycles them. The best-known garbage collected by HDL is the rancid fat-cholesterol-sugar mess stuck behind the artery wall—atherosclerosis. The HDL particles are actually shuttled back and forth through the cells that comprise the artery wall (the endothelium). Once behind it, they dock onto overloaded immune cells that are dealing with the atherosclerotic mess and unload the gunk. When "full," they transit back through the artery wall, and on to the liver for disposal. The "scavenger receptors" on the surface of the HDL particle that identify the garbage are aptly named.

It doesn't stop there, however. HDL is capable of scavenging all sorts of other bodily trash. Specifically it is extremely good at cancer prevention. In one study, increasing HDL by 10 mg/dl decreased cardiac risk by 50% and cancer risk by 36%. Now, as cardiac and cancer risk reduction goes, that is a very strong result, and a 10 mg/dl increase in HDL is not at all hard to achieve. Any modest improvement in exercise effectiveness will boost HDL by that much, frequently even twice that. As usual there is a catch. You have to get your body to increase the HDL. Pills can increase it too, but you don't get the benefit. If we look at HDL particles as a fleet of tiny garbage trucks, we are really interested in how many of them return back loaded, not how many are sitting around. The loaded ones are called mature HDL or HDL2b. This key HDL subtype, along with overall HDL, increase with effective exercise.

CAUSE OF DEGENERATIVE DISEASE
Atherosclerosis - Hardening of the Arteries

Various debris circulating in the blood tends to get caught behind the arterial walls when individual artery wall cells are in the process of being replaced. Very small LDL particles are an example of this debris, but other stuff is found there as well. Basically this debris quickly spoils (oxidizes). The spoilage is caused by circulating free radicals and is toxic. The ever alert immune system gets involved to stabilize the situation.

Cells from the immune system attempt to decompose the mess into something safe, but if conditions are right (poor diet and exercise), the mess will pile up. The combination of immune cells and the schmutz they are mopping up is called an atheroma. Two things can happen now, and neither are good. First, atheroma takes up room. If it takes enough of it, it can restrict or even block an artery. This is the usual cause of ischemia. Second, sometimes the atheroma bursts and spews a bunch of rancid debris directly into the artery. Arteries become smaller as they go along, so eventually the debris causes a clog. This can produce a stroke or heart attack.

In addition to the immune system repair attempts, circulating HDL, the so-called good cholesterol, will try to dismantle and remove the debris. It is quite adept at this.

Atherosclerosis is reversible, but this is difficult. It is easier to prevent. It can be attacked on several fronts.

- Reduce the amount of very tiny LDL particles.
- Reduce the glucose level.
- Reduce the level of circulating free radicals.
- Increase the level of HDL.

The size of the tiniest LDL particles is determined by several things. About 50% of the population has genetic good luck, and produces very few of them. Smoking will reduce particle size. This is likely the major reason why smoking causes heart problems. Trans fat reduces particle size as well. High triglyceride levels are also associated with small particle size. High triglycerides normally are due to excess sugar and starch. Exercise increases particle size. Bigger particles are better.

Circulating free radicals can come from many sources and turn out to be important in several body processes. They were demonized for years, and innumerable supplements were recommended to reduce them. (Actually this is still the case.) Tampering with the natural levels of the free radicals with supplements has led to problems and increased mortality. Exercise also lowers free radicals, and since this isn't fighting the body's natural uses for them, this method is beneficial.

Increasing HDL is a powerful defense against atherosclerosis. HDL and especially HDL2b ("mature" HDL) levels are largely driven by exercise.

With a well-controlled lifestyle, atherosclerosis can slowly be reversed.

The Lipid Group Score

Time for the report card. We will be looking at triglycerides and HDL You might notice that overall level of LDL cholesterol is not one of our measurements. You get an "A" if your triglycerides are under 100 mg/dl and your total HDL is above 65 mg/dl for men and 75 mg/dl for women.

An "A" means low heart disease risk and very good cancer resistance and is where you want to be. Specifically, triglycerides under 100 mg/dl means your body was able to use all the fat that came either directly from diet or from sugar conversion. The LDL particle size and percentages of small particles are obviously related. For a given level of LDL cholesterol, either you have a lot of little LDL particles, or you have a few big ones, which is what we want. The size is to some extent genetic. The size is reduced by smoking, high triglycerides, and trans fat, and is increased by exercise. Getting the size up to the safe levels is a very worthwhile goal, virtually a heart disease insurance policy.

A "B" score means triglycerides are under 150 mg/dl and your total HDL is above 55 mg/dl for men and 65 mg/dl for women.

If you got a "B," you should consider a lifestyle change. If you didn't get an "A" or a "B," you got a "C" and you need to strongly consider a lifestyle change.

If your triglycerides are high, the most likely causes are excess alcohol, sugar, or starch. Paradoxically, a high-carb intake causes high triglycerides (fat) and a high-fat diet will almost always reduce them. The relationship between high carbs, fat intake, and stored fat has been well established in the medical literature for at least 25 years, but you would never know it with all the advice to cut meat and cut fat to reduce high triglycerides.

Reducing triglycerides by a switch from carbs to fat will reduce the amount of the dangerous small-sized LDL particles.

HDL tends to be boosted more by exercise than diet. High HDL indicates your body is doing very effective garbage collection—basically an immune activity. It may be the physical aspects of exercise that actually permit the HDL to do its job. In any case, this is the reward for getting many things right, so keep a close watch on HDL.

When we say LDL cholesterol and HDL cholesterol, we are talking about how much cholesterol is found in the LDL or HDL particles. It's all the same cholesterol. There is no good or bad. The difference is that if cholesterol is found in LDL, it is floating about in the bloodstream and could (if small enough) end up behind an artery. If it is found in HDL, a rescue operation has occurred. Some cholesterol that was stuck behind an artery wall has been pulled out by the HDL particle, and is on its way out of your body. Now when your doctor talks of "good" and "bad" cholesterol, you will know what this really means. Doctors frequently dumb things down that have no need of it.

Did you get a scan? This is the best non-invasive test for atherosclerosis, as it looks directly at plaque. Well, almost directly. It actually looks at calcified plaque, which is one of the body's stabilizing reactions to plaque deposits. Calcified plaque tends to increase throughout life. For a sedentary overweight person, it could double as rapidly as every two years. For someone who exercises and eats appropriately, the doubling time can be stretched to 10 years or longer, or even halted or reversed. Calcification is a slow process. Hence atherosclerosis could effectively be in retreat with little change the amount of calcification.

THE STRESS GROUP

SUMMARY	STRESS MANAGEMENT GROUP
MEASURES	Chronic Stress and Inflammation
SCORING	"A" - Cortisol below 12 μg/dl, homocysteine below 8 nmol/ml, C-reactive protein below 1 mg/L and stress reduction activity 10 minutes or more per day. "B" - Cortisol below 14 μu/dl, homocysteine below 10 nmol/ml, C-reactive protein below 2 mg/L. "C" - Anything else.
RISKS	"A" - Healthy "B" - Some stress: internal, external, or both. "C" - Significant long-term cancer risk. Elevated glucose.
REMEDIES	"A" - No changes needed "B"- If internal, deal with cause. If external, add a stress reduction activity. "C"- If internal, deal with cause. If external, consider stress reduction and/or medication.
TIMING	Results are very rapid for externally generated stress. Internal stress may vary considerably depending on cause. Bacterial and viral infection - fast. Heart disease, more slowly.

External stress is usually divided into acute and chronic, though obviously there is considerable overlap. Life threatening-acute stress is, for most of us, most of the time, a thing of the past. Other than the threat itself, acute stress poses little or no health risk, largely because it doesn't last very long. It may even be healthy. This sort of stress is the fight-or-flight response. Acuity is peaked, blood pressure rises, blood sugar spikes, and the immune system gets ready to deal with possible wounds. Learning and memory are enhanced, presumably so the imminent danger will not be forgotten.

Stress that is continually occurring would be deemed chronic. This could result from a high-pressure job, a combat situation, relationship issues, a difficult caretaking activity, or other such things. The body handles chronic stress in a rather frightening way. Chronic stress suppresses the immune system, causes weight gain, impairs sleep, and raises blood pressure. These set off other chain reactions of undesirable events. We certainly do not want the immune system suppressed. Recall that cancer is essentially a staring contest between the immune system and millions of defective cells. Suppressing the immune system basically promotes cancer. The immune system tends to lose its effectiveness with age anyway, but stress greatly speeds up the process.

Why does the body have this unhealthy response to chronic stress? Our hypothalamus is in charge of this stress response, and in this case has help from two other ancient brains: the amygdala (fear) and the hippocampus (memory), as well as our modern consciousness. In our past, chronic stress would have involved a completely different and far more lethal cast of characters. Famine, roving wolf packs, hostile neighboring tribes, and other long-term problems would have instigated the chronic stress responses that are now so detrimental. But back then, it would have been a fatal mistake to kick back and relax. The long-term effects of chronic stress would have been the lesser risk. The immediate caution, alertness, worry, and fear had to be maintained or there would likely be no long term.

Internal stress can likewise have many causes, but inflammation is a common denominator. A viral or bacterial infection would be an example that in due course typically goes away. General lack of ideal homeostatic alignment would be another, but this one can persist for years or decades. If stress markers become elevated and stay that way, damage is being done.

We measure three things, all related to stress and inflammation, but in rather different ways. Cortisol is specifically and rapidly driven high by stress. It also rises in reaction to pathogens. Cortisol is generated by the adrenal gland under the control of the hypothalamus. Cortisol's quick reaction tends to mask what we really want to know, which is the average day-to-day stress.

C-Reactive Protein, or CRP for short, basically plays the role of a snitch. Any foreign material that needs to be gotten rid of is tagged by CRP and then destroyed by various immune system cells. Quite a lot of things could be marked: viruses, bacteria, dead or defective cells. A high level of CRP indicates that a battle is taking place somewhere. It could be a bacterial infection, heart disease, cancer, or, amazingly, psychological stress. Why is that amazing? Well, we would suppose that this sort of stress was something that mainly went on in the head. Why would CRP, something associated with garbage collection, get into the act? The reasons aren't entirely clear, but CRP does increase. It may be reacting to the elevation in cortisol. There is a known genetic variant which causes a higher than normal CRP. The goal here remains the same: get the CRP as low as you can. People with this genetic variant have an increased risk of disease, so care is advised.

Homocysteine is a complicated little beast. It is an intermediate product in an important biochemical protein-building operation. If homocysteine piles up, something is amiss with that process. Excess homocysteine may be instrumental in weakening the arterial lining (the endothelium), which could then lead to atherosclerosis. Because of this, it is now the new bad boy on the block. High homocysteine can indicate high stress, both internal and external. Vitamin deficiency can elevate it too, as can excess coffee.

In our day-to-day lives, we probably make a big distinction between external chronic stress, something usually psychological, and internal inflammation, something physiological. Our body apparently doesn't. This has at least one far-reaching implication. External stress, which we might suppose is "all in our heads," has serious impact elsewhere. It is causing the same sort of internal damage and destruction as a chronic internal inflammation. Further, this external/internal similarity makes it a little tricky to interpret the three numbers and figure out which type it is.

The Stress Group Score

You get an "A" if your cortisol is below 12 µg/dl, your homocysteine is under 8 nmol/ml, your CRP is under 1 mg/L, and you are meditating 10 minutes a day or more. If your cortisol is under 14 µg/dl, your homocysteine is under 10 nmol/ml, and CRP under 2 mg/L, you get a "B," and otherwise score a "C."

Now keep in mind that these are volatile numbers, especially CRP and cortisol. Just about anything could set them off: a rude driver on the way to your blood draw, a dispute about the bill, a masochistic phlebotomist, etc. If you can identify something like this, just continue your good diet, exercise, and meditation practices and measure again in three months.

If you conclude that there is no likely transient cause of elevated cortisol or CRP, and the grade is a "B" or a "C," some other information is needed. You will have an awareness of the stress level in your life. High stress would tend to drive cortisol more than the others. If this is the case, the cause is probably external chronic stress, and given the health implications of this, serious efforts should be made to reduce it. This would normally involve a concerted effort to deal effectively with the situation causing the stress, regular meditative activity, and possibly medication. High cortisol is very dangerous and must be dealt with.

If CRP stands out, this tends to indicate something internal. If you know or suspect you have heart issues (elevated blood pressure, elevated triglycerides, small LDL particles, etc.) you can reasonably expect CRP to go down as you undertake lifestyle changes needed to reverse heart disease.

High homocysteine could occur in either of these cases, and would likewise subside if they are rectified. If it doesn't, it could indicate an MTHFR deficiency.

In any case, if you can't get all the stress/inflammation numbers straightened out in 6 to 12 months, you are advised to pursue it further with the help of physicians, perhaps an endocrinologist, or if heart disease is suspected, a cardiologist.

Do You Have MTHFR Deficiency?

MTHFR stands for methylenetetrahydrofolate reductase, and a deficiency of this, often a genetic condition, will cause elevated levels of homocysteine. If homocysteine stubbornly refuses to go down, this could be the cause. Such a condition is common and can be determined by a DNA test.

Another common cause for high homocysteine is poor nutrition. Proper diet, of course, is the "cure" here.

There is no clear-cut remedy for MTHFR deficiency. You will need to consult a doctor, preferably one with good insights into this sort of situation. Traditionally B-vitamin supplementation has been a common treatment, but there are numerous complications that can arise from that. For instance, folic acid (B_9) can triple the risk of prostate cancer. This association between vitamin B_9 and prostate cancer was discovered by accident only about 10 years ago. There may be other such time bombs ticking away.

THE ANABOLIC GROUP

SUMMARY	ANABOLIC GROUP
MEASURES	Extent of renewal and the presence of an anabolic state
SCORING WOMEN	"A" - IGF-1 in the range 150 ng/ml ± 20, total testosterone above 20 ng/dl, HDL above 75 mg/dl "B" - IGF-1 above 125 ng/ml, total testosterone above 15 ng/ml HDL above 55 mg/dl "C" – Anything else
SCORING MEN	"A" - IGF-1 in the range 150 ng/ml ± 20, total testosterone above 500 ng/dl, HDL above 65 mg/dl "B" - IGF-1 above 125 ng/ml, total testosterone above 400 ng/ml, HDL above 45 mg/dl "C" – Anything else
RISKS	"A" - Healthy "B" - Renewal is moderate, cardiac protection is moderate "C" - Heart disease, accelerated aging
REMEDIES	"A" - No changes needed "B" - Consider more exercise intensity "C" - Do the recommended exercises. A "C" indicates you are not exercising or are doing the wrong sort
TIMING	Numbers should significantly improve in six months.

If the hypothalamus has concluded that it should conserve energy, it will quite effectively shut down a variety of processes that it thinks can wait, and will then guide the body into a catabolic state. There are a variety of reasons the hypothalamus might come to such a conclusion, many of them remnants of our Paleolithic days. Lack of food, preparation for winter, and migrations are three such. The hypothalamus is unaware that these have largely passed into history and interprets fat avoidance, excess sugar, and long walks as equivalent causes for catabolism.

Energy conservation, as it applies to the body, is a response to uncertainty or confusion, and carries with it none of the moral halo that accompanies cutting the gasoline or utility bills. The body wears out more rapidly from disuse than from use. It is designed to be active. Its notion of energy conservation includes a curtailment of repair activities. Neither new muscle nor new bone gets built, and precious energy-rich fat is clung to tenaciously. Another major energy guzzler, the brain, is likewise partly powered down.

We don't want any of this. It's a cold and bleak existence. It's neither healthy nor fun. Getting the whole of our anabolic machinery up and running again is, of course, up to the little dictator: the hypothalamus. But remember, the hypothalamus works for us if we take charge. The strongest way to get it to summon up the desirable anabolic mode is to eat a sensible selection of food, especially fats and proteins, and partake of frequent physical activity. By its ancient calculus, this must mean that successful hunting has become possible and it is time to spend, not conserve. This *hunting* mode turns on all the things we want turned on. It means building bone and muscle. Increased mental acuity. Increased creativity. Fat burning. Cellular repair and turnover. The immune system is powered up. This is the good life.

However, *hunting* mode does not mean we have to go out and kill cute little furry animals (nor risk life and limb dealing with any of the not-so-cute larger ones). If we are getting food and exercise, the hypothalamus will turn on anabolism. As clever as it is, it doesn't have the wit to figure out that we are essentially faking. Woe be it unto us if it ever sorts that one out. More likely it will learn how to thrive on potato chips first.

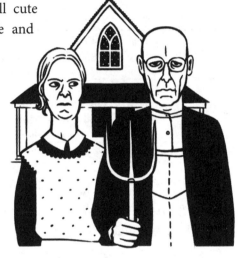

How can we measure anabolic **AMERICAN CATABOLIC** mode? This gets a little tricky because of the clever mechanisms the body invokes to perform these repairs. Rather than evolve some separate anabolism organ or system, it uses pieces of the body's extensive immune and repair system. The immune system is much more powerful and elaborate and gets engaged whenever there is any sort of trauma or wound—large or small. Involved in all this are commando units of white blood cells with all sorts of specialties: some fight the bacteria that accompany all wounds, some rebuild the cell support structure, some haul off the dead junk, some get the cells to start replicating, others tell the cells when to stop.

If a muscle or bone cell is worked hard, or even stretched, it is in a sense damaged, and this sets off some of the immune system repair machinery. Part of the activity is local. Damaged muscle cells want to repair and grow and prepare to do so, but this requires a blessing from the hypothalamus, which gets its information via two routes.

First, there are dedicated nerves that allow the hypothalamus to monitor physical activity. This is a lot more than just a nerve or two. The hypothalamus can figure out if the exercise was concentric (lifting, pushing, pulling, hunting, hard running) or eccentric (walking, jogging, migrating).

Second, cell walls from overworked muscles become stretched and porous. This allows various molecules to leak into the bloodstream that essentially say, "Heal me." The hypothalamus detects these too. If the hypothalamus thinks it appropriate (concentric = hunting), it will act and bump up several growth hormones, two of which we will measure, IGF-1 and testosterone.

Our somewhat beaten-up and overworked bone and muscle cells are also going to "express" a lot of receptors for these growth hormones. They have basically raised their cellular hands, calling for attention. The circulating IGF-1 will latch onto these receptors, which then cause, or more accurately permit, the cells to grow or divide.

Now isn't this a lot of physiological red tape? The damaged cell has to, in effect, get permission from the little dictator—the hypothalamus—to fix *itself*. Why would things be so elaborate? The tools the bone and muscle need for rebuilding are built-in. Why can't they just use them directly?

Well, there are (at least) two reasons, and they are big ones. The first one, which we have seen before, is energy conservation. Healing takes a disproportionately high amount, and if the hypothalamus thinks there is an energy shortage, or isn't sure, it's not going to permit "inessential" bone and muscle building. This is the reason bones break more readily in inactive people. This applies doubly to the elderly.

The second reason is this: the body is way too good at rebuilding. A newborn doubles her weight in three months.

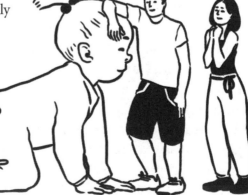

This is probably the fastest possible rate the body can build. If she kept this three-month doubling up, she would weigh in at over a ton on her third birthday, so this sort of thing clearly has to be managed.

So, in sum, the cells have almost completely given up their "right" to reproduce, thus leading to this more elaborate hypothalamically controlled system, piggybacking onto the immune system. More stable, more energy efficient, and vastly more complicated. The immune-repair system is second only to the neural system in terms of overwhelming complexity.

Testosterone is also raised in response to exercise, and whereas IGF-1 enables muscle building at particular sites that need it, testosterone is more of a general signal to build muscle everywhere. Women make a lot less testosterone than men, but use it mostly for muscle building rather than wasting it elsewhere.

The Anabolic Group Score

For men, score an "A" if your IGF-1 is in the range 150 ng/ml ± 20 (higher is dangerous), total testosterone is above 500 ng/dl, and HDL is above 65 mg/dl. Score a "B" if your IGF-1 is above 125 ng/ml and HDL is above 45 mg/dl. Otherwise a "C."

For women, score an "A" if your IGF-1 is in the range 150 ng/ml ± 20, total testosterone above 20 ng/dl, and HDL above 75 mg/dl. Score a "B" if your IGF-1 is above 125 ng/ml and HDL is above 55 mg/dl. Otherwise a "C."

Did you get a VO2Max? They are a bit hard to come by, but tend to cost under $100. They can also be estimated using your two-kilometer rowing time on a Concept 2 rower. Though not as good, these machines are at least widely available, being found in most gyms. VO2Max measures your ability to huff and puff. It's the maximum rate you can use oxygen. The higher the healthier, and it is a great exercise marker because many things must be operating well to get a good score. If your exercise is effective, your VO2Max will climb. This is a good way to monitor your overall progress.

HDL seems to pop up everywhere as sort of a wonder drug. We described its garbage collection function earlier. Though its claim to fame is cholesterol collection, it can go after dozens of other things and is apparently programmable. High levels of HDL mean the HDL garbage collection system is performing well.

Supplements
Bodybuilding Hormonal Supplements

Some bodybuilders supplement with IGF-1, testosterone, insulin, cortisol, and several other very powerful hormones. These are generally termed anabolic steroids. These do enhance muscle growth. They are banned in most competitive sports.

Use of these supplements is a controversial area. One frequently overlooked danger is product quality. Many of these products are not properly controlled and contain dangerous contaminants. There have been deaths from this.

However, even if quality supplements are obtained, their use is obviously doing something counter to the ideal hypothalamic regulation. The list of possible side effects is long. Enlarged heart, high blood pressure, and significantly increased cancer risk are just some. It is not hard to see why artificially increased growth-promoting hormone levels would increase cancer risk. Cancer is simply out-of-control growth after all.

Our opinion is clear. Don't do it. You would be playing with fire. Neither you nor anyone else can begin to understand all the subtle ramifications that can result. Trust your hypothalamus. Work out at the gym and let it decide what the optimal levels are. It will boost them too, but in a careful and controlled way.

When taking any sort of supplement, remember this: "If you take it, you won't make it!"

The body will usually nullify the effect of any supplementation by making less of any given hormone or other bodily chemical. It may stop making the hormone altogether, and later, be unable to resume the production.

ORGANS, IRON, AND BONES

The Liver and the Kidneys

We vertebrates differ markedly from crustaceans, having soft skin, internal bones, closed circulatory system, brains, and so on, but one organ we have in common is the liver. This may help explain why it is loaded up with so many functions. It performs at least 500 different ones, but the final tally isn't in yet. The liver has another feature that may come from crustaceans: it can regenerate itself, and is the only organ that can.

Here is part of the liver's repertoire:

- Storing sugar as glycogen
- Dispensing that sugar as needed later
- Making sugar from scratch from various amino acids
- Making cholesterol
- Making triglycerides from sugars
- Packaging lipoproteins
- Producing bile for digestion
- Breaking down of many toxins such as alcohol
- Storing various vitamins

- Producing blood plasma
- Producing several immune factors
- Producing clotting factors

It should come as no surprise that the liver is an organ you cannot do without. It is managed by the hypothalamus, but in its absence will muddle along, continuing to perform its many functions.

The quarterly blood panel measures ALT, AST, bilirubin, and GGT. All of these should be in their proper ranges.

The most common causes of liver problems are excess alcohol and hepatitis. Liver problems must be dealt with medically. The body will not function properly if the liver doesn't. If liver numbers are off, many other numbers will be off and probably will not have a lot of meaning.

MRSA infections will also send the liver numbers askew. Lyme disease as well. Binge drinking and acetaminophen are particularly deadly. The kidneys are also vulnerable to this combination. If you drink, don't take acetaminophen, and vice versa. Though the bottle carries a small warning, the complications can be far more severe than generally realized.

Unlike the liver, kidneys are a vertebrate invention and filter toxins and waste material from the blood, sending them on to the bladder for disposal. The kidneys are rich with tiny blood vessels, and by measuring one of the numerous items they are supposed to filter, creatinine, we can make an assessment of kidney function in particular and microvascular health in general. The "normal" range for creatinine is 0.7 to 1.2 mg/dl. Actually, anything over 1.0 indicates a problem. With improvement in exercise, especially anaerobic exercise, this number will drop, indicating improvement in microvascular health in general. Be sure to keep an eye on this number.

Is Your Iron Level Too High?

Iron by itself is toxic, but since cells need it, it is bundled into a non-toxic protein called ferritin. If ferritin is too high, it is not so "non-toxic" anymore. It can cause heart damage, liver damage, fatigue, rapid aging, and joint pain. Post-menopausal women often have elevated ferritin.

High ferritin can also be caused by an immune response to cancer or an infection. This would tend to be confirmed if high C-reactive protein were also present. Ferritin could be elevated in response to stress or due to hereditary hemochromatosis, a genetic disorder. Cirrhosis of the liver, diabetes, and arthritis could also cause elevated levels.

If ferritin is greater than 125 mg/dl, and all the other possible causes have been ruled out, consider giving blood once a year. If greater than 200, do it quarterly. (As medical procedures go, this is a very old one.)

Bones

If you got a scan and measured bone density, a number greater than 135 gm/cm^2 means your osteoporosis risk is low—for now. Other things being equal, you will lose bone density at 2% per year. A person with a density of 135 gm/cm^2 will be at the "fracture threshold" in about 15 years. This is where bones start to crush in, height is lost, and the back may start to hunch over. Calcium supplementation may slow this, but increase the risk of heart attack, so this is not recommended. However, safe prevention is quite simple. Proper load-bearing exercises, such as squats and deadlifts, will not only stem the loss of bone but will reverse it. New bone will be built. These lifting sorts of exercises are described in the EXERCISE section coming up.

What about All Those Other Numbers?

The blood work panels will have more measurements than described above. This partly reflects the automation practices of the analysis labs. There are two reasons to collect all these additional numbers.

First, if any are out of normal range (and test results will indicate this), it is imperative that a doctor see them. If you are working with a doctor, this will naturally occur.

Second, trends are very important, even trends within normal ranges. Trends mean something is changing and this bears further scrutiny. PSA, which tests for prostate cancer, is a good example. An increasing PSA, even within the normal range, can indicate cancer.

Also, when examining the various other numbers, bear in mind two things. First, many numbers are not that accurate. For example, usually blood tests are fasting numbers, but fasting levels don't tell the full story.

Second, the "normal" range on the report is pretty arbitrary. It may reflect what the labs commonly see, or perhaps some conventional medical wisdom. Do not necessarily assume these apply to you or are even all that meaningful.

WHAT CAN BE FIXED WITH QUANTITATIVE MEDICINE?

An important question you are no doubt asking is: "What's in it for me?" If I do all the changes you suggest, and fix my numbers, is that really going to modify my health? Will it really increase my longevity and prevent degenerative disease?

It definitely will. Individual results will vary depending on four things:

- Your personal genetic luck
- How old you were when you started the program
- How much trouble you were in when you started
- Your degree of adherence

If you start young and thoroughly comply, that long disease-free life becomes almost a sure thing.

Read the "Cohort" sidebars. Some of these people were quite sick. The vast majority of these people extricated themselves from various danger zones quite quickly and are on their way to permanent long-lasting health. We have little data on compliance, but suspect most of those who made less progress were not following the various protocols. It is not always easy to do so.

To be more specific, for the compliant, about 90% of the time, the suggested lifestyle modifications will change the numbers, and that will change the disease risk. There will be some stubborn cases and other lines of attack will be necessary, but for most, disease risk will be greatly reduced and disease-free life extended. Most people *will* experience these benefits:

- Elevated HDL and reduced cortisol will significantly reduce the risk of cancer.
- Driving down glucose, insulin, and triglycerides, is, almost by definition, a cure for adult onset diabetes. Driving down these same three will also tend to prevent the emergence of any dementias.
- Elevated HDL and effective management of triglycerides, coupled with a proper exercise program, will slowly bring down plaque buildup and greatly reduce the risk of arterial disease. It will begin to reverse atherosclerosis.

- Doing resistance exercise that involves big bones will prevent and reverse osteoporosis. If there is already loss of stature, that may partially reverse that too.
- Mental acuity and memory will improve.
- Quality of sleep will improve.
- Sense of well-being will improve.
- You will look younger—possibly a lot younger.
- In a medical and biological sense, you will actually *be* younger.

And sadly, there are a couple of items that usually do not return to their former glory, although some have reported an effect:

- Hair will not return to its original color, nor start growing again where it once grew.
- Hearing loss will not improve.

We have arbitrarily divided lifestyle into eating, exercising, de-stressing, and sleep. We will describe the specific effects that changes in each of these typically have on the key numbers. There is a lot of personal variation here, so the topics are discussed in somewhat broad terms. The idea is to choose modifications that suit your style, convictions, and likely compliance. Then try them out, measure again, and if necessary, modify further. Changes that improve health and longevity should not be a form of self-torture.

BIOLOGICAL AGE—TURN BACK THE CLOCK

Anyone who has been to a 40th or 50th high school reunion has seen the spread. Some seem fit as a fiddle, while others are shaped like one. Some are energetic, happy, etc., while others are not doing well at all. This is always cause for reflection and chatter, and is usually put down to genetics, or some other rationale. However, for almost the entire "class" the rate of aging actually reflects how close they stayed to ideal homeostasis and anabolism in that last 40 or 50 years, and has little to do with genetics. If you were to get a blood sample for each of the reunion attendees, you could plot "biological" age quite accurately. (Would certainly make for a memorable reunion, though you wouldn't likely be invited back.)

Here is what you could do though to estimate a biological age. Using the blood result from you fellow attendees, obtain the grade "A," " "B," or "C," for each of the four categories: sugar management, lipid management, stress, and anabolism. Take the current age, and for each "A" subtract three years, and each "C" add three years. The result is the biological age.

Those that got straight "A"s would have a biological age 12 years younger than their chronological age. The sure way to get those "A's is by using Quantitative Medicine. So here is a way to beat the clock, or at least slow it down.

Key Points
8 - STEP II - Quantify Yourself
- You can compute scores based on the various measurements.
- A homeostasis/anabolism score will indicate your overall health.
- A sugar management score of "A," "B," or "C," will indicate how well you are managing glucose and insulin.
- A lipid management score of "A," "B," or "C," will indicate how well you are managing triglycerides and cholesterol.
- A stress management score of "A," "B," or "C," will indicate how stressed you are, both internally and externally.
- An Anabolic score of "A," "B," or "C," will indicate the extent you are in renew and repair mode.
- Liver, kidneys, and iron are also key measurements.
- Knowing all your scores allows you to focus and direct your lifestyle choices.

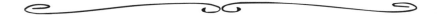

9 - STEP III - LIFESTYLE CHANGE GUIDELINES - DIET

THE HEALTH EFFECTS OF DIET

Dietary changes will have their greatest effect on the sugar management group of numbers, less on the lipid group numbers, and less effect still on the anabolic numbers. As far as disease prevention impact, adult onset diabetes and Alzheimer's would be the most affected, followed fairly closely by heart disease and cancer.

We will shortly get specific, but generally, if you got an "A" in sugar management, and you have been eating sugar and starch, you can continue to safely do so, but keep them on a short leash. The ability to metabolize sugar and starch tends to decline with age. If your numbers are sort of OK, a "B," say, cut carbs. Target the sugar first. Cut the sodas, the cake, then bread. For fruit, go for berries. If you got a "C," cut all these out. You are heading toward diabetes and need to reverse course immediately.

Insulin and Weight Gain

Insulin has many functions. One of the more insidious is this: if insulin is above 6 μu/dl, the weight-gain "switch" is on. No matter what you do, your body is going to try to conserve and store the food—especially carbs—as fat. You can starve yourself, which is as unpleasant as it is unhealthy, but as soon as you stop, your body will quickly replace any fat you lost. The way to trigger weight loss is to make dietary changes that will force your fasting insulin to a level between 3 and 6 μu/dl. This is fat-burning territory and is very healthy. If your insulin is higher, cut out starch, sugar, and fruit to drive it lower. Between 3 and 6, you will soon arrive at your healthiest weight. If you exercise, this weight will be lower still.

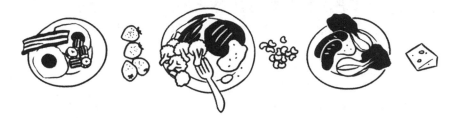

Six Meals a Day

Actually, three meals and three snacks. Each meal should have a protein portion from meat, dairy, or eggs, and two or three portions of vegetables. For each meal, the size of each portion should match the size of your palm, or a bit smaller. Vary the meat, sometimes red meat, sometimes white, sometimes fowl, sometimes fish. Take quality (grass-fed for instance) over quantity. Don't worry about "lean." You need fat, including saturated fat, and likewise, don't hesitate to butter those vegetables. And don't worry about cholesterol. Your body will manufacture what you don't obtain from eating, so there is no point in avoiding it. Eat the colored vegetables like broccoli, spinach, kale, peppers, tomatoes, onions, green beans, cauliflower, whatever you like. Bake it topped with cheese, or stir-fry it with tasty spices. Once again, quality over quantity. Organic if possible. (Beware: Not all organic food is created equal. Some is more organic than others. More information is available below in the FOOD SOURCING section.)

Take a snack between each main meal. It should consist of between two and four ounces of similar sorts of foods. Perhaps a cheese snack, or some nuts. Perhaps leftovers, or carrots or celery with a tasty (non-soy) dip. Or peanut butter This sort of thing, but no chips. If you eat bars, avoid the sugar-loaded ones. Better still, avoid the bars. Their ingredients tend to be the cheapest the manufacturer can buy and still come up with a plausible label. The third snack should be taken at bedtime and should be tiny. Again, don't worry about fat.

Now then, what about fruit, bread, potatoes, cake, pasta, sodas, and all that yummy stuff? This is the part of your diet that can get you into trouble, so here is where you need to focus your attention. The maximum amount will vary from person to person. For some, the maximum amount is *zero*. Others might be able to deal with quite a bit. However, you can determine a safe amount from blood tests. Of course you can make it easier by eating only real food: food that doesn't come in a package or can, and doesn't have a label. But if you are to avoid sugar, don't eat fruit.

We are about to show you how to determine a "personal sugar rule," which will give you useful dietary guidelines for dealing with sugar, fruit, and starch. There are four possible rules:

- Eat More Fruit and Starch.
- Hold the Line.
- Reduce Fruit, Sugar, and Starch.
- Fruit, Sugar, and Starch Are Forbidden.

But first, we need to deal with a special case: are you hypoglycemic?

Hypoglycemia

Hypoglycemia is an insulin management problem, and there could be many causes. If your fasting insulin is below 3 μu/dl and you aren't especially thin, hypoglycemia should be considered. In hypoglycemia, the hypothalamus seems to have an itchy trigger finger on the insulin gun. As soon as there is just a bit of extra glucose, it blasts some insulin with both barrels. This clears the glucose just fine, but overdoes it and doesn't leave enough in the blood, thereby creating a lack an hour or so later. That lack translates to a craving, which, if satisfied, restarts the cycle, and if not, leaves the person in a low-energy state. This pattern can be especially hard to escape.

There is a specific standard test for hypoglycemia. If your fasting insulin is very low, say below 3, or the above symptoms fit, you may well be hypoglycemic.

Hypoglycemia can be genetic, caused by bad diet, or due to other causes. However, it is easily managed. Eating six small meals a day of good nutrient-rich, low-sugar and lowstarch food will cure or at least manage hypoglycemia regardless of the cause. In fact, if you follow our dietary advice, there is little point to the test. The diet will cure hypoglycemia whether you have it or not. But bear in mind that you must eat the six meals (three meals + three snacks). Otherwise your glucose will sag between meals and you will crave sugar and be miserable.

If you would have scored an "A" if your insulin hadn't been too low, you can enjoy some fruit. But watch it. If you are craving sweets, cut that out too. If you got a "B" or "C," cut out all starch, sugar, and fruit. Your hypothalamus is just too sensitive to it.

Low insulin is not good. You will tend to have little energy, and little bodily repair will be occurring. Aging will not be retarded.

Your Personal Sugar Rule

The purpose of this categorization is to aid in developing eating habits that cause you to head toward the "A" sugar management.

If your fasting insulin level is below 3, and you are not hypoglycemic, your Personal Sugar Rule is "**Eat More Fruit and Starch**." Low insulin prevents the building of new muscle and bone. However, avoid junk. Eat healthy sugar and starch, such as northern fruits (berries, apples, etc.) and potatoes. A daily amount that seems reasonable should be chosen, and glucose and insulin re-measured after a month or so.

If you got an "A" in Sugar (insulin is between 3 and 6 µu/dl and fasting glucose below 80 mg/dl), then it is OK to continue eating the amount of sugar, starch, and fruit currently being consumed. The Personal Sugar Rule is "**Hold the Line**." However, low quality food, like cereal, should be swapped out for food richer in micronutrients, like northern fruits or potatoes. Breakfast cereals have little in the way of micronutrients beyond what the manufacturer added for "fortification."

If you got a "B" (insulin is between 6 and 12, and fasting glucose below 90) , then a reduction in sugar, starch, and fruit is called for. The Personal Sugar Rule here is "**Reduce the Fruit, Sugar, and Starch.**"

If you got a "C" (insulin is over 12 or fasting glucose is over 90, all sugar, starch, and fruit should be cut. The Personal Sugar Rule is "**Fruit, Sugar, and Starch Are Forbidden.**" This is a pre-diabetic condition, or worse. If these have already been cut and the numbers are still high, then more meat should be added and vegetables cut further. Dietary fat, including saturated fat, is ad libitum—all you want.

Try to follow your personal guidelines. The world doesn't stop turning if you make an exception, say, on your birthday, but the Quantitative Medicine experience has been that a couple of weeks of backsliding undoes several months of discipline. Unfair, we know, but that's how it is.

The Ideal Plate

From the nutrition and recipe book: *Eat Real Food or Else . . .*

The ideal plate contains:

- 1/4 Proteins
- 3/4 Micronutrient-rich vegetables
- Fats
- No sugars or starches (or cereal)

The proportions are by weight of cooked ingredients (a cup of raw salad is not the same as a cup of cooked spinach).

The "ideal plate" is designed to provide enough micronutrients and macronutrients. Proteins can be animal or vegetal. They include meat, fish, poultry, eggs, dairy, nuts and seeds.

It is assumed that vegetables are cooked or seasoned with fats. Protein generally comes with built-in fat. Fat is important and greatly contributes to satiety; in the vegetable portion of your plate, half of the calories might come from fat (this is, however, not much in volume).

Try to get all the ingredients from the healthiest, cleanest sources possible:

- Animal proteins come from healthy animals (grass-fed, pastured or wild) whenever possible.
- Vegetables that are particularly susceptible to contaminants should preferably be organic.

On the ideal plate, the protein sets the agenda. This doesn't diminish the importance of vegetables; it simply means that the quantity of vegetables is determined by the quantity of protein on the plate:

Whether you eat a 4-oz steak, a 6-oz fish fillet, or a 3-egg omelet, make the vegetable portion of the meal about 3 times larger than the protein portion.

After you have finished your plate, if you want more food, make sure the next serving has the same 3-to-1 proportion of vegetables to proteins.

The quantity of protein required varies from person to person and also depends on the activity for the day. Younger or older people, or athletes, might need more than the general population. However, the "ideal plate" offers a good dietary strategy for most people.

The exact quantity of fat for cooking vegetables is not important, just use a reasonable amount. The window for "reasonable" is pretty wide: within the context of our micronutrient-rich diet, the body can deal with excess fat fairly easily, but it cannot cope with deficiency.

Avoid sugars and starches (or cereals, which are also starches): they trigger unhealthy responses that make our body deaf to our hormonal signaling. This causes, among other things, overeating.

In a well-fed society, sugar and starches are useless empty calories.

Meal Planning and Composition

Specifically, three meals a day should be eaten, at the normal times, plus two snacks between the meals and a tiny one at bedtime. Breakfast should be the biggest meal. We are not suggesting portions here. Common sense should be used. Neither stuff yourself, nor leave the table hungry. One meat portion the size of your palm and two or three equal-sized vegetable portions would be about right for most people. By meat here, we mean any animal product, including eggs and cheese. Nuts and seeds are OK too.

Snacks should be made up of the same foods, and be about a third the size. Perhaps a half-cup of yogurt, and some celery with peanut butter on it.

With this diet, a person should not feel hungry, and would usually not overeat. Again: use common sense—eat moderate amounts.

Here is a typical daily menu for each of the four Personal Sugar Rules. This shouldn't be seen as a specific dietary suggestion, but rather a method for varying the sugar and starch (indicated in bold).

	Add Sugar and Starch	Hold the Line	Reduce Sugar and Starch	Cut Out Sugar and Starch
Breakfast	Bacon, eggs, broccoli with cheese **Muffin**	Bacon, eggs, broccoli with cheese **Berries**	Bacon, eggs, broccoli with cheese **Berries**	Bacon, eggs, broccoli with cheese
Morning Snack	Yogurt **Strawberries**	Yogurt **Strawberries**	Yogurt	Yogurt
Lunch	Fried fish, Sliced tomato **Zucchini** **French Fries**	Fried fish, Sliced tomato **Zucchini** **Kale**	Fried fish, Sliced tomato **Zucchini** **Kale**	Fried Fish Sliced tomato **Kale**
Afternoon Snack	Nuts **Sliced apple**	Nuts **Sliced apple**	Nuts **Sliced apple**	Nuts **Cheese**
Dinner	Steak Salad with artichoke hearts and hearts of palm **Corn on the cob** **Bell peppers**	Steak Salad with artichoke hearts and hearts of palm **Lima beans** **Bell peppers**	Steak Salad with artichoke hearts and hearts of palm **Lima beans** **Bell peppers**	Steak Salad with artichoke hearts and hearts of palm **Lima beans**
Bedtime Snack	Cottage cheese **Berries**	Cottage cheese **Nuts**	Cottage cheese **Nuts**	Cottage cheese **Nuts**

This is not a diet in the usual sense of something done to lose weight. Weight that was gained due to excess carbs will probably be lost. After some time on this diet, a person should arrive at their healthiest weight. Weight is regulated to a homeostatic set-point by the hypothalamus. The hypothalamus determines this set-point, and many will not be happy with the choice it made. It is difficult to go below this weight, as the hypothalamus will take strong action to maintain it. It will down-regulate energy, mental acuity, and the immune system. Someone attempting to force his or her weight lower will probably succeed at feeling miserable, but not at weight loss. Exercise will lower the homeostatic set-point, and will lower somewhat the amount of fat the hypothalamus feels should be stored.

What about Using "Energy Bars" for the Snacks?

This can be a nice time saver, but it is a bit tricky, and you are going to have to spend a lot of time reading the fine print on those bars. (And there is usually a lot of fine print to read.) The bar ideally should have a very low amount of sugar, a moderate amount of protein, and an even higher portion of fat. Few bars are constructed this way. Furthermore, the manufacturer has every incentive to economize on the ingredients. Avoid soy protein. Avoid low-fat and high-carb bars. Match it as best you can to your personal sugar rule. Energy bar manufacturers: can we have QM bars?

Carb Craving

If you were eating a lot of carbs and made a substantial cut, you may crave them for a while. It will get better after 6 to 12 weeks. Carbs and fat metabolize using different cellular chemistry, and the cells need a few weeks to fully adjust. If you experience difficulty, you can slow down and do it in stages, or just tough it out. There is no physical danger here. Your call. Not everyone experiences a problem. It may take up to three months for your body to completely adjust to the change, especially if it is a dramatic one. At that point, you can get another blood draw to verify your progress. (Alternatively, you can get a much cheaper draw that measures only the sugar group.)

Remember, don't cut fat. Fat does not make you fat. Carbs make you fat. And don't starve yourself—this won't work either. Skipping meals is a bad idea. Your hypothalamus is going to toss you into catabolism if you cut fat or skip meals, and that will defeat the purpose of the changes.

FOOD SOURCING

Organic Food

Our body is able to detoxify our food to a certain extent. However, it cannot deal with overwhelming concentrations and further, there are contaminants that the body cannot eliminate at all.

If on a budget, it may be best to try to focus on the ingredients that have the highest potential for concentrated toxins and try to go organic there.

- Root vegetables (carrots, beets, turnips, radishes) are efficient at extracting both nutrients and contaminants from the soil.
- Berries likewise hyper-concentrate anything in the soil, including contaminants.
- Dairy products. Though cows are pretty good at filtering out pesticides, they are not able to block added growth hormones and antibiotics. In fact, these are more concentrated in the milk than in the animal's blood.
- Some fruits can be peeled, but have to be peeled quite deeply to eliminate contaminants. The nutritional value in the peel, typically a lot of the total, is then lost.

Most organic food tastes better than non-organic. Taste reveals richness in nutrients.

Beware that the definition of organic varies from country to country, and organic may mean less than you might hope. One would certainly *hope* that such food is pesticide free or chemical free, but surprisingly, this is not actually the case. Certain categories of pesticides are allowed in organic production as well as certain powders and sprays. Two such pesticides approved for organic use are rotenone and pyrethrin. They are weak pesticides, so several applications are needed, meaning we get a greater dose of it. The effect of these on us really isn't known: however, rotenone is quite toxic to fish.

So again, a possible solution, other than growing it yourself, is to get to know the suppliers. At an organic farmers' market, you will likely deal directly with the grower and can find out exactly what is and isn't used to produce the food. Or grow it yourself. Then you can be 100% certain.

Agricultural Practices

Organic is far from the whole story. Other farming practices determine how rich the soil is, which in turn determines the quality and quantity of nutrients the plants can extract:

- Crop rotation (planting different crops in specific sequences on a given field) promotes soil fertility, nutrient richness, and natural pest control.

- Companion planting (growing mutually beneficial crops close to one another) promotes biodiversity.
- Diversity (farms with a varied mix) supports beneficial organisms that assist in pollination and pest control.
- Many common practices have undesirable effects, for example, fumigation and irradiation.

This is another argument for buying local ingredients, since it offers an opportunity to know your farmers and their growing practices.

GMOs

While consuming small amounts of GMOs probably does not present a biological danger to us, generalizing this agricultural practice carries serious implications:

- At our body's level, this means eating unnatural ingredients. Ingredients that change much faster than we are able to evolve. The long-term consequences of this are unknown. Though not strictly speaking a GMO item, trans fat would be a good example of unforeseen and rather disastrous consequences of meddling with Mother Nature.
- The technology involved in GMOs is such that the seeds come from a very limited number of sources. This impoverishes the variety of nutrients. GMOs accelerate a trend that started with agriculture, with ongoing selection taking away vitality from the food.
- At the environmental level, the impacts are huge. Plants are selected for some kind of resistance. This affects the ecosystem with unforeseeable consequences.
- At a society level, GMOs affect local farming and local nutritional practices.

ASSORTED NUTRITIONAL TOPICS

Dieting

This is a $20 billion industry, and one that has utterly failed to deliver the goods. The sales approach invariably involves some manipulation of your beliefs: perhaps an ad wherein a group of beautiful, slender, energetic people are happily enjoying some overpriced but undernourishing meal substitute. You try it. It fails, and you are usually made to feel that the failure is due to your own lack of discipline or that you need time to detoxify or some other pseudo-scientific mumbo-jumbo.

Don't fall for it. Here is your very exact diet reality:

- Any diet that uses calorie restriction will fail. Period. Your hypothalamus will completely compensate and leave you feeling miserable (catabolic) as well.

- You cannot lose weight if your insulin is high, even slightly high. High insulin is the body's signal to store food as fat. For some, but not all, carbs drive insulin up and cause weight gain. But for all, without exception, if insulin is high, food will be stored as fat, not burned.

- If your insulin is ideal, between 3 and 6 μu/dl, and you aren't undereating (i.e., you aren't hungry), then whatever you weigh is near your ideal healthy weight. Be proud of that. If that's not as skinny as you would like, there's basically little you can do diet-wise. However, exercise will lower your homeostatic set-point and tend to cause some fat loss. Your weight will probably stay about the same, as you will be adding muscle and bone density, but you will look trimmer.

Your ideal "diet" is whatever will drive your numbers to the right spots. You will need to design it yourself.

Don't Skip Breakfast

There is a widespread belief that skipping breakfast will cause weight loss. The belief has gotten a lot of press, but is based on very flawed research: the skipped breakfast was high-carb. High carbs versus nothing: two bad choices. Our proposed breakfast will provide the energy you need, but without weight gain.

Insulin Resistance

Are you insulin resistant? Check your sugar numbers. If your A1C is greater than 5.7% or your fasting insulin is greater than 15 μu/dl or your fasting glucose is greater than 100 mg/dl, you are insulin resistant. This will get worse and likely lead to adult onset diabetes. Cut the starch and sugar. We recommend you cut them out entirely until the sugar management numbers return to non-insulin-resistant levels. They almost always will, and you should have noticeable improvement in under three months. Insulin resistance is a serious warning signal.

What causes insulin resistance? Table sugar and fruit are broken down in the intestines to about 50% glucose and 50% fructose. Though there are other sugars, these are the basic two. Glucose is sometimes called dextrose. Starch is broken down in the intestines to 100% glucose. From there, all the fructose and glucose goes to the liver. Most fructose stays in the liver. However, glucose is treated differently. The liver first takes what it wants, then sends the rest to the bloodstream for general consumption by the cells.

In order to encourage the cells to use the newly available glucose, the body secretes insulin, which expedites the delivery by telling the cells to use that circulating glucose. Unlike a package from the post office though, the glucose can't be left on the doorstep. If it doesn't get taken up by the cells, it continues to circulate, and in response to this, more insulin is secreted. Obviously we have a vicious cycle here, but the body can only produce so much insulin, so things top out. This is insulin resistance. The cells are in effect "resisting" the insulin message. What's really going on is a supply and demand issue. Either there is too much glucose, or the cells don't want it, or possibly both. You can remedy this situation by meddling with the supply (less sugar/starch) and demand (more exercise). Ideally, you will do both.

Fructose doesn't *directly* cause insulin resistance, and since it is very cheap to manufacture, it was hoped that this would solve problems and thus the food industry gave birth to "high fructose corn syrup." Turns out, though, that it will indirectly cause blood glucose to soar, so it indirectly worsens any insulin resistance problem. The actual fate of fructose is this: first the liver replenishes its stored sugar supply, and then what's left is converted to fat. For storage purposes, the liver will gobble the fructose in preference to the glucose, so the unused glucose ends up in your blood. That's why fructose can increase blood glucose.

Are You Too Thin?

Recall that too thin may not be your healthiest weight. If your fasting insulin is low, say below 3 μu/dl, and your IGF-1 is low also, say below 100 ng/ml, it would likely mean that you are spending most of your time in a catabolic state. Insulin isn't solely about sugar management. It is also involved in transporting protein and other building blocks to the muscles. You cannot effectively build muscle with low insulin. Cells will not renew as well, meaning accelerated aging. Osteoporosis can become a serious risk and overall energy level will be low. The "cure" for this is to increase starches in your diet. However, not all starches are created equal. Choose the ones with the highest nutritional value. This would include legumes, corn, potatoes, squash, peas, and yams. Sugar and grain are still not a good idea.

Is Your Lp(a) High?

Lipoprotein(a), or Lp(a), is measured in the Quantitative Medicine panel. If it is higher than 15 mg/dl it needs to be dealt with. For about 8% of the population, it is above 30 mg/dl, and dealing with it becomes imperative. Lp(a) is a variant form of LDL. It is strongly genetic. It significantly elevates the risk of heart disease along with clotting risk.

Because of the clotting risk, those with Lp(a) above 30 should avoid NSAIDs such as ibuprofen, which also increase clotting risk. Naproxen appears to be a safe choice.

The Lp(a) particle is essentially a normal LDL particle with an additional protein attached to it. This addition is responsible for its clotting property and also makes the modified particle unpalatable to cholesterol-hungry cells. Hence it tends to accumulate and has more opportunity to get stuck in arteries, leading to atherosclerosis. There is no cure for this. Oddly, there seems to be no obvious evolutionary cause for elevated Lp(a) either, though one surely exists. Today, those with small amounts seem to do fine.

It is imperative to fight high Lp(a) with good high-intensity exercise and proper diet. It is possible to keep it under control.

There is not an enormous amount of research on Lp(a), which is odd, because many people are affected by it. Niacin and aspirin are sometimes proposed as treatment. These, however, have their own side effects, and the studies haven't been done that would elicit the overall benefit. Some studies indicate a greater prevalence of high Lp(a) in men than in women.

The particle size of the Lp(a) is related to LDL particle size, which is not surprising considering how they are constructed. Hence changes favoring the larger particle sizes would be effective countermeasures. This would mean reducing triglycerides via diet and regular, proper exercise. Not smoking and avoidance of trans fat are also important.

Though the risk of heart problems is elevated, it may effectively be counteracted by appropriate and disciplined lifestyle choices. However, it should be borne in mind that whereas some may avoid heart problems due to genetic good luck and only modest changes, this is not the case for those with high Lp(a). More information can be found in the "LIPOPROTEIN(A)" section in chapter 21.

Do You Have the APO-E4 Variant?

APO, short for apolipoprotein, is a family of proteins that coat fat particles (LDL, HDL, chylomicrons) so that they are soluble in blood. The coating for chylomicrons, the circulating fat from your last meal, is called APO-E, and occurs in three genetically determined variants, which are designated APO-E2, 3, and 4. Since genes come in pairs, one from each parent, people have a mix: half E2 and half E3, for instance. Those with APO-E4 present in both genes have a much higher risk of Alzheimer's, for reasons thus far unknown. Since strong evidence has emerged that Alzheimer's is a sugar metabolism problem localized in the brain (many researchers now call it type 3 diabetes), keeping sugar and insulin in healthy, safe ranges would be preventive. The Quantitative Medicine protocols are the most effective way to achieve this.

Are You Gluten Intolerant?

Gluten intolerance affects between 5% and 75% of the population, depending on which bestselling book on the topic you consult. Celiac disease is an extreme form of gluten intolerance and affects ~1% of the population. There is general agreement on this number. Gluten is found in wheat, barley, oats, and some other grains. Corn, quinoa, buckwheat, and rice, including "glutinous" rice, are gluten free. (Glutinous in the context of rice simply means it is sticky.)

Celiac disease is serious, genetic in origin, and damages the small intestines, and creates numerous gastrointestinal symptoms. Even if you have it, you might not know it. If you find you have difficulty digesting bread, you should get specifically tested for celiac. The cure is to avoid all gluten.

To be sure, TTG (tissue transglutaminase) and gliadin antibodies should be measured. TTG and gliadin will each produce two numbers:

IgA and IgG. All four numbers should be in single digits. If any are over 20 units, see a doctor, who will most likely recommend a gluten-free diet and some retesting. The approach we obviously favor is to simply give up gluten, especially grain. This will "cure" gluten intolerance whether you have it or not, and go a long way toward curing a number of other things. Gluten is often added to packaged products; food labeling may not be accurate enough to be a definitive guide.

CAUSES OF DEGENERATIVE DISEASE
Adult Onset Diabetes

This is also known as type 2 diabetes. It is more a syndrome than a disease, and is almost always curable. It is caused by high insulin resistance. Recall that insulin's job is to deliver glucose molecules to the cells. If the cells will not accept this, both insulin and glucose levels will increase. This state is called insulin resistance and if sufficiently severe, is termed adult onset diabetes. Ideally, glucose should be below 80 mg/dl and insulin below 6 µu/ml. In an insulin-resistant person, these numbers may be 130 and 15 or even higher. Typically triglycerides soar as well. All this circulating glucose and insulin is quite dangerous, promoting cancer, heart disease, and Alzheimer's as well as damaging the eyes, the kidneys, the fingertips and toes, the brain, and the heart. It lowers testosterone, impairs memory, and speeds loss of bone mineral density.

Adult onset diabetes is aging in the fast lane. The adult diabetic syndrome is so dangerous that anyone with significantly elevated glucose and insulin numbers should immediately and permanently cut out as much sugar and starch as humanly possible, start a serious exercise program, get the stress level down, and get enough sleep.

Most adult onset diabetes research is looking for a way to trick the biology of how a starch/sugar-overwhelmed system is incapable of coping. So far, none have been found, so little progress is made. Perhaps in another 50,000 years, we will have evolved some protective mechanism.

Adult onset diabetes is not genetic. You will frequently hear words to the contrary, but adult onset diabetes was practically unknown in our grandparents' generation and genetics simply cannot change that fast. It is largely due to high starch and sugar content in today's diets.

Starches and the Food Industry

Don't get confused by the food industry. They are spending $10 billion a year to do just that; to get you to eat something that is probably not good for you, something that by many standards is not even food. A fair amount of this advertising budget is targeted directly at our children, which would be appalling if we weren't so used to it. Not only do they flood the TV and the grocery stores with thousands of mostly starch-based, high-profit items, they also flood the medical research community with funding for thousands of papers proving their stuff is good for you. Actually, proving such a thing as that isn't easy, so they usually prove something else. More likely you'll see ads claiming their latest and greatest product is better for you than what they were selling you last year. Labs confirm it! These claims largely rest on the benefits of adding vitamins, anti-oxidants, whole grain, or whatever the latest fads recommend.

Use your common sense. If hunter-gatherers couldn't find it in their local forest, we probably aren't evolved to do anything useful with it. Actually, what is and isn't food has gotten blurry. The food industry constantly exploits this. A box of cereal isn't actually food in any traditional sense. It started out with something that could have served as food, but those origins are long gone, along with most of the nutrients. Even in its "whole" form, grain isn't much of a food and few pre-agricultural people bothered with it.

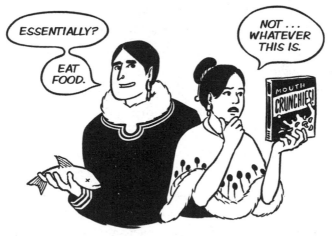

Don't get too caught up in this whole grain business. Yes, whole grain is better for you. How much better? Well maybe 10% less colon cancer compared to refined grain, or something along those lines. There seems no limit to the medical literature proving this again and again. The companies that sell processed starch (cereals, breads, chips, etc.) have a huge vested interest in keeping us hooked on the stuff, and have funded enormous amounts of confirming research. Yes, whole grain is better, but whole grain versus refined grain is *not* the real issue. The real issue is grain versus NO grain. How does that relate to cancer? Try finding anything out about that in the medical literature. Start by mulling this one over: hunter-gatherers don't eat starch, and hunter-gatherers don't get cancer.

Perhaps you should periodically hire a consulting hunter-gatherer and take him or her to the grocery store with you. He or she can quickly identify the real food. In any case, next time you are about to buy something in a box, that you intend to eat, ask, "Is this really food?"

In most countries, the high priests of nutrition are recommending that 50-70% of daily energy come from starches. (Whole grain of course.) This utterly delights the food industry. However, it should be borne in mind that the countries that most solidly and consistently *ignore* this dietary advice have the lowest rates of heart disease.

Cholesterol and Saturated Fat

You have probably heard by now that after a very prolonged exile from the American diet, cholesterol and saturated fat are back, and that it may be OK to just sometimes actually have a bit. Or maybe not. Why were these banished? There must have been some reason.

In fact, cholesterol and saturated fat were innocent all along. They were never proven guilty of anything. They were in effect framed by the aptly named Framingham Study, or rather its misinterpretation. They spent decades as the bad boys of nutrition, while the real culprits, sugar and starches, were busily starting an obesity epidemic, a diabetes epidemic, and promoting other degenerative diseases.

Saturated fat, from properly raised animals and vegetables is the healthiest fat. In second place is monounsaturated fat, followed by polyunsaturated. So don't worry about saturated fat. It's your body's preferred fat.

As you are well aware, trans fat is a complete no-no (unless it come from natural sources such as palm oil.) Trans fat is often lumped with saturated fat, especially by those with some sort of anti-meat agenda.

Likewise dietary cholesterol has no effect on your health. Your body will keep the internal amount regulated. It will use what you eat and make up the difference. This has been known for 25 years and is no longer disputed in any quarter we are aware of. Still the myth persists. Never mind. Enjoy all the cholesterol laden food you like.

Vegetarianism and Veganism

This subject is such a hot potato, we are reluctant to deal with it. By now, you've no doubt surmised that we are not big advocates. Let us try to separate two aspects of this topic that are frequently interwoven and cause much confusion: ethical considerations and nutritional value. Often grand nutritional claim are made by groups whose true agenda is sustainability or animal rights.

The ethical-political. Here the issues are efficient land usage, sparing animals, sustainability, religious beliefs, and other such considerations. These are personal beliefs and we are not commenting except to say that if you are choosing to be a vegetarian for these reasons, you are making a potentially significant personal health sacrifice.

The nutritional. If you chose vegetarianism or veganism solely for nutritional reasons, you were very poorly informed. To claim it is better for you from a nutritional point of view is a big stretch, especially veganism. Unfortunately, this big stretch is indeed often claimed, especially to garner support for the nutritionally unrelated side of the practice. Vegetarianism is not healthier for you; after all you are biologically an omnivore.

If a vegetarian will eat dairy and eggs (Lacto-Ovo vegetarianism), the needed dietary balance can be met, though it is difficult to obtain enough protein, and all too easy to obtain too much carbohydrate. A Lacto-Ovo vegetarian will need to keep a close watch on triglycerides and the sugar management group.

"China Study" is a book that purports to prove that all animal product is bad. This book is frequently cited. The book claims to be based on data on the lifestyles of Chinese people in 69 different counties. That collection of data is also called: "The China Study." We obtained the data and analyzed it, and rather surprisingly, the data proved quite clearly that veganism is bad for you. The people in the study that ate meat, including much maligned red meat, lived longer. Meat eaters also had lower rates of cancer. Those who ate less meat were less healthy and died sooner. Nuts and dark-colored vegetables were good, grains and light-colored vegetables were bad. If the China study data proves anything at all, it proves that our own dietary advice is best. It certainly does not prove veganism is good or animal product is bad, as is claimed in the book "China Study."

100% Animal Product is Not Good Either

As far as we are concerned, the ideal diet consists of eating both good quality nutritious animal and vegetable product. Neither is healthy in the absence of the other. A 100% meat diet will cause undesirable side effects, as will a vegan diet. Humans need both types of food. We are omnivores and are adapted to the mix.

Foods to Avoid

What are opposed is "factory" meat: feedlot animals or farmed fish. Though these animals can, in principle, be raised in a healthy and nutritious way, they seldom are, and real standards have yet to emerge. We are likewise opposed to most sugar and starch products. The sugar and starch do provide energy, but little in the way of nutrition. This includes grains as well, including whole grain. Fat is a safer and healthier source of energy. Fat is essential; sugar and starch are not. It is these considerations that guide our recommended mix of animal and vegetable product.

Calorie Restriction and Fasting

So far, both calorie restriction and fasting have fallen far short of expectations. One might think that since both were common in ancient times that there may well be a medical or health benefit, and in fact, for some period of time, Dr. Nichols looked into fasting. But as it turned out, the body, driven by the hypothalamus, always managed to compensate, and no benefit was seen in the blood draw numbers. Likewise, calorie restriction has not show any benefit is research studies done on monkeys. In a fasting or calorie restriction mode, the body goes immediately into catabolic mode. Repair is suspended, mental acuity diminished, and the immune system partly shut down, all, of course, for the purpose of saving energy. While this was a valuable survival skill in past time, all this conservation is not healthy, and not the direction we want to head.

Key Points
9 - STEP III - Lifestyle Changes - Diet
- A summary of lifestyle changes for diet, exercise, and stress reduction, suitable for posting on the fridge, is found at the end of Chapter 11.

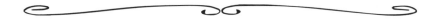

10 - STEP III - LIFESTYLE CHANGE GUIDELINES - EXERCISE

Proper diet, stress reduction, and good sleep provide an environment where cells can thrive. If any of these components are missing, the cells will be under duress and cannot be healthy. However, simply providing a healthy environment doesn't mean the cell is going to do anything useful with it, and this is where exercise comes into the picture. This is not a new notion.

> Nature implants no disposition in vain. It seems to be a catholic law throughout the whole animal creation, that no creature, without exercise, should enjoy health, or be able to find subsistence: Every creature, except man, takes as much of it as is necessary. He alone, and such animals as are under his direction, deviate from this original law, and they suffer accordingly.
>
> Glandular obstructions, now so common, generally proceed from inactivity. These are the most obstinate of maladies. So long as the liver, kidneys, and other glands, duly perform their functions, health is seldom impaired: but when they fail, nothing can restore it. Exercise is almost the only cure we know for glandular obstructions: indeed, it does not always succeed as a remedy; but there is reason to believe that it would seldom fail to prevent these complaints, were it used in due time. One thing is certain, that amongst those who take sufficient exercise, glandular diseases are very little known; whereas the indolent and inactive are very seldom free from them.

These words of wisdom, dating from 1832, are found in *A Treatise on the Cure and Prevention of Disease,* by one William Buchan, M.D. A similar message was given by Hippocrates some 2,000 years earlier.

In any case, we creatures of the whole animal creation would do well to take note and refrain from indolence and inactivity. And we have just the plan!

BIOLOGICAL POWER

We haven't talked much about cells and mitochondria. They are major topics in PART III. Degenerative disease prevention, mental health, energy level, slow aging—in short, everything—depend on the cells' biological power, their resources, and molecular machinery. Food is fuel; we want clean fuel. Stress and poor sleep compromise the cells; these problems must be avoided to the furthest extent possible. But exercise is what makes the cells active, makes them powerful and healthy.

This includes all the cells, not just muscle, but joints, ligaments, and tendons. Neurons (nerves) likewise improve their function. Even cells seemingly having little bearing on exercise, like those in the kidneys or liver (as noted by Dr. Buchan), benefit as well. As with most things in Quantitative Medicine, overall cellular health can be measured and optimized.

Mitochondria are tiny energy generators within the cells. In each cell, there are usually hundreds of them, sometimes thousands. They aren't really us at all. They have their own DNA and were once free bacteria. They were enslaved for energy generation purposes perhaps a billion years ago.

They generally do their job, don't rebel, and produce our energy directly from the fat and glucose we eat. But they extract a paradoxical and deadly sort of revenge: if they are not used, not worked, left idle, they will break down and poison the host cell. This deterioration of the cellular power production, and the subsequent toxic consequences, are one of the main causes of most of our modern health problems. But this deterioration needn't happen. The mitochondria can be kept busy and engaged, which in turn keeps them running smoothly and keeps them out of trouble.

EXERCISE AND YOUR NUMBERS

There are a range of exercises here, from easy ones that preserve and repair your joints to challenging ones that will preserve and repair just about everything else.

Physical activity has its greatest effect on your anabolic and lipid numbers, and a lesser effect on the sugar numbers. As far as disease prevention, heart disease, osteoarthritis, and osteoporosis benefit the most, followed fairly closely by cancer, adult onset diabetes, and Alzheimer's.

Exercise has innumerable benefits. A major one is its ability to increase HDL and especially the "mature" HDL—the "really good" cholesterol. Elevating HDL sharply reduces cancer and heart attack risk. Likewise, IGF-1 and testosterone, two major anabolic hormones, are also increased with exercise. These two (along with several others) greatly promote cell renewal and repair, and retard aging.

EXERCISE PROGRAMS

Most exercise programs emphasize weight loss, with the rest being mainly about bodybuilding. Our exercise program is like no other. You could say it emphasizes biological power—at least that is the end result—but it proceeds step by step, starting at the most fundamental level.

Our program is graduated from easy to strenuous, and its benefits track this progression. The more strenuous levels provide greater health benefit and disease prevention. You may or may not be a regular exerciser, but read through them all. Make sure you understand the concepts behind joint health maintenance and osteoporosis prevention, and are tailoring your exercises to encompass these. As you progress, attention will be focused on heart rate and its response to exercise. This is key to cardiovascular health. Finally, keeping the mitochondria busy and challenged provides the huge energy increases, degenerative disease prevention, and increased mental acuity that are the hallmarks of Quantitative Medicine.

This may sound a little complicated, but ahead is a step-by-step approach. Follow it carefully, and you will succeed. To summarize, here are the key points in the order in which they must be mastered:

Skeletal Health

The initial exercises aim at getting the joints into good shape, with full range of motion, strengthening the tendons and ligaments, strengthening the bones, and stimulating the neural-muscular paths. If you master these:

- You will completely repair and strengthen your joints, preventing or reversing osteoarthritis.
- You will improve your coordination and balance, causing new nerves to grow. (You may have once been taught that you cannot grow new neurons or nerves. This is incorrect.)
- You will strengthen your bones, preventing or reversing osteoporosis.

These items alone can benefit a good many people, and can be accomplished with a fairly easy program.

Heart Rate Variability

Many doctors recommend brisk walks and other modest approaches to exercise. While better than nothing, the heart and vascular system aren't particularly challenged. The heart will get into a groove. It will become efficient at dealing with the modest demand placed on it, but will be unable to accommodate increased workloads.

The modest elevation in heart rate means a modest increase in blood pressure and blood flow, but the cleansing and rejuvenating effects of a brief high pressure and high blood flow rate will not occur.

Running the heart rate up and down, intensely, but briefly, circumvents these problems. (And takes far less time as well.) Such activities strongly stimulate arterial repair and general heart-lung capacity. Heart attack instances plummet with such exercise, and, somewhat amazingly, cancer plummets as well. "Intense" sounds like work, and it is. However, the time is considerably shorter. A 30-minute brisk walk, for instance, might be replaced with three 30-second sprints up a hill.

The health benefits of this sort of exercise are hard to overstate. Repeated research has shown again and again that short but intense exercise practices are markedly more beneficial, with noticeable health improvements occurring within weeks.

Mitochondrial Health

In a state of ideal peak health, the energy-generating mitochondria are busy. Their efficiency goes up, as does their rate of proliferation. Such a state pushes every cell in the body toward its individual peak performance. This translates to better mental acuity and memory, slower aging, and a healthy and active immune system that completely overwhelms degenerative disease.

Attaining this level of health entails yet more dedication, but is available to all who are willing to make the commitment. Exercise sessions become more strenuous, but not necessarily longer. For most people, two intense 45-minute sessions per week, with a third milder one added for maintenance of balance, coordination, stability, and flexibility will do it.

THREE CAVEATS

Though it works faster than most exercise programs, ours is not a quick fix, but is instead a lifetime commitment. The system works, has been endlessly refined over the last 20 years, and for most, will deliver the promised results. Consider wisely what level of commitment you are willing to make. Be careful and be patient. Take note of these three caveats:

Avoid Medical Risk

Consult a physician before undertaking any of this. Tell him or her what you are intending to do and see if there are limitations you should observe. You may need to get some tests to determine this. Try to avoid having the doctor dictate the type of exercise. This isn't likely to be productive. (For decades, most doctors have recommended aerobic exercise. This is a poor form of exercise, and time consuming as well.)

Don't Overdo It

Joints and tendons take a few months to strengthen, but can take a couple of years to heal if you injure them. You will be building muscle strength faster than joint and tendon strength, so you will be in a position to injure yourself. Start slowly and build up. If you ignore this warning (and most people do) you will likely get injured, which will significantly slow your progress. Some soreness is normal. Some joint pain is normal. So you have to push yourself a bit, just don't overdo it. Pain should subside after two days at most.

This Works for Most People, but Not All

Some joint damage is permanent. This program won't reverse that. Some people can't build new bone and reverse osteoporosis. There may be other challenges. But for most people, and by "most" we mean 80% to 90% of all people of all ages, these programs are effective. If some element of the program doesn't seem to be working, see a specialist, or visit the website (QuantitativeMedicine.net) and see if there is additional information there. Most barriers can be overcome.

SKELETAL HEALTH

If you are a non-exerciser, this is a good place to start. Modest effort should yield noticeable results fairly quickly. If you already exercise, make sure you can do everything described in this section.

After 6 to 12 weeks of these skeletal health exercises, you may expect the following:

- You will have full joint range, with no, or at worst, little pain.
- Your balance and coordination will have significantly improved.
- Your energy level and mental acuity will have improved.
- Sleep quality will have improved.
- You will be preventing or reversing osteoporosis.

Let's start with the joints.

How Joints Work

Cartilage is the shiny hard material seen at the end of a chicken bone. In a working joint, it rubs against the cartilage of another bone. Sometimes there is a pad between them. The joint is enclosed in a pouch and lubricated with a slippery fluid. In spite of the lubrication and hardness, cartilage would soon wear out except for one detail: it's alive. There are living cells embedded in it that continually manufacture new cartilage. However, unlike all other cell types, the cartilage cells do not have a blood supply. The nutrients are instead found in the lubricating fluid. The cells comprising the pouch both make the lubricating fluid and generate the nutrients for the cartilage cells.

You will have healthy cartilage forever if you do two things:

- Spread the nutrient-containing fluid all over the joint.
- Compress the joint, by putting pressure on it, so that the nutrients get down into the cartilage.

If you don't do this, the cartilage-producing cells starve and won't make new cartilage. The old wears out, and can potentially wear through to the bone. This is osteoarthritis, a very undesirable situation.

To spread the nutrients all over the joints, move them through their full range of motion frequently, or as full a range as you can. To get the fluid down into the cartilage, make the joints do some work. Put some pressure on them.

Now it is crucial to note: you *have* to do this. Unlike a lot of other things, the body doesn't automatically take care of getting nutrients to the cartilage. It's simple and fast, but absolutely necessary that you take the time and trouble. Properly maintained in this way, joints will last a lifetime and a half. The only exceptions would be those damaged in some way, or overly stressed due to substantial obesity.

Let's Get Started

The knees are usually everyone's weak link, so start by seeing how far you can squat. Ideally you can get your fanny almost all the way to the floor with no pain, like our young lady here (actually, she's 95). If you can squat this deeply and come back up with no pain, you can probably skip the rest of this section. Just remember to frequently run your joint under full range of motion, while employing some mild weight or resistance.

If you do not have full range knee motion, here is a procedure to fix it. Start standing. Give yourself a pain level number from 0 to 10, where 0 is no pain at all, and 10 is excruciating. Whatever that number is, make a mental note of it as your *baseline* number.

Keeping this baseline number in mind, and starting from a standing position, no weight, squat as far as you can with no additional pain, then go a bit farther so that it hurts just a little (more). How much is "just a little"? About two "clicks" more than your baseline number. If 3 was your baseline pain, squat to about a level 5. Remember that spot and squat to that same position 10 times. Rest a bit, then do two more sets of these. What you have just done is lubricate and nourish your cartilage in areas where it was starving. It will immediately start building new, fresh cartilage.

The next day, your knees should hurt a bit and again the next day. If they already hurt when you began the exercise, they should hurt a bit more. The third day, they should be back to normal. Don't repeat this exercise until the knees are back to normal. If it took more than two days to return to normal, you went at it too hard. Wait till the additional pain has subsided, then start anew, but this time go for a lesser amount of pain. If, on the other hand, there was no additional pain the next day, or it only lasted a day, you need to press a bit harder and increase the range—range is key.

When you reach a point of full range, with no pain, and no pain the next day, add some weight. Use dumbbells or a barbell. Start light, continuing with the same procedure. Again, seek full range before adding weight.

Why all this elaborate pain business? Over two decades, Dr. Mike has tested various combinations of pain and recovery in order to fix joints. The above method has proven the fastest. Expect things to start happening quickly. There should be a noticeable improvement in a couple of weeks. Keep this up until you have gotten full range with no pain at all. You don't get to stop, but at this point you have reached an important milestone: your knee joints are in top shape. Remember, the joints won't take care of themselves. You have to lubricate and nourish them with full-range motion, and squeeze that nourishment into the cartilage by putting pressure on the joint.

Any other joints can be repaired the same way. Remember to go two notches above your baseline pain, with, again, two notches being the level needed for a three-day recovery.

Can't Joints Be Beyond a Point of No Return?

Possibly. You should get medical advice. However even a severely damaged joint can often be brought back from the abyss. Consider Dr. Mike's own experience: "Three years ago I damaged my knee in a mountain climbing accident An MRI, three years later, reported 'severe tricompartmental osteoarthritis, with areas of NO cartilage, and a large tear in the middle of the thinly remaining medial meniscus.' Knee replacement or exercise? I opted to give the latter a chance even in this severe case. After all, what did I have to lose at this point? So far, the exercises described above allow me completely pain-free walking and hill sprinting. I also have recovered full range, but with some pain, though less than before. Will I eventually need knee replacement surgery? Maybe, maybe not. One further point: as I knew how to renew a knee, I should not have waited so long."

What about Rheumatoid Arthritis?

Rheumatoid arthritis is an autoimmune disease, not a degenerative disease. A specialist is mandatory here as there are many effective treatments. However, once stabilized, the above "repair and maintenance" exercises would be equally important.

Neural Generation

While you are repairing your knees or other joints, why not add a few new nerves? It has been the conventional medical wisdom that you would get no new ones and were lucky to hold on to the ones you already had. Not true at all, though still widely believed. Again, it's a case of "use it or lose it." These next exercises aren't particularly strenuous either, but build balance, coordination, agility, and, as promised, new nerves.

First exercise. (You can do this between your squat exercises.) Stand on one foot. How long can you balance? Switch to the other foot. At first, your legs may feel a little wobbly. This is because the nerves needed to precisely control the muscles aren't activated yet. This doesn't take long, and fairly soon the shakiness will go away. Simple as this is, it is an excellent neural exercise. You are working out neurons all the way from your brain to your foot and back, plus the numerous little muscles that control stability and balance.

Pretty soon, you will become adept at this, and will be able to stand on either foot for however long you want. We are now going to add a new twist. Go find something about the size of a quart carton of milk and place it upright on the floor. Now then, while standing on one foot, bend down, however you can, and pick it up. Repeat with the other foot. If this hurts, you have discovered a new joint to work on. In this case, use something easier to reach. The whole idea here is to keep your balance while standing on one foot and bending over to pick something up. Keep this up till you can pick up coins from the floor. By that time, you will have built a lot of new neurons, and toned up quite a few small balance muscles. You can turn this into a game. You and your opponent each supply a roll of coins. Take turns picking them up. If you have to put a second foot down, you lose your turn and your shot at the coin. Don't play this with a kid. You'll rapidly go broke.

If you can hop 18" on one foot, you could play hopscotch, one of the best (and oldest) agility games on the planet.

Fancy Footwork

We will conclude this section with another fun agility-building exercise.

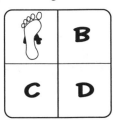

Get some masking tape and stick four pieces on the floor forming a one-foot square. A should be 12 inches from B, etc. Label them A, B, C, and D. Now, step back and forth on C and D, C-D-C-D . . .then shift to A and B, A-B-A-B-. . . then back to C and D and so on. Now do this pattern, C-D-A-B-C-D-A-B- . . . speed it up. It would look like this (the foot on the floor is shown, the other foot should be in the air):

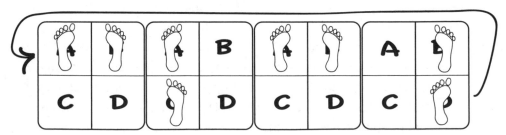

The faster you can go, the better. Up and back 10 times in 10 seconds is a reasonable target. Rest 10 seconds and go again. Once you get good at this (won't take long), change the pattern.

Standing on A and B, put your right foot on C, which should be behind your left foot, then the right foot back goes back to B, then your left foot on D and back. This pattern would look like this:

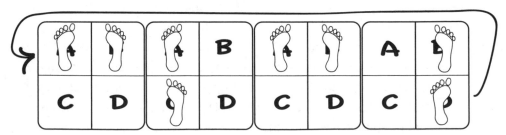

Or think of some new patterns, the more elaborate, the better. Just remember: when you go from awkward to easy, you have built new nerves, and that's the point. Staying with a pattern you have "mastered" is not of much use—those nerves have already been built.

We are going to move on to osteoporosis prevention, but by just doing the joint and agility exercises, you can in most cases prevent osteoarthritis, and greatly reduce the likelihood of falling. And all with exercises easily done at home, with practically no equipment at all.

Here is a possible exercise schedule

Monday - 30 minutes	Friday - 30 minutes
Stretch Joint exercises as needed, knees, hips, etc. Balancing exercises Agility exercises Ping-pong	Stretch Agility exercises Balancing exercises Joint exercises as necessary Speed bag Balance on wobbly objects Hopscotch

This is hardly any work at all—fun, really—and if you have been relatively sedentary, it will work wonders in a hurry.

At this point, you will be accomplishing the following: Your joints will be building new cartilage. You will be headed toward full, pain-free joint range. Your coordination will significantly improve due to new nerves being built. Muscles involved in balance will tone up.

The following areas will need further attention: Osteoporosis prevention will require exercises that stress the large bones. Reducing the risk of heart attacks will need exercises that vary the heart rate as much as safely possible. Driving all the cells to peak performance, and hence warding off all other degenerative disease, will mean a couple of 45-minute intense exercise sessions weekly. As you progress, these intense sessions would partially supplant the sessions proposed above.

OSTEOPOROSIS

Osteoporosis will be prevented or even reversed if the large bones, meaning the legs, hips, and spine, are stressed with the right exercises. The stress itself causes the bones to draw in calcium, and thus rebuild. In Dr. Nichols's cohort, over 90% of those in serious trouble built new bone, so this is firmly established.

Pills, however, won't work. Calcium supplements will slow osteoporosis, but only slightly, while at the same time increasing the risk of heart disease.

There are certain exercises that, if performed correctly, will put pressure on the bones, causing them to deform slightly. Under such stress, these bones then generate an electric field that draws in calcium and other minerals and physically initiates the bone-building processes. Nothing else, including calcium pills, causes this to happen. (This is another decades-old fact that has largely eluded notice in the medical community.)

The bones that must be stressed are the ones that tend to collapse in osteoporosis: the legs, hips, and spine. There are two exercises that stress all of these and we recommend you do them both frequently. Three sets of ten, each one, once a week would be best. Note that throughout, "three sets" really means four. Before doing any weight-bearing exercise, do a dry run. Do the same motions with minimal or no weight. This lubricates the joints and tests them as well.

If your knee joints aren't quite up to snuff yet, you can still start, but with limited motion. As the joint flexibility improves, increase your range of motion.

Start out like this. Sit in a straight-backed chair, feet on the ground, knees above your toes, lean a bit forward, but lean from the hips, with your back perfectly straight, or even arched back a bit. Then vigorously push yourself straight up. That hard push is important. That's the power move that stresses the bones and pulls in the calcium. Can you do this? If not, have someone assist you. Otherwise, do three sets of ten. If the chair is no problem, go into a squat. But don't go down to the "baseline plus two" level discussed in the joint health section. Stop right before that level, and drive up from there. Repeat. Proper form is essential; done well these exercises improve everything, done poorly these exercises can injure your back, hips, and knees. Form is key; it is the difference between graceful strength and debility and pain.

When this becomes easy, start adding weight. The weight needs to be borne on your shoulders or held in your hands, so that your spine gets involved. You can either put a bar across your shoulders or hold a couple of dumbbells. Don't overdo this exercise. The weight should present a bit of a challenge, but should not be arduous. It is hard to manage a bar at home, but a couple of dumbbells will work. At first, don't go for more weight, but instead go for more range and speed of execution. Then as soon as you can do full range without pain, add some weight. Weight and range are important, but attain full range first.

Deadlifts are the other osteoporosis-preventing exercise. Here too, you can use a barbell or dumbbells for weight. If you go to a gym, get a trainer to show you the right way to do these. It is easy to do them wrong and damage your back. Above all, NEVER undertake a deadlift hunched over. Your back must be straight, or slightly arched back, and tight. The lift is begun with the legs. Watch the exercise videos on QuantitativeMedicine. net. Form is very important.

Again—especially guys—there is a tendency to pile on the weight. Instead, keep the weight moderate, but challenging, and drive up rapidly. The explosive nature more effectively triggers the bone growth, which is our focus here. There are several other reasons to go for the explosive speed, which we will explore presently.

Do three sets of ten repetitions of the deadlifts and squats, with light, but somewhat challenging weight, driving up with power and speed. Do both deadlifts and squats each once a week, keeping the weight challenging, and you will probably never have to worry about osteoporosis.

You can also do things like climbing steps two at a time, with a powerful thrust, a great habit to get into. Besides stressing the big bones, this tends to keep the back aligned as well.

The full-body scan, discussed earlier, gives you a way to measure bone density progress. If you are near the fracture threshold, you will need to intensify your efforts.

Now your exercise schedule might look like this:

Monday - 30-minutes	Wednesday - one hour	Friday - 30-minutes
Stretch	Stretch	Stretch
Squats: 1 set of 10 repetitions	Agility exercises	Deadlifts: 3 sets of 10 repetitions
Free-play: do 20 minutes of something. Agility, flexibility, joints, weights. Don't get hurt.	Balancing exercises	Free-play: do 20 minutes of something. Agility, flexibility, joints, weights. Don't get hurt.
Spin on a stationary bike with low resistance for 5 minutes.	Joint exercises as necessary	Spin on a stationary bike with low resistance for 5 minutes.
	Speed bag	
	Balance on wobbly objects	
	Ping-pong	
	Hopscotch	

At this point, you will have great joints, and your agility and balance will be high. Nerves will be building. You will be preventing or reversing osteoporosis. You will be directly knocking out two degenerative diseases, and setting the stage for hammering the rest of them.

The areas that now need further attention are heart rate variability and biological power. That's it. Pull off these last two, and peak health is yours.

HEART RATE VARIABILITY AND BIOLOGICAL POWER

Most health sites, and many doctors, recommend mild aerobic exercise in varying forms and degrees. While better than nothing at all, it would be hard to characterize this form of exercise as particularly good. Brisk walking 2½ hours per week or jogging 1¼ hours per week are common.
There are also frequent recommendations to keep your heart rate below a certain level. The level is a relatively low one. Here are some typical numbers:

Age	Heart Rate Beats per Minute
55	140
60	136
65	132
70	127
75	123

Ostensibly this is done in the interest of safety, but it has exactly the opposite effect. To preserve heart health and prevent atherosclerosis, it is necessary to run the heart up and down through all its possible pulse rates, including its maximum. The maximum heart rate for a 65-year-old who exercises vigorously would probably be closer to 175 beats per minute than the 132 given in the chart.

These low heart rates correspond to a "standard medical practice" that seems to have a strange life of its own. There is absolutely no science, good, bad, or otherwise, supporting these low heart rates, nor has there ever been. It is some sort of superstition. There is no medical literature, past or present, that shows higher heart rates to be dangerous. On the other hand, there is a large body of science supporting the concept that varying the heart over its full range has huge health benefits and dramatically reduces heart risk.

Aerobic exercise is better than no exercise at all, but not by much. Keeping your heart rate moderately elevated for extended periods of time trains your heart and lungs to, well, stay moderately elevated, and, as you might suspect, this is only moderately beneficial.

However, moderate elevation of heart rate, even if prolonged, won't begin to accomplish the physical and cellular changes necessary to avoid degenerative disease and slow aging. More intensity is needed. The heart needs far greater variability, including brief periods of maximal output. The arteries and veins need the temporarily elevated pressure and rush of blood that accompanies it. Only by punching through the barriers that aerobic exercises impose can greater heart health be obtained.

How Safe Is This?

We are proposing running the heart to its maximum rate for short bursts. For which group of people might this be dangerous? Short answer: If you have no significant cardiac risk, it is completely safe. For most with cardiac risk it is safe. Further, such exercise vastly reduces overall cardiac risk for everybody. But with no trouble at all, you can find recommendations to limit your heart rate. For a 70-year-old, the usual limit is 127 beats per minute. This is very low, and the results from exercising with this restriction will correspond.

The American Heart Association has one-size-fits-all recommendations such as these on their website, but they also have a lot of good medical research there as well. In one paper, they investigated the safety of "maximal" exercise. Maximal exercise comes in many flavors, but will usually imply maximal heart rate, or at least a heart rate well above the lame standard limit. Out of 72,000 reported maximal tests, there was one reported cardiac death. In the last 10 years, none at all. This is safer that most daily activities, and of course, the reduction of cardiac risk resulting from such exercise will save many, many people, likely tens of thousands, from cardiac death.

There are three categories of people that should avoid maximal exercise:

- If you have valvular disease, some defect in the valves of your heart, more than usual care should be observed. In such a case, be guided by your last echocardiogram and your cardiologist's advice. He may be too restrictive, but no general advice can be offered here.

- If you have mechanically unstable coronary artery disease, sometimes the shear forces that are otherwise good for the heart might "shake loose" some of the detritus and trigger a clot and subsequent occlusion or blockage, leading to a heart attack. This sounds so vague as to warrant the usual generic and tepid advice to severely limit your heart rate during exercise. Please do not hear this point in that way; superstition is not necessary. If you have any family or personal history of heart attacks, you should nail down this risk by coronary calcium scoring and other additional measures to assess any such risk. If you and your cardiologist think this is a real risk, still don't keep your heart rate as low as the table demands, but do proceed with more than usual caution.

- If you have a known serious heart conduction defect that has been clearly shown to be triggered by higher heart rates, and is potentially life threatening, then certainly observe the heart rate limits your cardiologist suggests. This electrical problem should be respected, though even here we are more likely to recommend this be repaired than drugged.

How to Run Your Heart Up and Down

We suggest here that you replace long sessions of aerobic exercise with short anaerobic sessions of intense exercise. You can start slowly if you like. Paradoxically, in spite of the shorter time taken in interval exercise, the benefit is far greater. The heart learns to work over a variety of ranges, and the arteries get needed pressure and pulsing. HDL and the "really good" cholesterol, will correspondingly rise. Risk for heart disease will plummet, as will cancer risk. If you are undertaking reversal of adult onset diabetes, the rate of recovery will double. Heart rate variability is a major key to good, long-lasting, vibrant health, and the only way to get there is, as you might suspect, by varying your heart rate. The more variation, the healthier.

You should get a watch that will measure your heart rate, so you can track your progress. If a doctor has advised to limit your heart rate to a certain level, you will definitely need to have such a watch.

To run your heart up to its maximum, you need exercises that engage your legs and probably your back as well. An exercise using mainly arms, like swimming, probably won't work. Arm muscles simply aren't large enough to make the demands needed to elevate the heart rate.

Here are several possible methods. They would all be considered anaerobic, meaning your heart cannot keep up with the oxygen demand you are making. This is strongly desirable as it triggers processes in your body that will increase your ability to consume oxygen. Increases in oxygen processing correspond directly to increases in cellular and overall health. We will ultimately be recommending three exercise sessions a week: two demanding 45-minute ones and a light one incorporating the balance, agility, coordination, and joint health exercises discussed earlier.

Concept2 Rower. Most gyms have a couple of these. If not, they cost about $800 new, delivered, which is cheap for an exercise machine, so you could suggest that your gym equip itself with a couple. They aren't out of reach for home use either. The rower requires the use of legs and back, and can get the heart to a maximum rate in under a minute. These machines are quite safe, the sole caveat being to row with a stiff, erect back, and avoid hunching over. Don't start out trying to shatter any world records. Set up the machine for a 2,000-meter row, called the "2K." Try to maintain a somewhat challenging pace. By around 1,000 meters, you should be well "challenged," huffing and puffing, and finding it increasingly difficult to keep the initial pace. Complete the exercise as best you can.

Did you get a heart rate monitoring watch? Record your maximum rate, and how much it recovered in the 60 seconds after you finished. These are two key numbers you will want to track. A third key heart number is your resting heart rate. Measure this one lying in bed in the morning and before consuming any coffee. There is a fourth number of interest as well, which is the time it took you to do that 2K row. With this number, you can get an estimate of your capacity to use oxygen, called VO_2Max, either from the Concept2 website or directly from some of their rower models. More VO_2Max, more life, more health, less aging. It's the strongest predictive number we have, and the way to raise that number is <u>an</u>aerobic exercise.

After you have "mastered" the 2K row, you can try some intervals. Warm up for 2 minutes, then set the rower machine up for time intervals, 20 seconds of rowing, 10 seconds of rest. Just punch the buttons randomly till you find it or consult a local expert. Have the machine display watts. Give the first 20-second row all you've got. Anything left over can be done on the second row. If you have much left after the first two, you weren't trying hard enough. Remember, the whole idea is to place demands on the heart and body that they *cannot* immediately fulfill so that they will undertake all the changes needed to increase your biological power.

Hill Runs. If you are addicted to brisk walking, you might like this one. Briskly walk over to the nearest hill and run up it as fast as you can. If the hill is steep enough, you will start to run out of steam after 20 or 30 seconds. Set a "finish" line about 10 yards beyond your out-of-steam point and chug on. Walk down and do it two more times. These additional times will be harder as your body hasn't the time to replenish the energy store. This is desirable. You want your body to create more on-demand power capability.

WELL AT LEAST I'M BUFF!

If you weren't out of steam after 30 seconds, briskly walk to a steeper hill. If you really aren't enamored with brisk walking, you can just drive to that hill, but before the run, jog for a couple of minutes just to get the juices flowing (literally, if we are talking about joints), and get loosened up. Three 30-second hill runs don't seem like a lot (though they will, 25 seconds into them), but the benefit far exceeds brisk walking or jogging. Again, if you have an upper limit on heart rate, monitor it and make sure you do not exceed it. Be sure that all the joints you will be using are in top shape from the earlier exercises.

Wind Sprints. If you are in Kansas, or some other ultra-flat terrain, do this: Jog for about 2 minutes, then run at top speed for 30 seconds, then jog for a minute, sprint 30 seconds, and then once or twice more. Again, pay attention to maximum heart rate and joints.

Other Methods. You can devise your own. Got a bicycle and some open space? Pedal like crazy for 30 seconds, then coast for a minute. A treadmill could work: set it for maximum steepness. And, don't forget, there is nothing better than stairs. Find a tall building and barrel up those stairs.

BIOLOGICAL POWER

Remember, these exercises don't have a set goal. The whole point is to keep pushing your body to do more and more, to continually increase your biological power. And this newly gained power will only partly be spent on improving your anaerobic sprinting skills. Other things will happen. New, strong bone will grow. High levels of HDL, the artery cleaner, will be generated. Cartilage growth will be stimulated. Cells will be kept clean all over your body.

The various exercises about to be proposed will continue the transformation toward peak biological power. This is the final piece of our exercise program. To optimize this, we would suggest you choose from about a half-dozen key exercises, which we call Tier One, and execute them in a particular way. Don't pile on weight till you master form and full range movement. Weight is important, though: just do it last, after you have mastered everything else.

Whole-Body, Explosive, Concentric, Multi-Planar, Closed-Chain

This describes the principles that should be followed for all exercise, even climbing a flight of stairs or getting out of a chair. Doing exercise this way will maximize the benefit on several levels. Here is a description. This may sound a bit technical, but it isn't rocket science. It is more of a way to look at exercise, so bear with us. This is the final part:

- **Whole-Body** means that several things are moving at once. This improves neural function and coordination, and stimulates growth of new nerves.
- **Explosive** means pushing as hard and quickly as possible. This improves mitochondrial efficiency and number, which in turn slows aging and increases cellular health and strength—biological power.
- **Concentric** means a muscle is contracting when it is doing the work. If you curl a dumbbell, the exercise is concentric on the way up, and eccentric as you let the weight down. It's the concentric exercise that turns on anabolism, and that's what we want. Of course, a complete movement tends to involve both, so do the concentric part explosively, with a burst of energy, but do the eccentric part slowly.
- **Multi-Planar** simply means not merely working in a single plane, such as push/pull, or extension/flexion. This improves balance, coordination, and neural function.
- **Closed-Chain** means recruitment of the neurological chain: an exercise involving all the stabilizing small muscle movements. Tier One exercises like squats and deadlifts are examples of this. Most gym machines are not.

We'll give this sort of exercise an acronym: WECMC. To get the maximum effect from exercise, these elements need to be incorporated. This will cause the exercises to be done in a somewhat different fashion.

Tier One Exercises

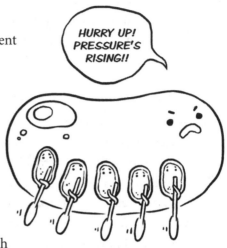

These are the most efficient exercises and should be done in a WECMC fashion. The following is a description of several such exercises. Watch the videos on QuantitativeMedicine.net to see how these exercises should be executed. Better, hire a trainer, at least for a few sessions. In any event, start with minimal weight until you have mastered the form, and then move up slowly. Don't rush, or you will tear a tendon or ligament, and these can take up to two years to heal. The concentric part should be explosive. The eccentric part, slow.

Squats. Squats are an ideal whole-body exercise. Go down slowly into the squat, and then explosively push up hard with your legs. The upward movement is concentric because muscles are shortening while working, the exercise is multi-planar, involving a complex series of motions, and is closed-chain, due to the sequence of neural-muscular activity and balance required. The explosive start and the whole body involvement are crucial elements. Form is important.

Deadlifts. Again, back stiff and arched, head up (head up position makes it easier to have the right form), grab the bar and get it off the ground by pushing up with your legs. Then straighten the back. Never let your back hunch over. Once you are confident with this exercise, try to increase the speed of the lift. This exercise can also be done in a "Sumo" position, with your legs wide, and arms between your legs.

Pull-Ups. If you cannot do a pull-up, use the assisted pull-up machine. Most gyms have one. Grab the bar, completely relaxed. Start the move with your upper back muscles, then power yourself up.

Snatches, Clean and Jerks, Power Cleans, and Kettlebell Cross Body Cleans are very good WECMC exercises. You will need to watch an instructional video or enlist the aid of a trainer.

Squat-Thrust-Throw with a Medicine Ball. From a squatting position, power up and throw a medicine ball straight up. Start with an invisible medicine ball, just to get the form. Catch the medicine ball or let it bounce once.

The 20/10 Rowing Intervals are also good WECMC exercises. To obtain the explosive motion, keep your back straight and torso tight. Drive back with your legs, and involve your arms only at the end of your stroke. Avoid the tendency to hunch over to obtain a longer stroke.

Lunges are good. Place your right leg forward as though taking a long step, but let your left knee go almost all the way to the floor. At this point, your right knee should be at a 90° angle. Now drive up to a standing position, bringing your left leg forward for the next step. Lunges are easier to do than describe—watch a video.

When doing these exercises, exhale on the power move (the concentric part of the motion), and inhale on the recovery move. Never hold your breath. On the rower, don't worry about it—just grab all the air you can.

CONSOLIDATING ALL THIS INTO A PROGRAM

Again we repeat: don't dive in. Start slowly for the following two reasons. First, muscle will build fast, but ligaments and tendons strengthen at a much slower rate. If you overdo it, you will soon have the muscular strength to tear them, and they tend to take up to two years to heal. Therefore, if you ever feel any twinges in joints, ligaments, or tendons, back off, don't tough it out.

Around 75% of the benefit from these exercises comes from using the right form, precision, and speed, and the remainder from hoisting all that weight up and down. We are not doing all this to build muscle (though this will happen). We are trying to increase your body's ability to recruit muscle (use the muscle it has), improve joint strength and range of motion, improve balance and coordination, and prevent osteoporosis. Bone and muscle development are natural consequences, but the entire process sets off a cascade of desirable bodily functions that go way beyond the "body beautiful" notion.

At this point, if you are doing all of the above, you are maintaining your joints and neurological health by doing some joint and balance exercises, you are preventing osteoporosis by doing squats and deadlifts, hopefully in an explosive way, and you are running your heart up and down in the Concept2 rower or some equivalent.

We would suggest that you incorporate six WECMC exercises by adding three of each to the two intense days. The best ones, the Tier One exercises, are squats, deadlifts, pull-ups, snatches, cleans and jerks, power cleans, kettlebell cross body cleans, kettlebell swings, and squat-thrust-throw with a medicine ball. A good trainer will doubtless have others. Trainers are quite imaginative in that regard.

Some other good exercises, though less effective, are the Tier Two group: lunges, leg presses, dumbbell rows, pull downs, and chest presses. Most of the other gym activity is Tier Three. Incorporating all these would yield a routine with two 45-minute intense days and a 1-hour coordination/flexibility day, looking like this:

Monday - 45-minutes	Wednesday-1 hour	Friday - 45-minutes
Stretch	Stretch	Stretch
Interval: Rower 20-10's	Agility exercises	Anaerobic: 2K row
Squats: 3 sets of 10 repetitions	Balancing exercises	Deadlifts: 3 sets of 10 repetitions
Kettlebell swings: 3 sets of 10 repetitions	Joint exercises as necessary	Medicine ball squat and toss: 3 sets of 10 repetitions
Pull-ups: 3 sets of 6 repetitions	Speed bag	Lunges: 3 sets of 20 pairs of lunges
Jerks: 3 sets of 10 repetitions	Balance on wobbly objects	Barbell cleans: 3 sets of 10 repetitions
Bench press: 3 sets of 10	Ping-pong	Any other exercises that suit your fancy: curls, random machines, up to you.
Any other exercises that suit your fancy: curls, random machines, up to you.	Hopscotch	
Spin on a stationary bike with low resistance for 5 minutes.		Spin on a stationary bike with low resistance for 5 minutes.

Note about sets of resistance exercises: Do one warm-up set, usually 10 repetitions, with very light weight, or none at all, but with as full a range of motion as you can manage. This both lubricates and tests your joints. Then do three sets with challenging but not too heavy weight, attempting to execute the lift explosively, cleanly, and quickly, while maintaining perfect form. This builds heart rate variability and biological power. Finally—optional—build up some muscle by adding more weight and doing a fifth set with just a few more repetitions. Do this with care, paying close attention to form and any joint/tendon pain.

For any exercise you do, determine which portions are the concentric part, where the muscle is contracting, and do that part explosively. For most exercises, there is a corresponding eccentric part where the weight is returned to its original position. Do this part slowly.

Tier Two exercises are good but are more restricted in movement. Examples would be the leg press, dumbbell rows, pull downs, and chest presses.

Tier Three is everything else, including most of the machines. It is possible to do the exercises explosively on the machines, though it will likely jangle the weights and attract unwanted attention. In most cases, the machine, not your own motion, determines the movement, so the complex, back-and-forth neural signaling is missing. Machines tend to isolate one muscle, so the sequence is lost as well. However, two machines that are quite useful are the "jammer" and the "viper." These are rarely seen. With the jammer, you push out and up from a crouched position. The viper is a rope-climbing simulation and is an excellent complex shoulder and arm workout.

A couple of points:

First, it is difficult to describe the proper form for doing squats and deadlifts. One absolute no-no is hunching your back over. Keep it straight, tight, and arched back as much as you can. Keep your weight on your heels. Breathe out when you are doing the lift, breathe in when recovering. Ideally, get a trainer at the gym to show you how to safely do squats, deadlifts, and other exercises. However, not all trainers know the right way either. Carefully watch the videos on the QuantitativeMedicine.net website. Start out with minimal weight, watching yourself in the mirror and checking your form. (Most gyms are full of mirrors so the clientele can admire themselves and one another.) If you can't do a chin-up, use the assisted chin-up machine.

Second, an important safety note: When you are about to hoist some large weight, there is a natural tendency to hold your breath. DON'T DO THIS. This puts an unnecessary strain on your heart. Inhale getting ready, and exhale while doing the lift.

PEAK HEALTH

Do the above, do them seriously and correctly, and you will attain peak health—your peak health. This is as healthy as you can be. This is the state where degenerative disease is repelled, where aging is slowed, where energy level is high, and where mental acuity is high. This is proven to work. One excellent measure of fitness is VO_2Max, which is the maximum volume of oxygen you can process.

Everyone who has undertaken the exercise methods and techniques we have just described and has tracked VO_2Max has seen a noticeable improvement in it. There is one, and only one, explanation: cells have increased their biological power. This, in turn, means two things: First, there are now more mitochondria. And second, the mitochondria are functioning better. The body will regulate the number of mitochondria up or down, as needed. It regulates down to save energy (food). Most of us don't need to worry about this anymore, so we want primarily the regulation upward. Additionally, mitochondria that are exercised are healthier. This is a great compound benefit of exercise. And this applies all over the body. Even in cells that are considered to be relatively permanent, like heart muscle and neurons, mitochondria are replaced every few weeks. True to their bacterial heritage, they reproduce by cell division, but unlike bacteria, this is a controlled process. (Interestingly, there appears to be a culling that goes on. Broken mitochondria aren't allowed to divide.)

What happens if we acquire and maintain a large and healthy supply of these mitochondria? The short answer: everything. Other than our joints, there is not a single process in our body that doesn't run on mitochondrial power, and the cleaner and more efficient this is, the healthier we are, the slower we age, and the longer we live.

Here is a stark example: Bats and mice are about the same size. But bats fly, and to do this, they need a disproportionately high amount of healthy mitochondria. What does that buy them? Mice live 2 years, but the tiny bat lives 20. And bats don't age. A bat that misses the nightly bug haul soon starves to death. Birds pull off the same trick. The larger ones outlive us. If we could fly, we would live to 250, but that's beyond the scope of this chapter.

Going for the Gold

The Tier One exercises, done in a WECMC fashion, will most likely improve your biological power to the maximal extent possible. The chart shows the six-month results from the initial group of patients that followed these protocols.

These were not Olympic trainees. Generally, these people were already sick or headed in that direction.

These 25 people were highly monitored, with quarterly blood tests, their heart rates monitored and recorded. Every exercise session was supervised by a trainer as well. Of necessity, many of them started slowly and step-by-step, as outlined above. Nonetheless, by six months all these people's health had dramatically improved. Most had reversed at least one degenerative disease. Some had reversed several. The trainer presence insured that the exercises were done, and done right, and the measurements verified the results, but it was the 25 people themselves who did all the work, who, in effect, cured themselves. This level of improvement is available to anyone who performs the exercises with the power and form required. It would definitely help to engage a trainer, but make sure the trainer has a good grasp of the exercise components. Just look at the results:

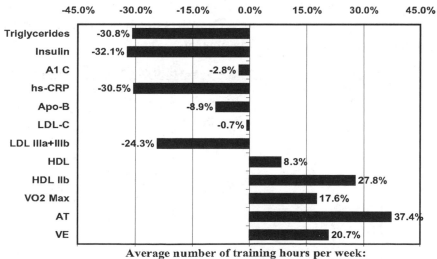

Average number of training hours per week:
Male: 2.3; Female: 2.7

The route to attaining and maintaining peak health requires some work, discipline, and dedication. It does not require inordinate amounts of time, though, and we are convinced that the benefits hugely outweigh the "costs."

The principal point is to keep challenging yourself. This, in turn, continually challenges your body to do more, and do it more effectively, maintaining and increasing your biological power. This does not mean spending half your life at the gym. What it does mean is keeping the exercises challenging. When you have mastered standing on a wobbly object with two feet, learn to do it with one. Employ more "WECMC" in the resistance-type exercises. Keep pushing yourself. If the demand is there, the body will respond.

ASSORTED EXERCISE TOPICS

Here are several generally useful exercise tips.

Interpreting VO$_2$Max and Heart Rate Numbers

You can either find a place that has equipment to directly measure VO$_2$Max (talk to your doc first), or use the indirect measurement provided by the Concept2 rower for the 2K row time. More VO$_2$Max means more health and more biological power. If you are using more oxygen in a maximal exercise, you are engaging more mitochondria to work better, and this is fundamental to all elements of health.

Heart rate can be recorded by the more expensive heart rate watches, or possibly by using some of the "smart" watches, which pair with smartphones. Here is a graph of a typical 45-minute intense session.

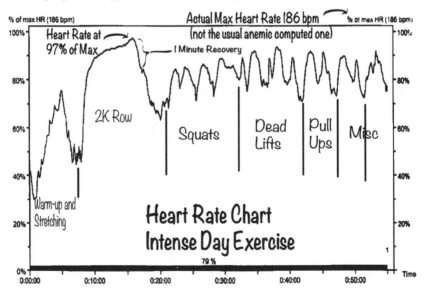

Spin Your Toxins Away

After some serious resistance exercise, your muscles will probably be sore the next few days. It's a "good sore," as they say, since you are building more muscle, but it may get a bit old. You can greatly reduce the soreness by doing this: at the end of your session, get on a stationary bike, set the resistance to "easy," and spin away for five minutes.

Picking a Gym

The most important criterion is that you feel comfortable and welcome. The main reason for doing so is health, and a gym that focuses on that is desirable. The YMCA gyms do well in this regard, plus they are reasonably priced and don't try to pressure you into long-term deals. Also, the YMCA trainers will show you the safe way to do an exercise, usually for free. For squats and deadlifts this is quite important.

If you like classes, by all means do classes. Many do not seem to emphasize resistance or interval training, but there are notable exceptions.

Strenuous classes like exercise programs that emphasize balance and heart rate variability are excellent.

One important machine to look for is the rower. The "standard" brand is the Concept2. Most gyms have these. The rower is a very safe and effective way to do interval and anaerobic-threshold exercise. However, there are many other ways, so lack of a rower needn't be a showstopper.

Another essential gym item would be a squat cage, which is a rack that allows you to load weights onto a barbell, along with safety rails to catch the bar should you fall or take on too much weight. Gyms usually have one.

Trainers

Unless the staff will instruct you for free, you should buy a few trainer sessions and have the trainer show you the safe way to do these exercises, especially squats and deadlifts. Not all trainers have the same ideas. Be sure to watch the exercise videos on QuantitativeMedicine.net too.

Trainers vary. Some primarily function as cheerleaders. Others provide serious medical benefits to their trainees (you).

Other than safety issues, you do not absolutely need a trainer. However, the exercise benefits will probably roll in twice as fast if you can find the right one. But how to proceed? First of all, find a trainer you can communicate with and who respects you. List the training protocols you are interested in and explain why. The prospective trainer should be interested and should not be dismissive. They should have some idea of what "whole-body, explosive, concentric, multi-planar, closed-chain" exercises are, as well as interval and anaerobic exercises. Generally speaking, they will be quite surprised that you have a definite agenda, as most of the people they deal with do not. If they seem to be unwilling to accommodate your agenda, or don't seem to be listening, talk to someone else.

You might proceed this way: Get your introductory safety session and chat a bit about explosive and interval exercise. See if this resonates. Maybe this will lead you somewhere. Barring that, go about the gym, doing whatever routine you have thought up, and keep a sharp eye on the various training sessions going on around you. You will probably be able to spot some trainers that are practicing the style we are looking for. A good trainer will come up with a huge repertoire of exercises, which will make the sessions more interesting, and will give all your various muscles and joints their day in the sun.

Normally gyms want you to buy a package of training sessions. Try to avoid this until you are happy with your trainer.

Alternatives

We have recommended that you join a gym, and that you use the rowing machine for both intervals and the anaerobic exercises, and use free weights for the rest. There can be endless variations on this. For intervals and the anaerobic exercises, anything that can run your heart up will work. Running or bicycling up a steep hill would be excellent. The gym machine that looks like a tiny escalator can work too.

Here's a venerable home program: the Royal Canadian Air Force Exercise Plan. This nugget dates from the '60s and is done entirely as calisthenics, no weights or equipment needed. It takes 11 minutes for men and 12 minutes for women. Here's a typical men's list:

- Toe Touching/Warm-Up: 2 Minutes
- Partial Sit-Ups: 1 Minute
- Leg Lifts: 1 Minute
- Push-Ups: 1 Minute
- Stationary Running: 6 Minutes

The female variant:

- Toe Touching/Warm-Up: 30 Seconds
- Knee Raising: 30 Seconds
- Arm Circling: 30 Seconds
- Partial Sit-Ups: 30 Seconds
- Chest and Leg Raising: 2 Minutes
- Side Leg Raising: 1 Minute
- Push-Ups (Kneeling): 1 Minutes
- Leg Lifting: 1 Minute
- Run And Hop: 3 Minutes

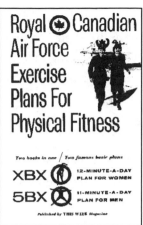

These are daily exercises and are graduated. They get harder as you go along, but they still only take 11 minutes. The full booklet is easily found online.

If you do not feel comfortable going to a gym, it is possible to set something up in your home. The Concept II rowing machine seems to have a street price of around $800 delivered. You can install a chin-up bar. If you can't do a full chin-up, consider pulling up from a supine position or using resistance straps.

Bar exercise is very popular now, and provides a good exercise routine.

Do something. Almost any reasonable exercise program offers significant health improvements over "couch-potato."

Famous Exercisers

Most Americans over 50 will remember fitness guru Jack LaLanne. He had a televised daily exercise show that started in 1953 and ran 32 years. He finally decided to call it quits in 1985 at age 71. There are online videos of his final show with Oprah. He is amazing. He looks 20 years younger, but you might expect that. However, he moves with the grace and agility of someone 50 years younger, and that is something to see. At an age where many are battling all sorts of mobility problems, this guy is bouncing around like a kid. He practiced what he preached, working out till the end, at age 95. In later interviews, he still had his vigor, looked years younger, and clearly had all his marbles.

Jack LaLanne was far from being the only physically fit celebrity who held it together way beyond retirement age. Fred Astaire at age 80 was challenged to dance on a Dick Cavett TV show and "improvised" something with remarkable fluidity and energy. No rocking chair for that guy.

Not everyone can have Jack's physique or Fred's dancing feet; these are gifts. But their health, vigor, and general youthfulness are available to all who are willing to keep active, eat sensibly, and take life as it comes. That part is a matter of decision and discipline, not a matter of genetic gifts.

SNACKS BEFORE AND AFTER EXERCISE

You can make some extra nutrients available for the muscles by having a snack 30 to 60 minutes before exercise. Likewise, such a snack 30 to 60 minutes after exercise can help the body repair and rebuild.

What sort of snack? Cheeses, apple, or nuts.

If Exercise Is So Damn Good, Why Do Many of Us Abhor It?

This has many dimensions. Clearly in times of scarcity, there is a survival necessity to conserve energy. In our wealthier modern times, this will seldom apply to most of us. Even so, whether or not to conserve is always up to the hypothalamus, and always in the context of its ancient worldview, so energy conservation remains a factor.

We are also social beings, having spent most of our evolution in tribes and bands. A tribe will not prosper if a substantial fraction of its members are non-productive. Are we beyond reproductive age? Hunting age? Perhaps gathering age? We live substantially longer than animals of similar sizes and so do our great ape cousins. But ultimately the tribes that survived were the efficient ones, not those saddled with large, unproductive sub-groups. We, the survivors' descendants, may have senescence wired in as it were, along with an aversion to energy-consuming exercise.

Modern times have upended all this. Most of us will get enough food. There's no longer an energy issue. If we have saved and behaved, we needn't be a burden for anyone. So there is no further need to turn all the dials down and wait for the twilight to end. We can, through sheer application of will, run up the cellular machinery to its possible peak potential. Run it as though we were young hunters in a time of plenty. What will happen? We will, in a sense, become young again. All these old cells still have plenty of sizzle left and will duly respond.

But this isn't how we are programmed. Isn't Mother Nature going to be peeved? Our choice. In the West, we live in a time of broad abundance. Maybe in 100,000 years we will have adapted to all this.

We can wait. We can choose the old ways and wind down. Or we can choose life now. We can ignite the processes that lie within. The processes of health and energy and acuity.

Once this is known and fully understood, ignoring it is as reckless as crossing a street blindfolded. The best way to go about the transformation is to measure, do a rigorous exercise program for six months, and measure again. If you did it seriously, it is almost a certainty that you have turned back your biological clock.

Some people like to exercise. Maybe 10%-20%. And there may be people that hate sugar. The sad truth is that we don't get to the promised land, at least not the one on this planet, unless we exercise (and manage the sugar too). So two things:

- You need to exercise.
- You need to make a lifelong commitment.

Many people, when first confronted with bad medical news, will go join a gym and with great zeal, pound away at it for, well, probably not all that long. There are good business reasons why the gyms try to get that one-year no-cancellation commitment.

We have tried to "package" the recommended exercises so that, though intense, they are over with quickly. You can get most of the benefit from these two 45-minute sessions. You can get a bit more if you do more, but you really can't get a lot more. Overtraining can be detrimental for a variety of reasons. You need renewal and repair time. Two 45-minute intense sessions plus an added session featuring balance, flexibility, and coordination are probably a reasonable upper limit.

Do something. The more it is like our recommendations, the better the result, but importantly, find a program you will actually do for the rest of your life. At this point you should have a good idea of what an effective exercise program should look like, and you have the means to test the results.

And remember, intensity is everything. Five hours of golf is not nearly as beneficial as 11 minutes of the Royal Canadian Air Force Exercise Plan. And you will go a lot further still with our 45-minute gym sessions. No matter. Do something. No exercise at all is a formula for disaster.

Do not get disheartened. A lifetime commitment is needed. As you slog through it all, keep telling yourself:

- Risk of heart attack is cut at least in half, maybe a lot more.
- Resistance exercise, done correctly, can completely prevent or reverse osteoporosis.
- Exercise raises HDL. This alone cuts cancer risk by as much as 50%.
- Exercise acts as an antidepressant.
- Exercise reduces the risk of dementia 50% or more.
- Exercise will cause the short-term memory regions of your brain to grow.
- Exercise raises IGF-1 and testosterone, thus increasing anabolism and cellular repair and renewal.

And enjoy the long, disease-free life you are creating for yourself.

Key Points
10 - STEP III - Lifestyle Changes - Exercise
- A summary of lifestyle changes for diet, exercise, and stress reduction, suitable for posting on the fridge, is found at the end of Chapter 11.

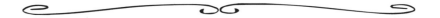

11 - STEP III - LIFESTYLE CHANGE GUIDELINES - SPIRITUAL DISCIPLINE

Stress reduction will, of course, have its greatest effect on your stress group numbers. By raising insulin levels, high psychological stress undermines sugar management as well. As far as disease prevention impact, cancer would be the most affected, followed by adult onset diabetes, Alzheimer's, and heart disease.

What's Killing All the Nurses?

Nurses are typically willing and accessible participants in health studies, and so a lot is known about them. They have about the same mortality as the general population, but two things stand out: they have about twice the rate of cancer, but about half the rate of heart disease. The exact reason for this puzzling difference is not really known, but we could speculate.

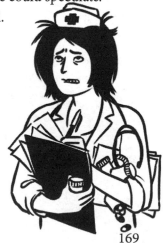

Nursing, by its very nature, is stressful. Nurses are continually dealing with medical situations, frequently serious and sometimes life threatening. Nursing also involves shift work, and this disrupts circadian rhythm and could also be a cause of cancer. This is seen in other professions involving shift work.

While shift work for nurses may be unavoidable, stress reduction techniques may be practiced. In fact, several hospitals have implemented such programs already.

CAUSE OF DEGENERATIVE DISEASE

Cancer

   Heart disease is in decline in the West. Though statin manufacturers are claiming full credit for this, there are many other reasons: reduced smoking, elimination of trans fat, exercise, and the low-carb movement being far more significant.

   Cancer, on the other hand, is on the increase. This is only partly due to greater longevity. The three most likely causes are stress, circadian rhythm issues, and pollution.

   Lifestyle change will not cure a cancer, though it will aid the recovery process. If you have a cancer, Western medical treatment is your best shot by far. Prevention, though, is possible.

   Some pollution is unavoidable as it is in the air and the materials that surround us. Pollution in food can, to some extent, be avoided by buying organic vegetables and grass-fed meat.

   It is well known that shift workers have higher rates of cancer. Thus quality sleep at regular hours is important.

   Chronic stress is another well known cancer promoter. In fact, a stress reduction program has shown a 50% reduction in cancer.

   Cancer is apparently quite rare in hunter-gatherers.

Chronic Psychological Stress Is Medically Dangerous

Stress is generally broken down into short-term and chronic (long-term). Some short-term stress may actually be good, as long as the cause of the stress does no harm. Chronic stress is a different matter.

The body does not seem to be well evolved to deal with chronic stress, but modern civilization seems to be well evolved to dish it out. All stress throws the hypothalamus out of homeostasis, but chronic stress holds it there. The principal hormones associated with stress are cortisol and adrenalin. Both of these are manufactured by the adrenal glands, which are perched, squatter-like, atop the kidneys.

As you might suspect, the hypothalamus is controlling all this, but it has advisors, basing its decision to order the release of these stress hormones on input from the neocortex (our conscious self), along with two other little "brains," one called the amygdala and the other the hippocampus.

The amygdala makes emotional decisions, and the hippocampus is involved in memory, particularly memory of traumatic events. From this, it is easy to see how quite a variety of things might initiate the stress response. The neocortex could perceive danger from its day-to-day view of things, or could as well imagine it, or misinterpret something normal as stressful. The amygdala can get into the act as well, generating a stress response that might not even register at the conscious level. Likewise, the hippocampus might remember some past real or perceived danger.

A cortisol measurement greater than 14 µg/dl could indicate chronic stress, a cause for serious concern. But cortisol is fast acting, and an elevated level could be due to many other things. Something stressful right before the blood draw, or even the draw itself, might trigger it. (This is called "white coat syndrome.") A high level could also be due to internal infection or heart disease. If you don't think any of these were factors, cortisol greater than 14 indicates a need for some sort of stress reduction activity. Cortisol is quite a volatile hormone, though, so some wild numbers will naturally occur. Your own sense of stress may be a more accurate measure. If in doubt, consider a second measurement. In fact, the more data points you have for cortisol the more likely you are to see the true underlying pattern, thus avoiding the transient and misleading extremes.

Even if your cortisol is less than 14, we still encourage you to consider a stress reduction activity. There appear to be many other significant health benefits that we are unable to directly measure. One NIH-funded study showed a 50% reduction in cancer and a 30% reduction in cardiac events following a stress management program. This is a lot of reduction. It is unlikely these results can be attributed to lower cortisol alone, but we are certainly very impressed with the results.

We do know that chronic stress carries with it a chronically high level of cortisol. Cortisol is "designed" to be one of the fight-or-flight hormones. It prepares the body for such moments by increasing available energy—blood glucose. It shuts down functions not immediately needed, like cell renewal and repair. It preps the immune system to deal with possible wounds, while simultaneously shutting down the parts of the immune system that are repairing or fighting degenerative disease.

This stress response is profound and intense, and is supposed to prepare us for life-or-death situations. We are pushed to the edge of our ability and acuity. In addition to cortisol, several other hormones are raised in preparation, but we cannot sustain this intensity long without physiological damage. But most situations today are not life threatening,

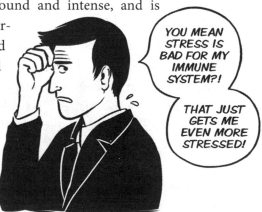

YOU MEAN STRESS IS BAD FOR MY IMMUNE SYSTEM?!

THAT JUST GETS ME EVEN MORE STRESSED!

and the body's interpretation is no longer appropriate. It could be that the body simply isn't taking any chances, but the consequences are not anything we want.

The cortisol-induced blood sugar elevation will cause fat to be stored, thus aggravating atherosclerosis and all the other high-blood-sugar problems. Impaired cellular repair means aging and loss of vigor. Lowered immune system function means cancer, and indeed, cancer is the most prominent problem associated with chronic stress. Cancer is a tug of war between your immune system and malfunctioning cells. If at all possible, get the cortisol down to a reasonable level. This is an area where anti-anxiety medication can play a role.

Many Approaches to Stress Management

Of course, the first order of business is to try to reduce the external stress. This is not always easy or even possible. However, we suspect that most people are unaware of the long-term health dangers. In view of this, some additional effort might reap rewards. A long daily commute may be aggravating, but only if you let it be. A stressful family member or co-worker might be receptive to something like, "I am getting stressed out by this, this, and that, and I am starting to have health problems because of it. Could you please consider a different approach?" This may not work, but it is well worth a try.

There are many books available on stress reduction. The popular online retailer, the one named after a major South American river, lists over 20,000.

There is also a direct step you can take.

Meditation Made Easy

Forget all the stereotypes. This is not about Buddhist monks and Zen masters, saffron robes and incense—at least not what we have in mind.

Almost all your waking moments, your brain is going nonstop. There is continuous internal chatter: "What is going on?" "Did she really say that?" "Is this the slowest checkout line on the planet?" "That cheesecake will send my glucose to the stratosphere." Typically, there are several such internal conversations going on simultaneously.

What we want you to do is go to a quiet, safe place and shut the chattering brain-computer off for 10 minutes. Just sit and think of absolutely nothing, or concentrate on one repetitive thing: a sound or a picture or a single simple thought. Do this for 10 minutes, once a day.

Advice for you beginning "grasshoppers": At first, your chattering brain-computer will only shut off for five or so seconds, at which time assorted random thoughts will come rudely barging into your idle consciousness and take over. Try again. Stare at a watch and see if you can go 10 seconds. When a thought tries to intrude, either push it back, or let it float away into some cerebral ether. Keep increasing the time. The ability will develop, and do so fairly quickly; it just takes a bit of practice. If shutting off the brain-computer seems too difficult, try instead to focus on a single simple object. A flame, perhaps, or your own breathing. Fully focus on that one thing.

Is spite of the troubles getting started, the health results from this practice are quite stunning. Recall the 50% reduction in cancer and the 30% reduction in cardiac events we mentioned earlier. These are huge benefits. A panoply of other bodily functions are positively affected as well; not as dramatically, but quite broadly—rather what we want. So persist!

Almost anything you can come up with that will temporarily shut off your computer-brain is OK. However, it should not involve significant physical activity. Jogging, for instance, would thwart the process. Walking would be OK, but not power walking or anything like that. When you walk or are outdoors, and do manage to quiet the brain-chatter, you will notice an odd thing. After a few seconds of brain-silence, your vision will undergo an interesting, though brief, alteration. Instead of the usual focusing on one specific spot, you will sort of zoom back and see the entire panorama. You will feel strangely connected to it. The experience is quite intense and hard to hold for more than a few seconds.

Ten minutes a day of brain-quieting activity confers many benefits beyond cancer and heart event reduction. First of all, you will be more alert, focused, and tuned in, as though you "rebooted" your brain-computer. Second, the intruding, stress-creating thoughts will become less frequent, possibly because their momentum was temporarily halted, or maybe the quiet time gave some of them a chance to find some natural termination. Third, this mental quieting gives the non-verbal part of your brain, the hypothalamus, the hippocampus, the amygdala, a moment to somehow be heard, to achieve some communication with the conscious part.

Avoid Obsessive Thought at All Costs

Another stressful item is obsessive thought, and the more obsessive that thought becomes, the more neural pathways it will forge. Neurons are literally getting physically modified, and they will get stuck that way, which is why it is so hard to shake the obsession. They will have to eventually be modified back or erased or reprogrammed to clear out that obsessive thought. For this reason, it is very important to try to derail obsessive thoughts before they can gain a toehold. Consider practicing this as some sort of mental inoculation. Don't let them get started. Refuse to let them into your consciousness. You aren't repressing them, you are preventing them from laying down neural tracks; this is quite the opposite.

Medication May Be Appropriate

It is important to get on top of any chronic stress. If your situation is such that you cannot pull the stress measurements into a low range, discuss anxiety-reducing medication with your doctor.

We seem to not have evolved much defense to chronic stress. This could either mean it didn't come up much in the hunter-gatherer world, or if it did, it was so serious that despite possible long-term consequences, the body's reaction was necessary for survival. Obviously, acute stress would be quite common in those eat-or-be-eaten times.

SLEEP

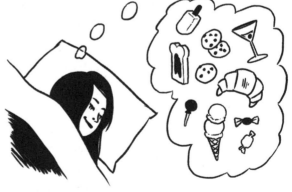

Day and night is, of course, our most fundamental life rhythm. Virtually every living thing on earth is synchronized to this. For all vertebrates, including ourselves, sleep time is repair time, so it should come as no surprise that sleep disruption has serious health consequences. We have already mentioned the nurses' higher cancer rate. That could be stress or could be shift work. In fact, shift workers in other professions experience similar increases in cancer risk.

Nine hours is ideal, though there is not a lot of harm with less, say, seven or eight. A full, deep, uninterrupted sleep is by far the most important attribute. You should dream and when you wake up, you should feel refreshed, not still sleepy.

Improved sleep patterns will have their greatest effect on your body's anabolic activity. By far the majority of necessary bodily repair occurs during sleep. If you aren't getting enough sleep, that repair will be reduced, or will not happen at all.

Dr. Mike's Philosophical Sidebar
A Simple Proposition

I've worked with people, sick enough people, over enough years to know that the quick and thrifty appearance of learning and of teaching will not sustain meaningful change over a long enough time and to the degree necessary to save and change a life.

We don't wake up sick with diabetes or heart disease or even premature aging from years of simply misunderstanding some jingoistic slogan. We arrive at such a point by long habit built of poorly remembered, if remembered at all, tweaks and nudges of information, misinformation, family dynamics, self-inflicted wounds of pride, discouragement and sometimes vain and groundless hope.

And the sad fact is, you cannot unpack such a past and path with a few pithy lines and a few good catchphrases: even good ones like "paleo diet," or "intense interval training," or "sleep is more important than sex," or whatever. But there is a way back; a sure way that will allow the unfolding of self-discovery, the emergence of self-mastery over time—and it does require time—that can be guided by an error-free methodology.

Folks, here is the claim: I have invented such an error-free methodology. Wow. Now if that is not hubris on steroids, what is?

Here is how it works:
- Step one: measure everything with a known and significant statistical value at predicting disease and aging.
- Step two: change something, any something. Eat differently, better, worse, who knows.
- Step three: remeasure to see what effect the change has had on the variables you are tracking.
- Step four: change something else, more and more intense variations of the same thing, or something altogether different.
- Step five: remeasure to see what effect the changes had.
- Are you seeing a pattern here? Now the kinds of things you change are drawn from three simple categories:
1. Eating behavior: content, type, and timing.
2. Exercise and activity behavior: content, type, and timing
3. Spiritual discipline: this includes sleep, time laughing, quiet time, prayer, meditation, Qigong, and so on.

Doing this as outlined is where to start; the next steps are seeing the results, believing the data, and acting on that data.

We have so thoroughly transcended seasonal rhythms that it is perhaps futile to address them at all. Northern hunter-gatherers would have to prepare for the lean winters by putting on as much fat as possible when food was plentiful, but we are largely free from any such constraints. Hunter-gatherers would sleep a lot more in the winter as well.

Maybe we do adjust our sleep seasonally. Maybe we are still tuned in to those ancient voices. It would be hard to hunt and gather on a stormy day. Is this why it is so easy to stay in bed when you hear that rain outside?

Key Points

9-10-11 - STEP III - Lifestyle Guidelines
- Lifestyle changes can make a great difference in your health, far greater than any currently available drugs.
- Most degenerative disease is preventable. Some is reversible.

EATING . . .
- Eating modification has the most effect on sugar numbers.
- Eat three meals and three snacks per day.
- People can tolerate varying amounts of sugar and starch. This has to be determined from blood tests. Establish your Personal Sugar Rule.
- Eat one portion of protein, two or three of vegetables.
- Energy bars may be used for snacks if chosen to have the correct ingredients.
- Check that you are not insulin resistant, not hypoglycemic, and not too thin.
- Do not worry about dietary cholesterol and saturated fat.
- It is difficult to thrive on a vegetarian diet, even one containing eggs and dairy.
- It is very difficult to thrive on a vegan diet.
- Fasting is usually not beneficial.
- Calorie restriction does not appear to work.

EXERCISE. . .
- Exercise will primarily affect anabolism numbers.
- Intensity is far more important than duration.
- Do joint exercises to prevent osteoarthritis.
- Do balance and coordination exercises.
- Do squats and deadlifts to prevent osteoporosis.
- Do anaerobic threshold exercise (interval rowing, etc.) to increase heart rate variability.
- Do explosive resistance exercise (squats, deadlifts, etc.) to increase anabolism.

STRESS. . .
- Try to minimize day-to-day stress.
- Practice 10 minutes of meditation per day.

SLEEP. . .
- Get at least 7½ hour of sleep.
- Quality is important.
- Lack of sleep has serious health consequences.

Copy this page and place it in a prominent location.

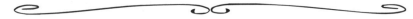

12 - ADDRESSING THE RESULTS

Quantitative Medicine is an iterative process. Quantify yourself. Get measurements, and compare them to the known desirable numbers. Then select a direction to head, a lifestyle change to undertake. Make it and reassess. This is a lifetime process. Even though you drove your numbers to ideal levels, they will change as you age. You will have to keep measuring and modifying to stay in your health "groove."

How fast will the body react to lifestyle changes? For some areas, almost immediately; others could take months or longer. As usual, there will be considerable variation from person to person, but here are some estimates.

Sugar management issues that are short of full diabetes will respond in as little as three months. Triglycerides, insulin, and fasting glucose should move significantly toward an ideal homeostasis in this time. We would suggest you decide on a very specific program, hold rigorously to it for three months, then retest for just the sugar management numbers.

As an example, suppose your fasting glucose was 100 mg/dl and your triglycerides were 140 mg/dl. These are not all that bad, but they are not ideal either, and may be indicative of an undesirable trend that needs reversing. Further suppose you cut out all starch and all sweets for three months, while still eating fruits. So a diet of meat, vegetables, and fruit, but no bread, pasta, cake, cookies, etc. At three months you retest the sugar management numbers. Your numbers should be noticeably different. Fasting glucose should be below 90, triglycerides should be below 100. They may be better than this or worse. However, you will now have "quantified" yourself. You know how much the numbers shifted in response to your lifestyle change.

Possibly you did really well and got a fasting glucose of 75 mg/dl and triglyceride level of 90 mg/dl. Congratulations. On the other hand, if you did not get below 80 for glucose and 100 for triglycerides, you didn't cut enough, and the fruit will probably have to go, along with alcohol. Or perhaps you could still eat berries and cut something else—berries are metabolized relatively slowly. You get the idea. By experimenting, you can push the numbers toward, and eventually into, the ideal ranges. Since this needs to be a lifelong change, take it easy and give things time to adjust.

The lipid group works somewhat differently. Triglycerides, as we just saw, move rather quickly. The HDL and LDL numbers depend on both diet and exercise, and take longer to change, perhaps six months, but possibly as little as three.

The anabolic group is mainly responsive to exercise and should show a lot of improvement by within six months.

The stress group of numbers responds very quickly. Success in stress reduction will show up rapidly, at least at the subjective level. Stable and lower cortisol could take many months to reach.

Adult onset diabetes involves an entire syndrome of problems and it might take as long as a year for things to reach an ideal homeostasis. However, there will be immediate and measurable progress.

There are many overlapping processes at work in a change of lifestyle. Using this book as a guide, each individual will have to take an educated first guess at which lifestyle changes will be needed to drive the various key numbers to ideal homeostasis.

LIFESTYLE CHANGES AND EXISTING DISEASE

We have mentioned degenerative disease throughout, but mostly in a preventive context. This is not a book about treatment. If you know you have a degenerative disease, or the testing indicates you might, you should be under the care of a practitioner. That said, it is important to know the effects that lifestyle changes have on these various diseases, and whether or not the change is likely to have much effect on existing disease, or whether it is primarily for prevention.

Achieving ideal homeostasis and anabolism will block all degenerative diseases. The effect on preexisting degenerative disease varies:

- Adult onset diabetes will be reversed and cured.
- Alzheimer's will be slowed, and in the early stages even partially reversed.
- Atherosclerosis will be halted, and slowly reversed.
- Cancer in principle will be slowed, but if a tumor has resulted, it must be treated. Future cancer risk and risk of recurrence of a treated cancer will both be reduced.
- Osteoporosis can be stopped and reversed. Loss of stature will, in some cases, reverse also.
- Osteoarthritis can be reversed in some cases.
- Aging will noticeably slow.

Everyone has different propensities to various diseases. However, the root causes of these diseases are all the same, and if the ideal homeostatic set-points are attained, along with a stable anabolic state, the progression of these diseases is greatly reduced, if not reversed.

The methods needed to attain these ideal states vary considerably from person to person. Everyone needs to find their own ideal health formula.

However, the protective effects of ideal homeostasis and anabolism are common to everyone. And equally, everyone can effectively pursue these goals. Discipline and perseverance are necessary, but this is true for most worthwhile things, and most people have familiarity with such undertakings. Achieving these health goals should lead to a long and healthy life.

IF THINGS DON'T PROGRESS AS EXPECTED

The measure and modify Quantitative Medicine approach works well for 80 to 90% of the population. However, sometimes it is slow, and sometimes it doesn't work at all. Here some common problems:

Difficulty with Carb Reduction

Ease of adjustment to carb reduction varies from person to person. Cells can run on glucose, fat, or even protein. However, the actual mechanisms to convert those nutrients to energy are quite different, and cells tend to adapt and lock-in to the ones they are accustomed to seeing. When the nutrient base changes, the cellular processing machinery must change as well. This WILL happen, but not instantly. We have no cases where people were completely unable to process fat. Rather, it's a question of time. For some, it is almost immediate, but for others, it can be quite difficult. If the cellular adjustment is slow, you will feel low-energy and malnourished during the transition. The fastest way is to just tough it out. However, you can make a slow transition as well if you prefer.

TESTIMONIAL

My Personal Experience with the Quantitative Medicine Nutritional Advice

My friends Charlie and Lien seemed to belong to some strange cult and were insistent that weight gain was carb-driven. They said crazy things such as, "Eat as much fat as you want, but don't touch a carb."

I had never been overweight, but once I got into my 40s, my weight started to creep up. I tried various diets and swam regularly, but this did not help. Taking the advice of Charlie and Lien, I decided to cut carbs completely to see if I could get results. Unfortunately, the results were not good! I felt simply awful—always hungry, tired, and weak, particularly after exerting myself. My conclusion was that I was a person that simply had to have carbs.

I consulted with Charlie and Lien, who asked their doctor for advice on my behalf, and was told that the transition to a no-carb diet could take up to six weeks. As it had already been four weeks, I decided to tough it out for two more. However, after six weeks, I was still craving carbs and feeling awful. The doctor's response was to hang tough, it will happen. Grumpy and hungry, I decided to persist. I managed to make it to the eight-week mark, and although I still felt hungry most of the time, I had lost some weight. This gave me enough of a reward to continue.

Finally, after several months, my cells had figured it out! My cravings for sugar and starchy foods like bread and pasta are now a thing of the past. I am no longer hungry all the time. My weight has stabilized at a point that satisfies me and, best of all, I finally feel terrific—full of energy and happy to be slimmer. I no longer like the taste of excess sugar and find that a little goes a long way.

- Kate Goddard

Glucose Declines, but Not Enough

Here, fasting glucose drops, but sticks at a high number. For most people glucose will drop below 90 mg/dl. This includes adult onset diabetics. (If you were diabetic, and got to that level, or even below 110, consider yourself cured.) For people with quite high glucose who cut out starch and sugar, the number will fall quite rapidly. Somewhere between 90 and 120, the fall might slow down or stop altogether. The first line of attack in this case should be to cut the carbs further. You can safely cut them down to zero if you want, but more practically, shoot for below 50 grams per day. Also, it may take a few months. However, after six months, if your fasting glucose is still above 90, take a look at your A1C, which is an indication of your overall glucose. If it is 5.2 or less, you have probably done all you can. A fasting glucose of 110 and an A1C of 5.2 are not all that bad. If you maintain it, your risk of degenerative disease will be fairly low, but don't let up. And, as a rule, with A1C in the ideal range, the fasting glucose will eventually fall as well.

Less Weight Loss Than Desired

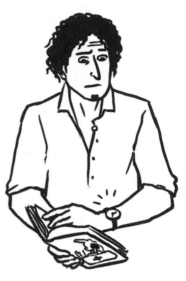

There was some initial weight loss, but not as much as desired. Fat, like so much else, is regulated by the hypothalamus. The hypothalamus will burn it until you reach its idea of your ideal weight. Its idea may not jive with your own, but it is trying to put you at the optimum weight for health purposes. Recall that the healthiest weight range is normal through overweight, and that if your insulin is not too high, your body will regulate your weight to its healthiest value. It may not be in your best interest to make heroic attempts to lose more weight.

Cutting or Quitting Alcohol Causes Carb Craving

Such a craving can result in surreptitious compensatory overeating. Possibly some things are being eaten that weren't in the past. Chips, pretzels?

Exercise Aches and Pains

In perhaps a majority of cases, the advice to go slowly and strengthen ligaments and tendons is ignored at first. However, it is a lesson quickly learned. If exercise is causing increased back and shoulder pain, the cause is usually excess enthusiasm, meaning failure to implement the training sequence.

Start over. First get all the joints working full range, and then gradually increase the load. If you tore or pulled some tendons or ligaments, go easy. They will take time to heal. You should work them lightly, and it's OK if they hurt a bit the next day, but that additional pain should be gone two days later.

Add weight slowly. Strengthen the ligaments, tendons, and bones first. Then the heart and lungs, and finally, the muscles. Muscle adapts easily, and insufficient attention to tendons and ligaments will result in injuries.

In a Nutshell

- Measure your 16 or so key numbers.
- See which ones should be improved.
- Figure out which lifestyle changes should improve them.
- Make the changes and measure again.

Some people are already in ideal ranges. Obviously as long as this persists, nothing needs to change. This comprises around 10% of the general population and around 90% of the hunter-gatherers. For many people, there will be a single problem group, perhaps sugar management, lipid management, or osteoporosis. This permits a focus, which, for most people, seems to speed up the change.

If many things are wrong, all of the lifestyle modifications may have to be rigorously followed. Adult onset diabetes tends to push everything out of ideal homeostasis, but the improvements will be equally broad and dramatic.

If discipline and perseverance are present, Quantitative Medicine seldom fails. It is a complete health management system.

Key Points

12 - Waiting for the Results

- Response to lifestyle change varies considerably.
- Sugar numbers should move significantly in three months.
- Lipid numbers take three to six months.
- Stress numbers can improve almost immediately.
- Adult onset diabetes can take up to a year.
- There are numerous special cases.

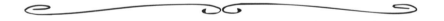

PART III - THE SCIENCE OF QUANTITATIVE MEDICINE

WHO ARE WE? HOW DID WE GET HERE? WHY AREN'T WE WELL?

13 - INNER SPACE

Quantitative Medicine's basic principle is simple enough in concept. Measure someone's health, i.e. quantify it. Then make necessary changes to correct those measurements—to move them to the ideal zones. Measure again to monitor the progress and check for any needed mid-course corrections. The measurements define your health. If they are optimum, your health will be too. If you improve them, your health improves. They are locked together.

What to measure and its interpretation were the topics of PART-II, but little justification for all those measurements and adjustments was given. We will undertake to remedy this now in PART III. We weren't deliberately withholding information in PART II. It was mainly an issue of complexity. We need to delve into the working of the body at the cellular level and address how all those pieces interrelate if we want to have a deeper understanding of why we get sick and specifically why we get degenerative disease and finally, how to counter it.

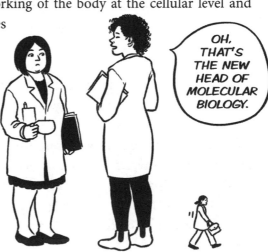

OH, THAT'S THE NEW HEAD OF MOLECULAR BIOLOGY.

For those who want that explanation, here is PART III. Here we delve into molecular biology and our own evolutionary past and try to see how it all came to be, why are we what we are, and why we respond the way we do. If you are only interested in measuring and making the changes that will arrest and reverse degenerative disease, PART II is all the information you will need.

For those wishing to move forward, we have a lot of underlying science to cover. It is tiny science indeed. We generate energy from sugar and fat by manipulating individual electrons and protons. It doesn't get much tinier than that.

To explore the body's mysterious and complicated workings, we could take the medical school approach and start enumerating all the parts, bones, muscles, and so on, but this is a fair amount of drudgery and doesn't really get us much closer to the all-important why?

In fact, to explain how Quantitative Medicine works, it is far better (not to mention more fun) to "evolve" a human from scratch. We will start with primordial soup and finish with a working human being, complete with brains, picking up the various parts as they become available.

The only problem with this approach is that rather than following a nice well-marked road, it will be more like crossing the murky waters of Lake Unknown.

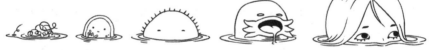

Lake Unknown is vast, and we will be hopping from stepping-stone to stepping-stone. Sometimes we will have to hop pretty far. There's just a lot that is not known: a lot of missing links, and places where evolution seems to have simply jumped way ahead. Still, it's what we've got.

So we will start from the very beginning. Once we get our human evolved, we can specifically examine why he gets sick, and see what actually transpires to cause good, healthy cells to go astray, for all degenerative disease starts and stops at the cellular level.

Finally, we explain why the cure works: how relieving cellular stress allows the well-evolved repair mechanisms to clean up and renew.

With our Quantitative Medicine toolkit, we will be able to precisely measure health, particularly cellular health.

So let's get ready for the first hop. It's a really big one…

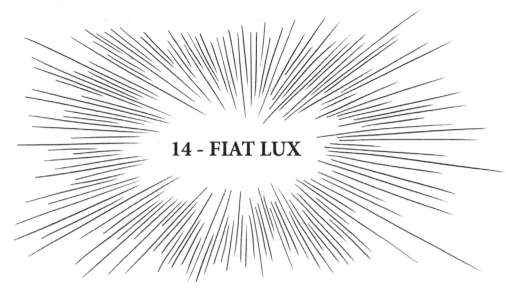

14 - FIAT LUX

Let there be light. Thirteen billion years ago there was nothing, and then in an instant, an entire universe, or at least its beginnings. The Big Bang was a colossal blaze of pure energy. And nobody really knows how or why it happened. It just did. But "it" happened in such a way that there could be matter, atoms, elements, and the like. We take the existence of atoms for granted, but they too are mysterious. Why are electrons so much smaller than protons? Why are atoms attracted to each other? Why is there gravity? There are dozens of other such fundamentals about which we are entirely clueless.

The Big Bang itself produced huge clouds of hydrogen and little else. These clouds coalesced into the original stars. No planets yet. No elements either, aside from hydrogen and some helium. These two gases clumped together, developed enough internal pressure to ignite, and become stars of varying sizes. Stars of all sizes are still forming. Some others are dying, and a few have blown up.

The larger the star, the shorter its life, with the largest of them lasting only a million or so years. Above a certain size, a star will finish its existence in a colossal explosion called a supernova. This grand finale has a marvelous side effect: it produces, via fusion, all of the heavier elements. Aside from hydrogen and helium, the material for the entire rest of the universe was manufactured this way. This includes our own personal collection as well as everything around us. This is still going on. Smaller stars, like our own, don't explode. They just slowly fuse into a couple of additional elements. The larger ones collapse into black holes. Our own star, the sun, is of fairly modest size and isn't quite large enough to end up as a black hole. It will die, leaving a large lump of coal, its remaining atmosphere drifting away as a nebula-like cloud. We have about five billion years to worry about this. Good thing.

But we are getting ahead of ourselves. Let's zoom in to around nine billion years after the Big Bang—four billion years ago. A lot of the initial fanfare has subsided, and thanks to the supernovae, we have all the heavier elements we are going to need. We wouldn't have evolved very far with hot gas alone, except perhaps as politicians. Our own corner of the universe had been fairly quiet for all those billions of years, but finally, just enough gas and rubble had accumulated for things to start to happen.

OUR LOCAL LUX

Five billion years ago, our solar system wasn't quite solar yet, still just a rotating disk of gases and debris from various supernovae. Gravity managed to gather enough hydrogen together in the center of this disk to ignite, and the sun was born. A new baby sun, less energy than now, but still plenty. Most of the remaining rubble and gases formed the planets; other bits and pieces became comets and asteroids, strewn about here and there.

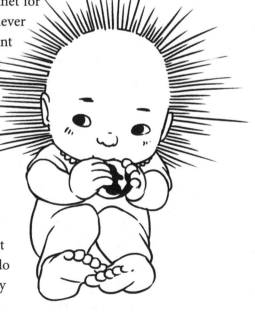

Earth muddled along as a new planet for around 200 million years, but we will never know what went on because an errant planet the size of Mars slammed into it and basically blew it up. Some of the original Earth was permanently lost to space, some coalesced to form the moon, and the rest settled back to form what could be called Earth-II. And away we go. Days were shorter then, and a lot hotter. Was there water? Probably not much after that collision, but some was evidently acquired. How do we conjure up life on this hot, steamy barren rock?

We're going to cheat a bit and peek at the answer. We find that all life as we know it is built mainly from a couple of dozen amino acids. A good next step would be to acquire a supply of these. Amino acids are fairly simple molecules, primarily concocted from a small set of atoms, mostly the Big Four—oxygen, hydrogen, carbon, and nitrogen—but sometimes sprinkled with sulfur or selenium. Thanks to all the supernovae, these elements are plentiful. Time to put them together. But how? There's no living thing available yet to do the assembly.

Could there be a way to get the amino acids from natural processes? Researchers Stanley Miller and Harold Urey took a shot at this in the 1950s. They created a contraption that would plausibly simulate conditions on early Earth: a lot of heat, clouds, a watery soup loaded with the six necessary elements, and finally, a key ingredient—lightning. Success! They got the whole kit. Out of this hellish brew, all the amino acids needed for living things were formed.

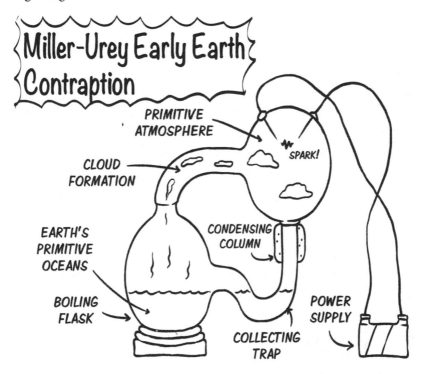

That's progress, but it's one thing to have the construction materials, and quite another to put them together. On to the next step.

RNA WORLD

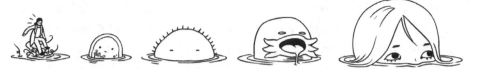

We just leapt to the next stepping-stone on our journey across Lake Unknown, and landed in RNA World. We really don't have any solid evidence that there ever was such a thing. All creatures now have both RNA *and* DNA, and even the simplest creatures are very complicated, but let's explore this lost world anyway.

RNA is a string of nucleotides. There are five types of these. They aren't all that complex, consisting of just a couple of dozen atoms. They are called adenine, guanine, cytosine, uracil, and thymine. We will use their official initials: A, G, C, U, and T.

RNA uses A, G, C, and U. For DNA, T replaces U. None of these five are all that complicated, and they can also be created from scratch with a slightly modified Miller-Urey Early-Earth contraption. So now we have a supply of material for both RNA and proteins. What next?

We will have to take another big leap. Somehow, these nucleotides got strung into something useful; something that could even replicate. We would suppose that once this sort of thing had started, it would rapidly spread, so we could imagine a world of tiny, stringy RNA sea creatures. We "know" (because we cheated and looked ahead again) that bacteria and everything else are full of these strings of RNA, and we know they are the key to life. But where are they now, the ones that were creatures in and of themselves? They're all gone! Did the bacteria eat them all? We suppose so, but we simply don't know. Seems reasonable that there just had to be an RNA world. In fact, some scientists have cooked up some RNA that can make copies of other RNA, but not of itself (yet).

THE GADGETRY OF LIFE

If amino acids are the building blocks of life, then the RNA strings that assemble the blocks are surely life's gadgetry. In early RNA World, we've got assorted nucleotides, with some of them stuck together as strings.

How hard is that? They usually represent the strings using the official letters. RNA uses C, A, G, and U. (DNA swaps T for the U.) So CAGGAGUNNU would be an RNA string. However, they usually aren't simple strings; they loop around and stick to themselves, forming quite elaborate structures like this, which is one of the simpler ones found in cells . . .

The nucleotides form strings and start attaching across to their complement: C<=>G and A<=>U.

"SIMPLE" RNA

Or this . . .

"NOT SO SIMPLE" RNA

Incredibly complex, goes all the way back to bacteria.

This RNA has between ten and twenty thousand nucleotides and is a complete programmable protein factory.

. . .which is part of a ribosome, a very important gadget indeed. It looks like two large heaps of spaghetti, and you would rightfully wonder how you could get something useful out of such a tangled mess. For this step, we are going to have to take another big leap across Lake Unknown to another stepping-stone.

Ribosomes

A ribosome is a huge wad of RNA strings and is a biological contraption without peer. It is a programmable digital protein factory—literally. Proteins are the building blocks of life and are strings of amino acids. If you have a ribosome and want a certain protein, you simply tell it the sequence of amino acids you want, and it will make up the protein. You can get anything you want, as long as it is cooked up with some combination of the 21 amino acids. In this sense, it is a general-purpose protein-making machine. Instead of needing thousands of different RNA gadgets—one for each necessary protein—we have just this one universal programmable version. Ribosomes are one of the most astounding things in all of molecular biology. Whoever would have thought that we are cooked up out of a myriad of tiny, digitally controlled protein factories?

How do you "program" a ribosome? This is the most amazing thing ever.

Those of you over 50 may remember when computers used punched tape. The tape had various patterns of holes in it, and the computer would read it and do something useful. This is exactly how a ribosome works. The "punched tape" is a strip of RNA.

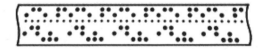

Remember the nucleotide letters A, G, U, and C that make up RNA strings? The ribosome reads the RNA "tape" three letters at a time, and from that, makes one amino acid. Each little group of three letters is called a codon. For instance, if you wanted to make a protein consisting of one molecule of the amino acid serine, then two of proline, then one leucine, you would need to feed a four-codon RNA "tape" into the ribosome machine. Each codon consists of three nucleotides, and so the tape for our protein would be represented AGU-CCC-CCC-CUC, where AGU is the codon that specifies the amino acid serine, CCC is the codon for sroline, and so on. This is no abstraction. It literally works this way. An RNA "tape" with the protein sequence is fed into the ribosome, which then "reads" it three letters (one codon) at a time and assembles the correct amino acid, tacking it on to the growing amino acid string.

So how cool is that? We now have RNA synthesizing the stuff of life, and it is using other RNA to tell it what to synthesize, and the whole process is digital! (As you've no doubt guessed, we have these ribosomes, and have them by the truckload. But we are getting ahead of ourselves.)

Now to go from four nucleotides gotten from our Early-Earth contraption to the amazing ribosome, a complete programmable protein factory, is, you will surely agree, quite a big leap. Do we have anything in between? The smoking gun would be an RNA "something" that could reproduce itself. Some viruses are pure RNA, and all viruses can replicate, but they cheat: they hijack cellular replication machinery to pull it off, so that doesn't count. Some scientists have cooked up an RNA gadget that can produce some RNA, albeit shorter bits, so maybe this is part of the missing steps. What would RNA creatures eat? No clue here, of course. There wasn't much on the menu. There was sunlight, various sorts of minerals, and, of course, their fellow RNA creatures.

DNA

We are about ready to depart RNA World. Next stop will involve DNA, which always gets top billing, while RNA does all the work. That's life. DNA is just a filing cabinet. It has copies of all the RNA tapes we will ever need. For all practical purposes, DNA is made from matched pairs of RNA strands. Cells can easily convert DNA to RNA and vice versa. With the DNA filing cabinet, we are all set to make something. DNA has the blueprint. If we want to make toenails, for instance, the formula is in the DNA somewhere. The RNA tape for toenail-making is obtained by copying the right stretch of the DNA, then off to the ribosome, and presto, out comes the toenail.

We have some tools in our evolutionary toolbox now. We know how to make proteins. Just get RNA strips from the DNA and run it through a nearby ribosome. We'll now have to hop a few stones in our Lake Unknown, but let's see what else could be made.

THESE BUILDING BLOCKS ARE STILL IN USE

Live began—bacterial life anyway—around three billion years ago. The amino acids and nucleotides then available turned out to be versatile enough to construct every living thing that would ever evolve. This seems quite remarkable in and of itself. Beyond patience, nothing new was needed. However, as the complex living structures evolved, they became far more conservative: sequestering, preserving, and protecting their DNA.

Bacteria, on the other hand, are endlessly experimenting. Evolving consentingly. Snipping up and swapping DNA with one another with little regard to the consequences. Because of this, the bacteria are extremely adaptable, and manage to thrive in amazing extremes of conditions. But even with all this, it is the same list of amino acids and nucleotides. At this level, bacteria and all grander creatures, including ourselves, stand on common ground.

Given this "mandate" to cook everything from a couple of dozen amino acids and five nucleotides, it is tempting to speculate that it's literally universal. Elsewhere in the universe, the same atoms are available in similar proportions. We already know that. Given all the variety that has evolved here, how could there possibly not be similar and recognizable life elsewhere?

Key Points
14 - Fiat Lux
- Both amino acids and RNA/DNA nucleotides can form spontaneously in the primordial soup.
- RNA creatures must have evolved first, though none remain.
- RNA structures can become very complex. One, the ribosome, can make strings of amino acids from "digital" RNA "tapes."

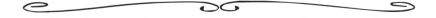

15 - BACTERIA WORLD

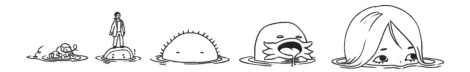

After about a billion years of primordial soup, a new living creature came about. Not a very intelligent one, but very resourceful, and very, very complicated. We would suppose there must have been predecessors that were simpler, but since we can't find them, we have to conclude they all got eaten.

Bacteria, and a very similar type of creature called archaea, constitute Bacteria World. These are called prokaryotes. Ourselves, all other multi-celled living things, animals, plants, fungi, or algae, as well as some single-celled creatures, are called eukaryotes. That's it. Every living thing, at least on this planet, is either a prokaryote or a eukaryote.

ADVANTAGES OF DNA

DNA stores information. It never does any work. In principle, RNA could store the same information, and we are guessing that it once did. So why bother with the additional complication of DNA? There are two strong reasons.

DNA is a double strand of complementary RNA-like strips. Complementary means that where one strand has a T, the other has an A, where one has a C, the other has a G, and vice versa. Our double strand then looks like:

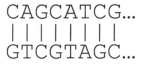

CAGCATCG...
| | | | | | | |
GTCGTAGC...

If one strand is damaged, it can be repaired by matching it up to the complementary strand.

This system works amazingly well. DNA is preserved through generation after generation. Species separated by tens of thousands of years have DNA matching well enough to have fertile offspring. The poster boys for this are the camel and the llama. These two animals can produce fertile offspring even though they have been evolving separately for four million years.

The other DNA advantage has to do with sexual selection, but that will have to wait, as sex hasn't been invented yet.

WELCOME TO BACTERIA WORLD

Alien visitors from another planet would be advanced beyond anything imaginable. Before visiting us, they would do a Life Form Scan to see what was about down here. They wouldn't want to catch anything. The report, which we had translated into English, looks like this.

LIFE FORMS: Planet dominated by microscopic living beings. Found everywhere and extremely numerous. Microscopic beings have constructed numerous larger life forms which they inhabit. Microscopic beings' combined weight exceeds that of all other life forms. Microscopic beings can metabolize a wide variety of material and may be able to metabolize us. Avoidance recommended.

By three billion BC, bacteria had covered the earth. They had gobbled up RNA World and were busily devouring just about everything else. One category ate rocks, another petroleum. What would we be like if we had evolved from them? Many metabolized methane or CO_2. Earth didn't start out with any oxygen; CO_2-breathing bacteria produced oxygen as a waste product. And, as the report states, the bacteria outweigh everything else and outnumber we eukaryotes by around 10 trillion to 1. We host more bacteria than we have cells of our own. Though much tinier, their combined weight is three pounds. They can and do live almost anywhere and on almost anything, including, of course, us.

We don't want to dwell on bacteria. We just want to see which pieces of them we can use, and then we'll move on to multi-celled creatures.

Bacteria are the most primitive creatures now living. We'll credit them with several innovations that are still with us today:

- DNA. Bacteria have DNA. It's arranged in a loop rather than a strand, but it's otherwise the same DNA.
- Energy. Bacteria run on ATP molecules, the universal life energy currency.
- Metabolism. Bacteria can create ATP from sugar using two different methods, and can also make ATP from protein and fat.
- Bacteria use RNA to do all the work. RNA tapes are generated by reading sections of the bacteria's DNA. RNA-based ribosomes generate needed proteins from amino acids.

We will use all of these to evolve our human. Let's take a closer look at these newly acquired features. (We already know about DNA and RNA.)

Every living thing uses a molecule called ATP for energy. It powers our muscles, our brain, everything. The organism may be metabolizing sugar, fat, methane, or rocks, but ATP is the result. All the numerous processes going on in a cell use ATP as their energy source. ATP looks like this.

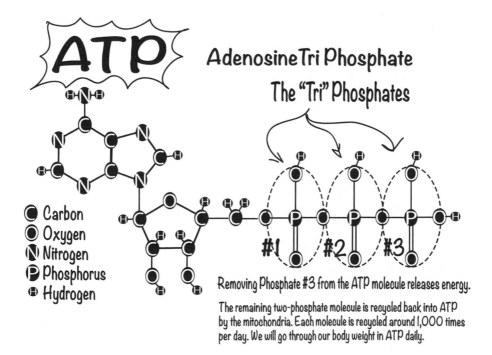

ATP — Adenosine Tri Phosphate
The "Tri" Phosphates

- Carbon
- Oxygen
- Nitrogen
- Phosphorus
- Hydrogen

#1 #2 #3

Removing Phosphate #3 from the ATP molecule releases energy.

The remaining two-phosphate molecule is recycled back into ATP by the mitochondria. Each molecule is recycled around 1,000 times per day. We will go through our body weight in ATP daily.

We have two methods to produce ATP: a quick inefficient one, and a slow very efficient one. Using the quick method, one glucose molecule can produce two ATPs by fermentation. When using this method, muscles will feel like they are burning. The slow, efficient method uses yet another elaborate contraption called the "Krebs cycle-electron transport chain-proton motor." This can produce 38 ATP from a single glucose molecule. That's 19 times better, a very nice improvement, but immensely more complicated—yet invented by bacteria.

We eukaryotes can't pick up everything we need from a bacteria. Here are some key differences that will have to evolve later:

- Our DNA is in strings, not loops.
- We keep our DNA in an inner nucleus for protection. Intermingling with stray DNA is not permitted.
- We have sex. Each parent contributes half of their DNA.
- Our outer membrane is single layer, not double layer.
- Our cells have various organelles, which perform a variety of functions, bacteria don't have these.

HOW TO MAKE ATP

Since we need it ourselves, let's see how the bacteria generate ATP.

The Easy Way—Fermentation

The first method, fermentation, is simple, and evolved first. You will agree with this after you see what the second method entails. Anyone that ever tried to home-brew beer or make wine knows that the fermenting mash or crush is warm. Same chemical reaction.

$$C_6H_{12}O_6 + 2\ NAD^+ + 2\ ADP + 2\ Pi \longrightarrow$$
$$2\ CH_3COCOO- + 2\ NADH + 2\ ATP + 2\ H_2O + 2H^+$$

The $C_6H_{12}O_6$ is sugar. That plus a couple of other items produce the CH_3COCOO and two ATPs. Not much ATP, but importantly, no O_2 was needed, so this is a handy reaction to have at your disposal if you have no oxygen available. This is the case for us after a burst of activity. Early Earth had no oxygen in the atmosphere, so this would have been the only choice.

For beer and wine makers, the CH_3COCOO, otherwise known as pyruvic acid, goes on to become alcohol. In us, in the absence of oxygen, it goes on to become lactic acid, the exercise "burn."

The Hard Way—Krebs Cycle+Electron Transport+Proton Motor

For those bacteria not satisfied with the easy fermentation method, evolution cooked up a procedure 19 times more efficient and about 500 times more complicated. And guess what: it involves an electric motor— really! A lot of bacteria have taken this up, even though it is very complicated. It involves a multi-step process that ends up pumping a bunch of individual protons across the inner cell membrane. Bacteria have an outer, fairly porous membrane, but their inner one is quite tight.

The protons that are pumped into the space between the two membrane walls have, as do all good protons, a positive charge. Here is our electricity. Because of this charge, they are drawn back to the inner parts of the cell, but to slip back in, they have to pass through yet another cellular gadget that is stuck in that inner cell membrane. The gadget's name—ATP synthase—rather gives away its function. When the proton slips past it on its way back to the inner part of the cell, it forces it to spin. Yes, spin! It's the only wheel-like thing in all of life. It's a tiny motor driven by a waterfall of electrically charged protons returning to the inner part of the cell. That ATP synthase is not just loping along at one or two spins a second, either; this thing is turbocharged. The ones in your heart spin at around 3,000 rpm. That's about how fast a car engine is spinning at 70 mph.

But shovel in more protons, and the motors will spin on up to over 20,000 rpm. The car engine would self-destruct at less than half this. And, unlike car engines, the proton motor is almost 100% efficient, with no polluting byproducts at all. Just imagine, what's powering us 24/7 is several hundred trillion little proton motors, all humming along at several thousand rpm. Incredible. Feel the whirr? This spinning motor can be used for other things. The bacteria flagellum, a little tail used for propulsion, spins like a propeller. It is connected directly to a proton motor.

The motor itself, ATP synthase, is one of those massively elaborate molecules like the ribosomes talked about earlier. How ATP synthase evolved? No clue.

We're not done. There is a fair amount more to this ATP generation. To get the motor to run, we need to pump protons to the outside of the inner cellular membrane. This is done by a sequence of chemical reactions called the electron transport chain. Each "link" in the sequence runs on the stuff resulting from the previous link-reaction, and at each step, a few protons are shoved out of the inner cell. To drive the electron transport chain, we need to feed the first of the four reactions with NADH, yet another molecule.

A different group of reactions generates the NADH. This group is arranged in a cycle, called the Citric Acid Cycle or the Krebs Cycle. Like the electron transport chain, each step uses the results of the previous step. At one point of the cycle, additional fuel is added in the form of another molecule, Acetyl-COA.

This sequence, Acetyl-CoA->NADH, NADH->proton pumping, and protons flowing through the proton motor is very, very complex, and is the same for every life form that uses this elaborate sort of energy generation. Acetyl-CoA is a "universal fuel." The glucose, fat, or whatever you ate is converted to Acetyl-CoA and fed into the Krebs Cycle-Electron Transport Chain-Proton Motor energy generation system.

Whew—that's a complicated one. If you step back from it, it's quite unimaginable how all these pieces could possibly have evolved from mutations and DNA sharing and so on. We did have to take a really grand leap across Lake Unknown to get to this stepping-stone, but the gifts the bacteria have given us, the digital protein factory and the super-efficient energy generator, take us a huge step ahead.

We are rather versatile in that we can create Acetyl-CoA from carbohydrate, protein, or fat. Plants take it a step further, and can generate it from sunshine and CO_2, but before we move along, look at the list of things that various bacteria can "eat."

- Sugar, fat, and protein
- CO_2 and sunshine
- Iron
- Nitrogen compounds
- Sulfur compounds
- Methane
- Petroleum compounds
- Pesticides
- Ammonia
- Rocks

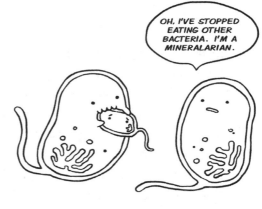

There's even one that eats uranium. Yum! Whatever it is, somewhere, somehow, some bacteria have probably figured out a way to eat it. Of course, the most readily available food supply would be other bacteria.

RECEPTORS AND TRANSPORTERS

Bacteria have to interact with the world around them, and lack eyes, noses, and mouths. Instead, they have receptors and transporters, and, as you would expect in Bacteria World, there are a huge variety of these, each specialized to a specific chemical or nutrient. Cells from all living things follow this same scheme, so we will need these pieces as well.

Receptors

We imagine bacteria as smooth little beings of indeterminate shape, some equipped with a rotating flagellum. In fact, they are more like punk-rockers, studded with hundreds of different receptors and transporters, all sticking through the cell membrane. The outside parts of the receptors sense chemicals in the external environment. It could be a nutrient, some necessary biochemical, or, for an invading bacteria, some bits of us.

The receptors are very specific, sensing an exact match with a certain chemical. They actually match up their molecules to the external chemical and latch on to it. The matching gives the cell the ability to be quite accurate in its selection, rather like a specific key fitting a specific lock. The external "keys" are called "ligands." There are thousands of different ones. Once the key is in the lock, the inside part of the receptor will launch some specific cellular activity.

Examples in our own cells would be insulin receptors, which tell the cell to grab some circulating sugar to eat, or the IGF-1 receptors, which tell the cell to launch any needed repairs.

The individual cells, whether bacterial or human, have considerable control over their receptors and transporters. They can be "turned off" or even removed. A human cell that has no need of repair, for instance, will turn off (will not "express") its IGF-1 receptor. The cell can simply remove the receptor, or can leave it in place for future use, but block its interior action.

Some receptors are slow, operating via chemical pathways. Others are fast, operating by more electrical ones.

Transportation through the cell membrane carries the process one step further. A transporter is a receptor combined with a means to pull the biochemical across the cell membrane. This could be inbound, as in the case of nutrients, or outbound, for waste disposal or transmission of chemical messages. Transporters come in several flavors as well. Some molecules can get in and out of cells without any specific mechanism.

A cell needs a variety of molecules, some very small, O_2 for instance, and some quite large. All cells, bacterial or eukaryotic, have an outer membrane made of fat. The membrane is porous, and some molecules get in through these pores. This is called diffusion, and is the easy way, requiring no precious cellular energy—always desirable. For diffusion to work, three criteria have to be met. First, the molecule obviously has to be small enough to get through the pores of the cell membrane. As it is oozing through, it runs into the fatty cellular membrane material. To get past that, it has to be soluble in fat. Oxygen and CO_2 are good examples of this. Finally, something has to be pushing it along. This means that the pressure behind it must be greater than the pressure it is facing. The pressure difference is called the gradient. Cells also have tiny channels which permit some molecules that are not soluble in fat, water for instance, to pass through.

We can exhale CO_2. The partial-pressure of CO_2 in our lung cells is around 12%, whereas the partial-pressure in our atmosphere is extremely small, around 0.04%. Thus our waste CO_2 can easily diffuse out. However, if the external concentration rises to a similar number, we can no longer get rid of the CO_2 by diffusion, and are in mortal danger. Although diffusion is a means of transport, it's not really a "transporter" in any active sense. When water is diffusing, the process is called osmosis.

Transporters

It's fine that water, oxygen, and CO_2 can get in and out of a cell, but what about molecules too large to fit through the pores, or molecules that won't mix with fat? Here we have to resort to some sort of gadget stuck through the cell membrane. This is our "transporter," and like the receptors, it is specialized to attach to specific molecules. It offers a tunnel through the fat of the cell membrane, so that problem is solved. Within reason, it can be whatever size it needs to be in order to move its special molecule through, so the size problem is out of the way as well.

This leaves the gradient. Is the molecule going with the gradient (from high pressure to low pressure) or against it? If the molecule is going with the gradient, then the transporter only has to open a "gate" and let it through. No energy used for this case either, or at least not much. If the molecule has to go against the gradient, uphill as it were, the transporter has to physically move the molecule through. This will need energy.

Transporters that open and shut a gate are called passive, and those that push the molecule up a gradient hill are called active.

The transporters that take the glucose (sugar) from the blood into the cell are a good example of the passive sort. The most important one actually has two gates, acting like a double door. The outer one opens and lets a glucose molecule into the middle of the transporter. Then it closes, and the inner one opens, releasing the glucose into the cell interior. The reason for this additional complexity is probably so that the cell can regulate how much glucose it lets in.

An example of an active transporter would be the process of getting the glucose into the bloodstream in the first place. These sorts of transporters are found in the intestines and liver, where they have to shove dietary glucose "uphill" into the blood.

Using transporters and receptors, cells can communicate with one another, and do. Even bacteria do this. Biochemicals excreted from neighboring bacteria allow a communication of sorts, with resultant group behavior. Flurries of messages like "Reproduce, there's a bunch of food available," or "Flee, there's penicillin about," would produce the expected group behavior. This could lead to some interesting sorts of specialization, where some members of the bacterial colony find the food, some watch for dangers, and other members do the reproduction. This actually does happen, but it's not on our evolutionary path, so we'll move on.

UNEXPECTED USES OF MEDICAL TECHNOLOGY SIDEBAR
Your Personal Bacteria Collection

One potentially cancerous element in the environment is our personal biome. Did you even know you had one? Or if you did, were you aware that it is different from everyone else's? Your personal biome is the collection of microbes that inhabit your skin, lungs, and digestive tract. We are not talking about a few dozen or so germs. You are awash in these creatures. Your personal bacteria collection outnumbers your own cells 10 to 1. They are tiny, of course, and collectively weigh only about three pounds. (You are bacteria free—sterile—on your insides, where bacteria can't directly reach.)

For the most part, our personal biome is harmless or even helpful, but this is not always the case. Many possible residential bacteria can be cancerous in and of themselves, or increase susceptibility. The most notorious of this lot is H. pylori, responsible for stomach cancer and widespread in China.

Can you do anything about your own biome? You can certainly mess it up. A course of antibiotics is a weapon of mass destruction. Likewise, antibacterial hand soap or antibiotic-laden meat (most factory meat) will destroy large portions of your biome. However, if you do not smoke and eat a sensible diet, your biome will likely be a beneficial one

A person's biome is so individualized that it is already being used forensically. A careful criminal may not leave any fingerprints at the scene of a crime, but unless he commits the act in a hazmat suit, he will leave his biome behind. Further, he will have picked up the biomes of people he recently visited, as well as any potential victims, thus leaving both a trail of his past movements and marking his getaway path.

Apparently a one-night stay in a hotel room is enough to thoroughly populate it with your personal biome. This lingers until the next guest, so the scent, as it were, remains hot for a while.

Supposedly the deflated football scandal of the 2015 pro football playoffs has been solved using forensic biome methods.

Of course, "biomic" evidence isn't used in court—yet.

BACTERIAL METABOLISM AND DEFENSE

One would imagine bacteria happily floating about, dividing, evolving, and so on, but this is the wrong picture. The world ethic was (and largely still is) eat or be eaten. Since bacteria are constantly and rapidly evolving, both what they could eat and how they could avoid being eaten were constantly improving. Bacteria don't really have anything like an immune system, but they are far from helpless, possessing a wealth of defensive techniques. They can change form, hide their identity, cluster, become toxic, and so on.

One item of interest in the bacterial arsenal is their means of defense against viruses. (Bacteria even have to worry about that!) Bacteria are able to manufacture certain enzymes that can destroy these invaders. This is the start of the immune system arms race. As we evolve along, the immune system will evolve too, picking up bits and pieces here and there, becoming more and more complex.

One bacterial defense mechanism of great importance is mutation. Bacteria are quite promiscuous with their DNA, which is not sequestered in a nucleus. Bits are constantly getting added and deleted, and each change is a variant bacteria. If conditions change, this sort of random DNA shuffling can produce more "fit" bacteria very rapidly. We eukaryotes, by contrast, are very slow. Our DNA is tightly and precisely preserved.

OUR BACTERIAL HERITAGE

Once we take a microscopic peek at the interior of our own cells, it is astonishing how much resembles the bacteria and archaea that it emerged from. To begin with, our entire system, with DNA as the blueprint and RNA as the workforce, originated in bacteria. The chemistry here is identical. Same molecules. Furthermore, two of the most complex molecules known, the RNA ribosome and the ATP synthase enzyme, were invented and perfected by bacteria. These are completely essential to life as we know it.

A host of other cellular machinery also came from bacteria. One excellent example is receptors and transporters. These are found throughout the body and perform the same functions as in bacteria.

Bacteria are also credited with the amino acid construction method, common to all living things.

Our diet mimics that of the bacteria, or at least some of them. We metabolize fat, sugars, and proteins. These capabilities were also developed in bacteria.

We have even retained the anti-virus defense that bacteria managed to evolve: virus-destroying enzymes known as defensins.

Perhaps we should have a Bacteria Appreciation Day. Or perhaps thats a bad idea. They have also caused us a host of problems.

One major difference from the bacterial way of life is the sanctity of the DNA. Bacteria will swap DNA randomly, add bits, remove bits, constantly changing. Multi-celled creatures (and some more complex single-celled ones) sequester it in a cell nucleus, continually protecting, repairing, and preserving it.

We now have what we need from Bacteria World, so it's time to move on. We have quite a way to go, and a few more leaps across the stepping-stones of murky Lake Unknown, but the leaps are perhaps getting a bit more manageable. At this point, we know how DNA works, how body parts are built, how cells generate energy, and how they interact with their outside world. We are halfway there.

Key Points
15 - Bacteria World
- Bacteria have DNA.
- DNA is redundant and therefore less susceptible to damage.
- Bacteria are everywhere, vastly outnumbering all other life forms, and equaling them in weight.
- Some bacteria can convert oxygen and other materials into energy with very high efficiency.
- The Krebs cycle was a bacterial invention.
- ATP is the universal energy molecule, used in all of life.

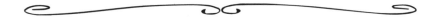

16 - THE GRAND MITOCHONDRIAL DEAL

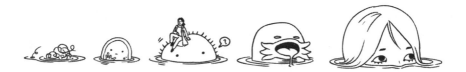

Life is currently divided into three domains: Bacteria, Archaea, and Eukaryota. This is a relatively recent development. Bacteria and archaea were lumped together prior to around 2005.

BACTERIA AND ARCHAEA

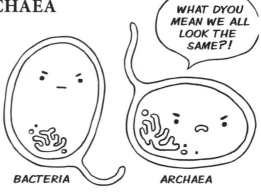

WHAT DYOU MEAN WE ALL LOOK THE SAME?!

BACTERIA   ARCHAEA

Bacteria and archaea look the same: microscopic single-celled creatures with circular DNA and so on. Apparently there is a significant genetic difference. Their ribosomes work somewhat differently, the cell membrane is different. This may not seem like a huge deal, but it apparently is to those who worry about such things. For us, it does have impact: we appear to be a hybrid of the two.

THE BIGGEST LUNCH DEAL EVER

Little decisions can have major consequences. Around a couple of billion years ago, an archaea, out for a leisurely swim, decided to take a lunch break, and something along the lines of the following transpired . . .

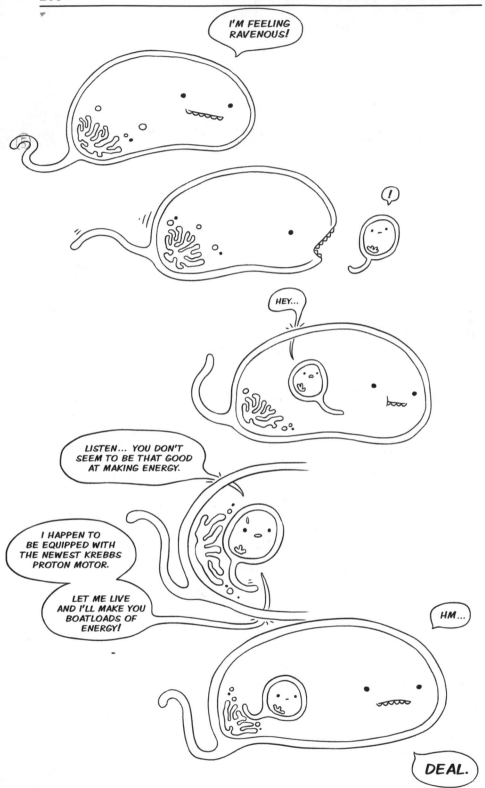

. . . they shook flagella on it, and thus was born the first eukaryote. The newly enslaved bacteria got renamed mitochondria.

The mitochondrial slaves made good on their side of the deal, dividing and dividing, and producing quite an excess of energy. The newly born eukaryote also divided, each time splitting the mitochondrial crew among the new progeny.

What a colossal deal. The eukaryotes grew and prospered, eventually becoming multi-cellular, with elaborate, multiple strands of DNA. The stalwart mitochondria remained true to their heritage, hanging on to their own separate DNA genome, duly maintaining it in its bacterial-like loop. It's still that way. All higher forms of life are "infested" with these mitochondria. They are not us, though we wouldn't get very far without them. Analysis of their genome suggests that all eukaryotes are descended from that one lunch deal. This includes us, plants, fungus, and the tiny world of one-celled protozoa. This could mean that it only happened once, and we are all descended from that single strange lunch bargain long ago. Or maybe not. Plants, in addition to mitochondria, also have chloroplasts, another enslaved bacteria.

However, the rarity of this symbiotic capture speaks volumes about the prospect of finding life elsewhere. This planet had been a bacterial (and archaeal) soup for 3.5 billion years, with uncountable encounters like that described above on a daily basis. Yet the "deal" only happened once. It must, therefore, be very unlikely indeed. So when we are finally visiting the faraway galaxies, we may well find an abundance of slime worlds, and little else.

But let's get back on track here. The lunch deal theory is but one of several, each with its strong and weak points, but however it came about, we now have a single-celled creature with other creatures inside, generating energy. With all this extra energy, what can be evolved? Even the simplest eukaryotes have these new features:

- Sex. Reproduction from parents is now possible.
- Nucleus. Eukaryote DNA is now protected in a nucleus. No more genetic hanky-panky, like those swinging bacteria.
- Other organelles. The excess energy supports other gadgetry within the cell: chloroplasts (plants), Golgi apparatus, and others.
- DNA is no longer a single, circular chromosome, but is pairs of DNA strands.

- The cell membrane is now single rather than double. The mitochondria, however, stay true to their bacterial heritage and retain the double-membrane structure.
- As cells get bigger, the need for intracellular communication and management grows greater.

SEX AND DNA

Bacteria have one DNA based chromosome, configured as a loop. We have 23 pairs, configured as strings. Other eukaryotes have different numbers of pairs: some ants have 2, some ferns, over 500. However, we all have pairs, bacteria don't. Even the simplest protozoa has pairs.

Pairs of DNA mean sex. One half came from each parent. So does this mean those single-celled protozoa have genders and their "special" moments? Sort of. For many of them, there is a distinct male and female. Some have combined that into the same animal. Some are genderless, becoming male or female depending on the situation. For some species, there are more than two sexes, the maximum known being seven. (That's variety!)

There are also eukaryotic reproduction methods that don't involve sex, such as cloning. Some of the tinier eukaryotes reproduce by cell division when the environment is good, but turn to sexual reproduction when times get tough and some adaptation is needed. This makes sense. Sex is expensive. It takes two parents to make one creature, whereas bacteria, using division, can reproduce without a partner.

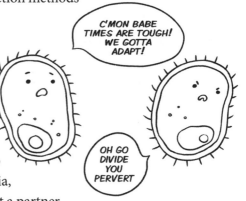

Given the tendency of most creatures to produce 10,000 progeny in hopes that one will survive, perhaps this cost is irrelevant.

Why sex? Cell division is complicated enough. Some quite elaborate cellular gadgetry has to duplicate the DNA loop, separate the two pieces (they are usually a tangled mess), and then pinch the cell into two pieces. Although quite a few old-fashioned eukaryotes still prefer this, it is the sexual method that really caught on. It's a lot more complicated. Step one, not at all trivial, each parent has to create a special cell with only half the genome in it, one from each pair of chromosomes. The sperm and egg are familiar examples of this. So now there are two half-cells, called gametes. Step two, these two have to get together somewhere, form a new complete single cell, build a nucleus around the DNA, and construct the rest of the cell from scratch.

It's even more complicated than that. When the parents are creating their eggs or sperm, rather than just picking one chromosome or the other from the available pairs, they further shuffle the chromosomes, obtaining something not exactly like dad or mom. This is a lot of additional trouble, but it must be important, because it happens from protozoa on up. This genetic card shuffling is called recombination.

This has its advantages and disadvantages. Given the large number of possibilities available by simply selecting one chromosome from each pair, you would wonder why further shuffling is necessary. Just selecting one of the chromosome pairs produces 8,288,806 models of sperm and eggs. Combining the two would get that squared. You would think this 13-digit number would be enough, but apparently not. The shuffling of individual pieces gives enormously more variety. We suppose this would maximize adaptability. However, if adaptability is all that desirable, it would seem a bit odd that the eukaryotic DNA would be sequestered away in a little fortress, safe from the licentious DNA swapping that goes on in Bacteria World.

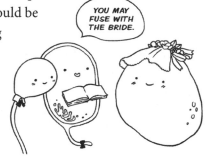

YOU MAY FUSE WITH THE BRIDE.

This brings us to the topic of natural selection. Almost all school texts talk about a random cell mutation, maybe from a cosmic ray, that conferred some survival benefit and so on. This is the hard way. First of all, that mutation has to occur in a gamete (sperm or egg), and second, that gamete has to reproduce. If you further consider that most random mutations aren't helpful at all, you can see that this is a very, very long shot. There weren't domestic foxes. So this means that in the several million years that they have been around, the right random mutation never occurred.

What they don't tell you in those schoolbooks is that almost all natural selection is sexual. Instead of waiting for that lucky gamma ray, just have a child. The shuffling or recombination can produce change, including beneficial change, in a hurry. How much of a hurry? Some Siberian researchers bred foxes, and for each generation picked the most placid ones for breeding the next. Within a few decades, they had perfectly human-friendly "dog-like" foxes. This obviously leaves random mutation in the dust, and largely, such sexual selection has done most of the heavy lifting, evolution-wise. (We suppose schoolbooks may tend to avoid certain topics altogether . . .)

NUCLEUS AND NON-LOOPING DNA

These are yet more eukaryotic features, and it's not clear why they are better. The bacteria are winning the survival race, both by weight and by numbers. However, we are certainly winning the complexity contest. So stringy nuclear DNA seems to be prerequisite, as all eukaryotes have it. How did these two features come about? We are again peering into Lake Unknown. The nucleus obviously offers some protection, and also provides a central location for anything needing an RNA "tape." We don't really know. Anyway, it works. The larger single-celled protozoa are visible— barely—and are 200 times longer than bacteria.

So how far along are we now? From bacteria we can metabolize various nutrients for energy and needed cell materials. From the leap to the eukaryotes, we pick up the mitochondria, stringy DNA in the nucleus, and, of course, sex.

We also don't know where the single cell membrane came from, since all the bacteria have a double one.

We are making progress, but once again, we are finding a big stretch of Lake Unknown lying ahead.

METABOLISM AND DEFENSE

Our newly minted protozoa had only a single possibility for food: bacteria. Not to be outdone, the bacteria decided to broaden their culinary horizons and add this new creature to their menu as well. That, of course, meant war. Both bacteria and our new single-celled eukaryotes were going to have to come up with yet another new bag of tricks to survive the threat of one another and thrive.

The protozoa had a substantial advantage. With all its new complexity and available energy, it could support a much more elaborate and complex defense system.

First of all, it retained the virus-attacking enzymes that were already evolved in the bacteria. It then came up with several new ones. It evolved little molecules, aptly named defensins, that could pull all sorts of nasty tricks on invading bacteria or viruses, such as snipping up their DNA or poking holes in them.

Nonetheless, the bacteria could mutate very fast, so no matter what the protozoa came up with, there was likely to be a bacteria somewhere that could outwit it, or rather out-mutate it. We'll move on now, but keep the very useful defensins.

SIZE

Because of the specialization and compartmentalization, eukaryotic cells have the potential to be much larger than bacteria, and larger they are indeed. A typical eukaryotic cell is perhaps 30 microns across. Someone with sharp vision can see 100 microns. Bacteria are around three microns across. So this is 10:1. Of course volume and weight would tend to go with the cube of this, so here the eukaryote has a 1,000:1 advantage. In fact, the several hundred mitochondria floating around in the typical eukaryote cell have remained bacterial size.

But why are bacteria so tiny? Actually, we have over-generalized here. There are big ones—big for bacteria, that is. There is one, an inhabitant of fish's gut, weighting in at 800 microns, which is large even by eukaryotic standards. Not to be outdone, there is a eukaryote, micromonas, that has managed to miniaturize itself down to two microns, making it a tad smaller than the typical bacteria. To reach this tiny size, micromonas has shed a fair amount of the eukaryotic kit. There seemed to be no need to go to all this trouble. Micromonas is a common ocean algae. Pretty spacious headquarters. But about the bacteria. Size is, of course, the result of survival of the fittest. Thus, their size is best because it is best, a wholly unsatisfactory answer. A better question is "Why are single-celled eukaryotes so much larger than (typical) bacteria?" We don't know that one either.

MITOCHONDRIA CHANGED EVERYTHING

Available, abundant energy enabled us to grow, become multi-celled, eventually become human. But it came at a price. The mitochondria still carry a lot of their bacterial heritage. They do not have the DNA protection or repair facilities present in the eukaryotic cell.

Slowing aging and retarding degenerative disease depend largely on mitochondrial health. Perhaps this is over half the story. To keep mitochondria healthy requires, interestingly, using them. The life span of a mitochondria is about three to four weeks. If they are worked, they run cleanly and replicate well. If they are not worked, they tend to stop right in the middle of their energy generation cycle, may die, and may take the host cell with them. This seems a little paradoxical, as most machinery we are familiar with lasts longer if used lightly. Exercise keeps mitochondria busy, and this may be its principal benefit.

Cellular health is also required for mitochondrial health. A cell that is contaminated with toxins, or perpetually overloaded with sugar will not be a very clean environment.

With a short life span, there is a lot of opportunity for reproduction errors to accumulate. This generally does not happen, and there are processes at work to select only the most pristine mitochondria for replication. How this is done is another unknown.

Key Points
16 - The Grand Mitochondrial Deal
- Eukaryotes formed as a symbiotic fusion of bacteria and archaea.
- All animal, plant, and fungal life forms are eukaryotes.
- There are single-celled eukaryotes: protozoa, for example.
- Eukaryotes have additional energy. Sex evolved, along with organ specialization and large size.

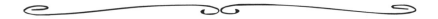

17 - SPECIALIZATION

Where are the two-celled creatures, or three, or four? There don't seem to be any. There are groups of single-celled creatures that work together. These are "colonies" and aren't the evolutionary direction we want to head. Even bacteria can (and do) act as a cooperative group.

One well-studied colony-like creature is volvox, a type of green slime. Such slime has some degree of specialization and may give some clues as to how the process works.

Blissfully, we are not descended from, or even closely related to, this green slime. However, this serves to illustrate that multi-cellularity isn't such a tough evolutionary road. There are at least eight different multi-celled creatures that pulled it off in different ways. What we don't know is how they did it. Obviously a multi-celled creature has to have specialization. Otherwise it's just a colony. We won't worry too much about how it developed. We would rather pry into a very knotty problem that arises yet again: reproduction.

MULTI-CELLULAR REPRODUCTION

So far we have single-celled eukaryotic creatures that reproduce sexually. When a pair of these produce a progeny, they have essentially produced another complete adult. It doesn't need to grow.

If the creature is multi-cellular, a huge complication sets in. When the multi-celled parents get their single-celled baby, not only does it need to grow, the various cells need to divide and need to know what to grow into. This is a tough one. Consider a human fertilized egg. First one cell, then two, then four cells, and so on. In a few weeks, some of these cells have become a heart, others are working on limbs, etc. How do the cells know what to become? This is a tremendous leap.

STEM CELLS

We do have a few clues. There is the idea of stem cells, and it's been in the news for the last several years as a possible source of replacement organs. Stem cells

BAH, THAT WHOLE MULTI-CELLED THING WILL NEVER TAKE OFF...

can, in various ways, grow into cells with specific functions. Once they have made this commitment, they are said to have "differentiated." But not all stem cells are created equal. What they can or can't do varies. The number of different sorts of cells they can differentiate into is called, amusingly, their "potency." Obviously that fertilized egg is top dog in the potency department. You can get an entire human being from that one cell. These cells are usually called "totipotent." (We suppose an "omnipotent" cell could become anything: a woman, a giraffe, a toad, a palm tree, etc.)

The other categories of stem cells are more specialized, and are of primary interest to us. These are the less potent "adult" stem cells. They can be ranked accordingly: pluripotent, multipotent, oligopotent, and finally, the least potent, unipotent, which can only generate itself. A cell that couldn't divide at all would be, we suppose, impotent.

Only totipotent and pluripotent are considered to be true "stem" cells, but the pecking order extends on downward. The pluripotent cells differentiate into multipotent cells, then oligopotent, producing just a few types. These lesser cells can still replicate, so they are sort of "junior stem cells." Their official name is "progenitor cells." The end-of-the-line cells cannot replicate or differentiate at all. Your skin, at least the part you can see, is in this state.

Stem cells can vary their rate of renewal. In normal times, they will regenerate new tissue at a regular rate, but if there is a need, healing of a wound for instance, they can move at a much faster pace.

All the body's tissues that are routinely replaced use the stem cell-progenitor cell hierarchy. This includes the liver, the skin, the stomach, the intestines, and many other items. For instance, the skin you can see is at the final step in the replacement chain. It can't replicate and is fully differentiated. New skin is getting created underneath by stem cells (actually the junior versions). The progenitor cells that are creating that new skin stay put, keeping as far as possible from harm's way, and replicating themselves as needed. It is good that they are well protected. If they get damaged, there is the possibility of producing damaged daughter cells. Most cancers have this sort of origin. Since the stem cells are well preserved, the replacement tissue is almost as good as new. But not quite—we do age.

As a stem or progenitor cell differentiates, forming one of the specific cells in its repertoire, it may go through stages, losing "potency" at each stage. Alternatively, a stem cell might divide, forming a copy of itself. Typically, these sorts of cells do both, building up a supply of identical stem or progenitor cells till the need arises, then differentiating into the required replacements.

This is a pretty clever repair system. Instead of trying to replace worn-out cells with copies (which would themselves be worn out too), just toss the worn-out cells and get the nearby stem cells to "differentiate" and make brand-new ones. Of course, we need to take some care to preserve the stem cells, since they are the source of all these new cells. Further, these stem cells can typically differentiate into several different types of cells. So for all the repairable tissues in the body, there tend to be special stem/progenitor cells that are sort of the master keys for all the other cells. One type of progenitor cell might make various sorts of skin cells, others make the intestinal cells, and so on.

You may have heard that the body totally replaces itself every seven years, or something like that. This is nonsense. Frequency of cell repair varies from fast—intestines replace every four days— to never—neurons and heart muscle cells, for instance. (Actually, "never" means "hardly ever." It turns out that recent research finds heart muscle cells replacing about once every 50 years, and there are instances of new neurons. So "never" sort of means "not on a regularly scheduled maintenance program.")

THE "PHONE" TYPE CELL HAS A TURNOVER RATE OF AROUND A YEAR, SITUATING IT BETWEEN THE BONES AND STOMACH.

Here is the standard replacement schedule:

Cell Type	Turnover Time
Small and Large Intestine	4 days
Skin	2-3 weeks
Mitochondria	3 weeks
Red Blood Cells	4 months
Stomach	7 days
Pancreas	40 days
Bone	3 years
Fat Cells	8 years
Heart Muscle	50 years
Lens	Never
Neurons	Never
Tattoos	Never

This chart glosses over quite a few important details. Take the small intestine as an example. The lining of the intestine takes a beating. It is a highly acidic environment and has to deal with everything we eat. It gets replaced about every four days. But the intestinal lining is composed of several different sorts of cells, and replacing 20 feet of this every four days is quite a project. The progression from progenitor cell to actual working intestinal cell is a virtual assembly line.

It turns out the intestines have little cave-like things called, interestingly, crypts. The protects the progenitor cells from the flow of the caustic and unpredictable intestinal "stuff" (usually called lumen) and, unsurprisingly, are the home of the intestinal progenitor cells. From this lair, the progenitor cells divide and migrate toward the "villi," which are larger finger-like things that protrude into the caustic lumen flowing by. It is these villi that take the beating. As a progenitor cell proceeds toward the villi, it starts to differentiate. This is a continuous assembly-line sort of process. The progenitor cell will differentiate into one of four very different types of cells. One of the cells absorbs nutrients, and the other three secrete different digestive juices. The absorbers are the most numerous and called enterocytes. This is really quite a neat trick, because the four cells don't look at all alike, and perform distinctly different functions. You wouldn't guess they had the same "mother" cell.

So now we have a handy way to go about growth and repair. Just get some stem cells that can make all the needed cell types, stash them away in some safe strategic location, and they will do the rest—somehow. Of course, if you want to repair a machine, you will turn it off first, if you can. The stem cells know this and do most of their work in the middle of the night.

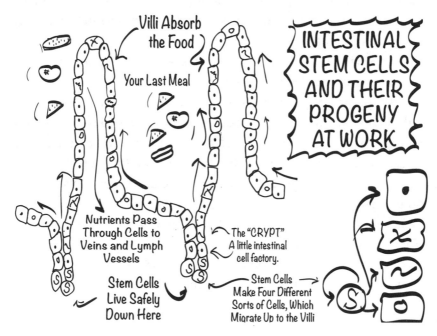

Other stem/progenitor cells have different manufacturing strategies, but they all seem to be hierarchical.

Tattoos last forever because the ink is injected down into the protected progenitor cell area, which doesn't turn over like surface skin cells.

From this sort of hierarchical structure, we can get a bit of insight into how a newly fertilized egg might operate. After some divisions, the outer ones could tend toward skin type stem cells, inner ones toward other sorts. They can differentiate into more specific cells later on. Doesn't explain much, but it's a start. Once you begin looking at the details, it's hard to think of anything more amazing.

Despite the organizational convenience and efficiency of the stem cell repair system, dangers lurk. The stem cell "potency" is the key. Stem cells are the guys that can divide and morph. If this gets out of control, there is a risk of cancer. Indeed, most cancers are the result of this. A fully differentiated cell typically has no ability to reproduce, so no matter how defective it is, it probably isn't going to do much harm.

SPECIALIZATION

Multi-cellularity makes specialization and compartmentalization possible. In a single-celled creature, there is some organization, of course, but by and large, things are simply floating around. The cells clumsily lurch and wiggle about, some with flagella.

With specialization, many new features are possible: organs, limbs, digestive systems, muscles, even brains.

The simplest "true" multi-celled animal is a tiny worm-like thing called a nematode, with exactly 1,031 cells, no more, no less. With these, it manages to make a mouth, a throat, an intestine, several muscles, some nerves, and sexual organs, which is a lot of the full kit. Notably missing are a respiratory system, a circulatory system, immune system, and various organs.

Nematodes emit a flash of blue light when they die. No one knows why.

There must have been simpler multi-celled creatures. The nematode couldn't simply jump into existence with all those different cell types and functions, but this is yet another missing link.

Organs

Several organs vital to humans originated long before the arrival of vertebrates. The standout is the liver. Crustaceans have livers, and they perform roughly the same tasks as our own, aiding digestion, filtering, manufacturing cholesterol. Insects, however do not seem to have a liver, so we'll give a hat tip to the lobster and his ilk for contributing this valuable organ.

The heart is a somewhat different story. Insects and crustaceans don't have a closed circulation system. An open circulation system means that the blood and nutrients simply slosh around. But there is a muscular organ that aids in this, making sure that sloshing is thorough. This would surely be a starting point for our own heart, but we don't really know. If so, the insects get credit for that.

Crustacean blood is blue instead of red. The color comes from oxygen carrying copper, which tarnishes blue in the process. We use iron. It tarnishes too. Think of rust. Insects don't have blood, at least not the type that transports oxygen and CO_2, so crustaceans get credit for that. How the switch was made from blue blood to red, and why, nobody knows.

MEDICINE OF THE FUTURE
Suspended Animation

The simple but inefficient fermentation cycle requires no oxygen, and all our cells are equipped to use it. Would it, therefore, be possible to survive without oxygen, by just using fermentation to barely keep the cells ticking over? The answer might be yes. It is a little tricky, though: if the cells are suddenly denied oxygen while things are running full tilt, they tend to self-destruct. However, if you can slow things down in advance, it appears to be possible. It hasn't been done in humans yet, but it may soon (not for space travel, but for another, more useful, application).

Researchers have successfully put pigs and dogs into suspended animation. They use various techniques. They may chill the pig way down, then have it breathe hydrogen sulfide. The pig appears to die. The heart stops and there is no measurable brain activity. The pig can remain like this for several hours. Then they reintroduce oxygen and the pig recovers, seemingly 100% intact. Other researchers use other methods, but the idea is the same. Slow the body first, then cut the oxygen.

Now the proposed use for this with humans would be in cases of severe accidents. In many such instances, victims die on the way to the hospital despite frantic lifesaving efforts. If the first responders could put the victim into a state of suspended animation instead, they could take him to the hospital without further worry. He could be operated on in a proper operating room without all the drama. The surgeons could take their time, and the victim would obligingly "chill" till they were ready to operate. A hospital in Maryland is planning to try this on victims who otherwise would have little chance of survival.

IMMUNE SYSTEM

Eukaryotic cells still have the chemical warfare defenses that are present in the simplest bacteria, but with cellular specialization, a completely new approach was added. A group of cells evolved whose sole function is to act as a police force. These are known as white blood cells or leukocytes, and come in over a dozen different types. They are all daughters or granddaughters of a single stem cell type: Hematopoietic Stem Cell, or HSC. Such stem cells are quite well protected, residing inside bones, which is a good thing too—we have a lifelong need of healthy, functioning immune cells.

The leukocytes are mobile. Most cells are attached to something, such as other cells or some sort of cellular scaffolding. Leukocytes will follow chemical scents—called interleukins—which are normally given off by other leukocytes. In some cases, normal cells will secrete these as sort of an SOS. The leukocytes could certainly use a flagellum, but no such luck. To get around, they normally hitch a ride in the bloodstream, but once they have landed at the scene of the crime, they move by deforming themselves. This movement is akin to the bound victim in the whodunit who inches across the room to the telephone and dials for help with her nose. The scientific term for such inching about is diapedesis.

Leukocytes are formidable bacteria killers. They will typically engulf a bacteria, then poison it. Few bacteria can survive this. One well known exception is the tuberculosis bacteria, which turns the tables inside out and actually reproduces inside the leukocyte, eventually popping it. This hijacking of the immune cells makes tuberculosis quite hard to get rid of.

Most bacteria are destroyed if identified. However, the identification procedure is another chink in the armor and represents a very tough problem. Ideally, the immune system will identify anything harmful—bacteria or viruses, bad cells, or even inert objects—and once identified, will attack and kill them, or at least wall them off. However, it must not disturb any healthy cells and must also ignore all the necessary circulating hormones and other vital chemicals. This is a tall order, and made immeasurably tougher by the numerous devious and clever ways bacteria and viruses disguise themselves to evade detection. The staph bacteria can not only survive and reproduce inside a leukocyte, it can also, in effect, change its spots, having a modifiable outer membrane prevents that blocks the leukocytes from locking on to it.

The immune system works only on the "inside." Generally this is where blood flows. Your skin is obviously "outside." However, anything that has direct contact with stuff from the outside world is also "outside." This would include your stomach, intestines, and lungs. These surfaces are all teeming with bacteria, much of it useful. All these surfaces have bacteria-proof barriers. Inside, things are sterile, meaning, in principle, no bacteria or viruses at all. (Some, like the chicken pox virus, can hibernate undetected, emerging years later as shingles.)

The immune system works amazingly well, but it is commensurately complicated. However, it is key to cellular and general health, so we need to dig deeper.

The immune system is broadly divided into "innate" and "adaptive" systems. Vertebrates have both. Our 1,031-celled nematode has neither, but it seems the innate immune system evolved soon afterwards, because almost all non-vertebrates have a pretty sophisticated one. The innate immune system defends against any invader. The adaptive immune system, a vertebrate-only feature, permits memory, so that a pathogen, once seen and conquered, is remembered and readily defeated again. Without the adaptive feature, you would get the same disease over and over. This is indeed the case with non-vertebrates.

Cellular Police Force (Innate Division)

Let's take a close look at the innate immune system. The first new feature is a system of toll receptors, which can identify a variety of bacteria, fungi, and other foreign objects or invaders. "Toll" means wonderful in German, such was the impression this discovery made. Several of the various leukocytes are armed with these. Once a toll receptor recognizes a foreign invader, it triggers some sort of attack. This can vary. It might power down the cell to prevent a virus from hijacking its reproductive machinery. It might trigger apoptosis—programmed cell death. In many cases, it signals for help from other immune system cells. There are several types of toll receptors, each able to spot various attributes of invading viruses and bacteria.

The repair function, the healing of a wound, for instance, is also considered part of the immune system.

The innate immune system has three basic cell types, all daughters of the HSC stem cell types: engulfers, poisoners, and "natural killers."

Engulfers are called phagocytes (cell eaters). There are three subtypes here. A large one that can engulf a lot of bacteria (macrophage), a smaller, very mobile one (neutrophil) that tends to be a first responder, and finally, in mammals, a marker one (dendritic cell) that identifies the pathogen.

The poisoners are called basophils and eosinophils. Basophils are responsible for allergic reactions. Eosinophils specialize in bacteria, and carry toxins that will destroy them.

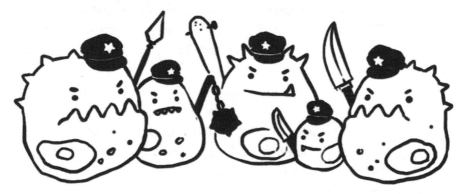

Finally, the most sinister of the lot, and perhaps the most interesting, is the Natural Killer cell. This one will kill any normal cell in the body that it thinks is compromised. Kind of like the police blowing up the house to get the bad guy. Now here's the really amazing part: How does the natural killer cell "know" whom to kill? It turns out that each "normal" cell has to hang a specific complicated protein, called MHC, on its surface. MHC contains a lot of DNA, peptides, and other identifying information, rather like the security-check questions you go through when you do some online credit card transaction. Happily, the credit card company doesn't kill you if you get these things wrong. The natural killer cell is not so forgiving. If the MHC is wrong, or not there at all, it kills the cell. If the cell has been invaded by bacteria or viruses, it will likely display the wrong MHC, but perhaps more importantly, if the cell is cancerous, the MHC may also be wrong as well. Hence, natural killer cells are also the front line against tumors. Since tumors are made up of our own "stuff," most immune cells don't see them as anything out of the ordinary.

So far, we have six cells in the innate immune system. This is an ancient collection: insects, worms, crustaceans, and other complex invertebrates all have a similar system. When we get to the vertebrates, we'll keep these six and add several more to form the adaptive immune system. This is going to get a lot more complicated (as if it weren't already).

Interleukins

As you can easily imagine, out-of-control immune cells could be highly dangerous. For this reason, there is a coordinated chemical communication system. These chemicals, which are secreted and detected, are called interleukins, so named because the white cells themselves are called leukocytes. There are a couple of dozen interleukins with a variety of functions: some are generated by cells needing help, and others are generated by the white blood cells themselves.

The first responders, the neutrophils, migrate out of the bloodstream toward a wound or infection. They follow a chemical scent, typically an interleukin, that is secreted by the actual cells in distress. Once hot on the trail, a neutrophil is said to be activated, and in this state will excrete interleukins of its own to call in more neutrophils and other white cell reinforcements. If a neutrophil encounters a bacteria, it will engulf it and kill it.

The types and levels of the circulating interleukins provide a good overview of any infectious battles that may be going on. These are monitored by various organs, which can respond by greatly increasing the size of the white cell army. But it's more nuanced than that. Some interleukins promote various sorts of white cell generation and differentiation. Others serve to regulate. This elaborate chemical communication system is found in most multi-celled organisms, though not the tiny nematode.

COMMUNICATION

Communication is present in the simplest bacteria, both internally and between one another. It is usually chemical, with various processes acting in response to some chemical that they detect or secreting the chemical when they need something. It's not always chemical: temperature and light can also be sensed, and some signaling is electrical.

Bacteria communicate among themselves more than you might suppose. They can signal one another to increase or decrease reproduction in response to various situations, or to hide in various ways if a predator is afoot. Single-celled eukaryotes take off from there. Once the jump is made to multi-cellular, an additional problem of intercellular communication arises. If the sender and recipient are nearby, it may suffice to excrete some key chemicals. However, two other communication systems not found in the single-celled species are added to the mix: nerves and circulation. Our nematode already has nerves: exactly 302 neurons. (Nematodes appear to value precision.) Nematode neurons go point to point. This is different from ours, which branch and interconnect extensively. Actually, size imposes no requirement for neural systems. The largest eukaryotes, trees, have no nerves at all, though they all have circulatory systems.

As multi-cellular creatures get larger (a nematode is about the size of a comma on this page) a couple of new problems kick in. First is nutrient distribution. In a tiny nematode, food and oxygen can reach nearby cells by simple diffusion, but for a beast to get any larger, a delivery system is needed. Though absent in the nematode, hearts soon developed, but without a closed circulation system. These hearts simply sloshed the fluids around, rather like a fan in a room. Insects and crustaceans, like lobsters, have such systems.

These animals are much more complex, with senses of sight and smell, limbs and pincers. Food processing organs like the liver are now turning up. Neural development has soared as well. The lobster has 100,000 neurons, a cockroach over a million, and a real all-around oddball, the octopus, has 300 million, more than many mammals.

We now have most of the pieces that make up vertebrates. Looking at our inventory, we have cells with DNA and energy sources, a basic design that is usable everywhere. We have sexual reproduction, which includes all-important sexual selection. We have multi-cellularity with cellular specialization. We have an innate immune system with six different types of white blood cells. We have neurons to tie things together, and some primitive forms of circulation. Specialty organs are starting to develop. We have a nice stem-cell-based hierarchal organization for cell renewal. Clusters of neurons enable memory and learning. We are almost there.

Two pieces acquired at this juncture are key to good health and degenerative disease avoidance. The innate immune system is the first line of defense against cancer, and will destroy any cells that are malfunctioning. The second key feature is stem cells. These cells, kept, insofar as possible, out of harm's way, stay healthy and are able to generate the working every-day cells that wear out. Keeping the stem cells in good shape require a clean diet and exercise. Mitochondrial degradation and damage to stem cells probably account for 95% of degenerative disease.

Key Points
17 - Specialization
- There are no two-celled creatures. The simplest, after the single cell, is the nematode at 1,031 cells.
- Reproduction for multi-celled creatures is considerably more complicated.
- The fertilized egg, which is a single cell, must generate all the cell types.
- A stem cell can generate a variety of types of cells. They can reproduce by division as well. The fertilized egg is a stem cell.
- Once a stem cell becomes a specialized cell, it is said to have "differentiated."
- Progenitor cells are like stem cells, but produce fewer cell types.
- Some cells last a lifetime, and some are frequently replaced.
- Innate immune cells developed in early multi-cellular creatures.
- The immune system recognizes and kills many bacteria and viruses.
- Immune cells communicate via chemicals called interleukins.
- As plants and animals grew in size, communication between different regions became a problem. Neurons evolved as a solution for animals.
- The simplest multi-celled animal has neurons.

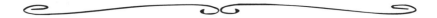

18 - VERTEBRATES

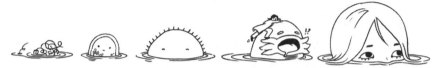

For aesthetic reasons, we would like to redo the grand flow of evolution. Up till now, all is well. We have all this wondrous complexity, incredible miniaturization of impossibly elaborate functions; all in all beautifully evolved biological systems and creatures, and at last we are ready for our first vertebrate, and therein lies the issue: at the start of the vertebrate parade, a parade in which we proudly participate, couldn't evolution have come up with something less horrifyingly ugly than the hagfish? Really. There are gorgeous butterflies, dragonflies, and so on, so why this monstrosity? Why not a bird, a beautiful tropical fish, even a shark, anything but this:

We suppose we must take what we can get. Anyway, on closer inspection, there's already something fishy: the thing has no vertebrae. A "vertebrate" with no vertebrae? You'd think that would disqualify it, but the high priests of taxonomy have made an exception largely because it's got all the other requisite pieces. Plus its DNA credentials look solid. It's got a heart, gills for lungs, a liver, kidneys, a fairly elaborate hypothalamus, a , a spinal cord (though no spine), teeth, a tongue, a sense of smell, and the requisite sexual bits.

THIS BOOK ISN'T HELPING MY SELF-IMAGE...

So once more, we have taken another leap over Lake Unknown. This slimy thing is much more complicated than a lobster. When did it lose its hard shell, and where did it get all those new organs,

227

organs we have as well? Again, we cannot find any trace of intermediary species, just suddenly: hagfish. So we suppose those intermediate species were all eaten. But somewhere in the evolutionary process, the crustacean-like outer shell was jettisoned, so likely not much of a fossil record.

This happened about 500 million years ago. In due course, hagfish became fish, and the rest, as they say, is history. We have seemingly reached the shore on the other side of Lake Unknown. There are still gaps, but they aren't major. We came ashore, we evolved. We now know a lot (albeit with some broad missing links), and have almost all the pieces needed to construct our human, so let's take a look at the new equipment that got added in this vertebrate step: the hypothalamus, the hippocampus, the closed circulation system, and several other innovative pieces of biological gear.

CLOSED CIRCULATION AND ITS BENEFITS

Instead of washing all the cells with the necessary nutrients, the vertebrates feature a closed blood-distribution system. This entailed an additional major development: a huge network of blood vessels and capillaries would need to deliver the nutrients to practically every cell. However, there was a huge payoff: limbs, organs, eyes, etc., could now be remotely located, and animals could grow a lot larger and become more specialized. Further, the arteries and veins could constrict and dilate to control the flow. Thus the stomach could get additional blood when it needed to digest, muscles when physical activity was called for, and so on. As usual, more complex, but it opened the door for organs, complex brains, larger sizes, and other significant benefits.

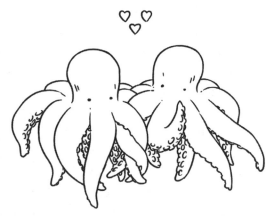

Again, we don't find the transition animals. There are, however, a few invertebrates that have closed circulation systems, notably the octopus. And as if confirming the benefit, the octopus has a pretty decent brain as well, a brain larger than all the fish and reptiles, and quite a few of the smaller mammals. The octopus has three separate hearts. Though not on our evolutionary path, the octopus does prove that we don't have a monopoly on all these new developments. And the octopus is ancient too, on the scene well before the hagfish, though it has been evolving as well.

The octopus's well developed brain is apparently a somewhat different design. It has no division of cerebral function like that found in the vertebrates. Starting apparently with the hagfish, we have the cerebellum in charge of movement, the hypothalamus as master of metabolism and hormonal control, the hippocampus for memory, something akin to the amygdala, and a thalamus acting as a neural switchboard. Essentially everything but the neocortex. (In all fairness to the octopus and our various feathered friends, there does seem to be substantial problem solving-ability and other sorts of intelligence exhibited with their existing neural equipment, so perhaps we are overlooking something.)

THE VASCULAR SYSTEM

Most people, even many doctors, view the heart, arteries, veins, and capillaries as an ordinary plumbing system, and indeed there are certain attributes in common with the one that brings water to our home and takes away the waste. But there are major differences too.

First, the body's plumbing system has to be leaky. The nutrients in the blood must get out of the bloodstream and into the hungry cells. Second, the system can't be shut down for repairs: after a few minutes without oxygen, cells die, so maintenance must be done while the system is running.

Arteries

Let's dissect an artery. It is more complex than a simple piece of pipe. It has four layers. The inner one, called the endothelium, is made up of a single layer of very thin skin-like cells. This important layer is a bit fragile. Next is a thin crosshatched elastic layer, which is not made of cells, called the basement membrane. Surrounding this is a layer of muscle cells. What are muscle cells doing in an artery? They wrap around the "pipe" and squeeze or relax to control the blood flow. Veins have them too. Finally, there is a tougher outer layer, again made of non-cellular material. Actually the non-cellular layers consist of a layer of elastic material and a layer of tough structural material, so you could equally say that the artery has six layers. The blood and other fluids flowing through the artery or vein are collectively called the lumen.

The capillaries have only the two inner layers, allowing them to be in intimate contact with the cells they are servicing.

The lymph system, which, among other things, acts as an add-on to the vascular system, is composed of lymph vessels and capillaries that are practically identical in construction to the veins.

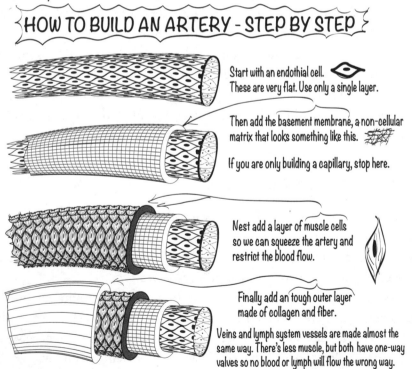

HOW TO BUILD AN ARTERY - STEP BY STEP

Start with an endothial cell. These are very flat. Use only a single layer.

Then add the basement membrane, a non-cellular matrix that looks something like this.

If you are only building a capillary, stop here.

Nest add a layer of muscle cells so we can squeeze the artery and restrict the blood flow.

Finally add an tough outer layer made of collagen and fiber.

Veins and lymph system vessels are made almost the same way. There's less muscle, but both have one-way valves so no blood or lymph will flow the wrong way.

The Endothelium

The inner layer, the endothelium, is composed of a mosaic of endothelial cells and is very complex. The endothelial cells themselves are incredibly flat. If you enlarged one so that it was the size of a postcard, you would have a pretty accurate 3D model. The scaled-up endothelial cell would be about that thick. Where the endothelial cells join, they overlap, as there's hardly any edge. The side of the cell that is in contact with the blood has a slippery coating called the glycocalyx. Microscopically, glycocalyx looks like short fur. We expect the endothelium to be largely impermeable until it branches its way down to the capillaries.

Capillaries

In the capillaries, the endothelium has to be leaky, albeit in a very controlled fashion, as nutrients have to be delivered to the hungry cells. The tiny capillaries have shed their two outer layers in the process, leaving only the endothelium and the basement membrane. In some regions, notably the liver, the endothelium is actually missing in places, opening large gaps, which will put the blood flow (the lumen) into even closer contact with the adjacent cells.

The capillaries are now about the same size as the cells they are tending, and are in fairly intimate contact with this.

The nutrient "load" is delivered in a variety of ways. Some of it, oxygen, for instance, can diffuse right through a cell wall. Oxygen is carried by hemoglobin, a molecule that largely fills the red blood cells. In an oxygen-deprived area, O_2 molecules diffuse out of the red blood cells and into the oxygen-starved ones. CO_2 has to return to the lungs, and the now-empty hemoglobin carries at least some of it back. Other sorts of nutrients are engulfed by the endothelium, ferried across in little bubbles called vesicles, and then released to the hungry cells on the other side. In some cases, mall tubes develop through the endothelium, and some molecules traverse these. Some endothelial cells have little windows that allow certain molecules to diffuse right through. Finally, several of the smaller molecules can go around the endothelium, via the junctions where endothelial cells join.

In like manner, assorted molecules exiting the cell find their way into the capillaries, which will soon combine into veins.

The Lymph System

Cells are sloppy eaters—about on par with a two-year-old. Around 15% of the nutrients are spilled, but there is yet another part of the circulatory system that mops up the mess: the lymph system. It does this with its own set of capillaries, which are stopped off at one end. These capillaries are porous, and capture the spill, which is mostly plasma. The capillaries branch into lymph vessels, and eventually dump into a large normal vein.

No new inventions were needed here. The lymph capillaries and vessels are made just like veins, using endothelial cells, basement membrane, surrounding smooth muscle, basically the whole bit. The lymph vessels squeeze to pump their contents. You would think this would squish the stuff both ways, but lymph vessels, like veins, also have numerous one-way valves.

Cleaning up the spill is evidently more important in the brain. Here the lymph vessels surround the veins, forming a sort of double tube. This tidy arrangement eluded detection till 2014. The discoverers named this the glymphatic system. The G is for the glia—helper cells to the neurons.

The intestines send most food straight to the liver. Fat seems to be a major exception. The intestines package fat into large lipoprotein particles called chylomicrons and send them into lymph vessels. These then also end up in circulation and are quickly consumed by hungry cells.

The immune system seems to have set up residence in the lymph system as well—in particular, the lymph nodes. These are bean sized and scattered all over the body, but especially prevalent in the armpits and groin. These are the sites that the cells of the adaptive immune system (soon to be introduced) scamper off to when they happen to recognize some sort of pathogen.

The spleen and thymus are considered lymph system organs. The spleen appears to be a warehouse for immune system cells, and the thymus actively generates a type of adaptive immune system cells and gives them their name: T-cells. The tonsils are also part of the immune system. When the authors were children, these were routinely snipped out under general anesthesia. At that time, the tonsils' purposes were unknown, and therefore why not get rid of them? They have a well researched function now, though. They are the first line of defense against ingested bacterial and viral pathogens. So, tonsils turned out to be useful after all. Hopefully the "if in doubt, snip it out" era of medicine is passing.

THE ADAPTIVE IMMUNE SYSTEM

Another feature missing in the hagfish and its close cousin, the lamprey eel, is the adaptive immune system. This would soon show up in the jawed fish. It was added on top of the existing innate one and is even more complicated!

The "reason" for the development is this: The innate immune system can recognize quite a few bacterial and viral pathogens, but this recognition is more or less fixed, cast in the innate system's white cells. With their assorted toll receptors, they can recognize a more or less specific spectrum of bacteria.

If bacteria would stay put—genetically speaking—this probably would have done the job. But, of course, bacteria and viruses mutate all the time, continually picking up new DNA and discarding old. As soon as some bacteria came up with a new trick that eluded the innate immune system, vulnerability to infection dramatically increased. Of course, the innate immune system could, in principle, have evolved more and more toll receptors, but whereas bacterial DNA can evolve in a hurry, we eukaryotes are glacially slow. This was not a contest we were going to win.

By contrast, the adaptive immune system can recognize every molecule in the universe, or so it is claimed. This includes bacteria and viruses, as well as other toxins, like rancid LDL. In a human body, the adaptive immune system can recognize around 10 million sorts of patterns. How it does this is another of those "gee whiz—how could this ever have evolved?" moments.

Cells of the Adaptive Immune System

The adaptive immune system is a bit complicated. Recall that the innate system consists of engulfers, poisoners, and natural killers.

Engulfers, also called phagocytes, are cell eaters. There are three subtypes here. A large one that can engulf a lot of bacteria (macrophage), a smaller, very mobile one (neutrophil), that tends to be a first responder, and finally, in mammals, a marker one (dendritic cell) that identifies something as a pathogen.

The natural killers look for markings on a cell exterior and will destroy the cell if these markers seem a little fishy.

The adaptive system brings three more cells into the mix:
- B-cells. These are antibody managers.
- Helper T-cells. These dispatch and coordinate.
- Killer T-cells. These kill bacteria, and can kill our own cells.

The B-cell or T-cell designation has to do with where the cells "mature" and causes a lot of confusion. Things are a lot clearer if we look at what they do. B-cells are in charge of antibodies. You have heard of antibodies. More in a minute. Helper T-cells are like managers or dispatchers. They don't directly kill pathogens, but speed up and focus the response in a variety of ways. Killer T-cells do exactly what their name implies. All three of these cells have antibodies stuck on their surfaces, forming receptors, and they roam about the body looking for some invader that matches (called an antigen).

Antibodies

An antibody is a little Y-shaped protein that matches patterns on a pathogen (also called the antigen, for **anti**body **gen**erator). They can either be stuck onto a B-cell or T-cell, where they are used as receptors, or they can circulate freely. They detect bacteria and viruses, but other things as well: toxic chemicals, damaged tissue, and the like. Needless to say, there is a huge, almost infinite variety of such patterns possible, so the human body generates a huge amount of B and T cells, and then "programs" them to specialize by using one of the 10 million different antibodies as a receptor. So in a sense, there are 10 million different types of B and T cells. At any given time, there are around 10 billion such cells in circulation, so this means duplication, and around a thousand cells will carry the same antibody for each of the 10 million types. A thousand isn't a lot of defense against a rapidly dividing bacterial invasion, but the body has a solution to that, and what a solution!

Adaptive Defense and B-Cells

As soon as one of the B-cells matches an invading bacteria, it scurries off to a lymph node and starts replicating very rapidly. Each of the replicated cells is slightly different, so as to fine-tune to an exact match. The various new B-cells that match the invader best then start spewing huge numbers of antibodies into the

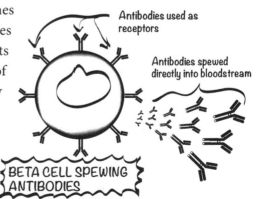

Antibodies used as receptors

Antibodies spewed directly into bloodstream

BETA CELL SPEWING ANTIBODIES

circulatory system. These are free antibodies and circulate about the body attaching to invading bacteria, thereby neutralizing them and marking them for destruction by a passing macrophage.

Immunity

The B-cells aren't quite done. Some of them differentiate into B-memory cells, which typically last a very long time. Should the pathogen show up again, the memory cells are ready to lurch into the above high-speed replication cycle immediately.

T-Cells

The B-cells are primarily looking for pathogens in the blood or other things outside of the cells. However, if the body's cells themselves have been invaded, the T-cells get involved. The T-cells have the same huge variety of antibody receptors as the B cells, but seem to be far less trigger-happy. In fact, unless some "proof" is presented that a cell is infected, the T-cells do nothing. The killer T-cells look for an antigen match within the cell, specifically the MHC protein. Once either of the T-cell types are activated, they go into a massive replication mode similar to the B-cells. After the replication, the helper T-cells secrete various interleukins, which draw other immune resources to the vicinity. The killer T-cells kill the infected cell by poisoning it. (Actually, they inject an enzyme that causes the infected cell to commit apoptosis—cellular suicide.) Like the B-cells, both T-cell types produce some memory versions that last a very long time.

This whole T-cell/B-cell campaign tends to take 5 to 10 days to kick in. This is why colds and similar diseases usually last about that long. Until the T and B cells arrive and finish things off, all the defense is in the hands of the innate immune system.

What Does All This Have to Do with Degenerative Disease?

A lot. We will soon delve into this question. However, the two principal areas of interest are atherosclerosis and cancer. Here are a couple of previews.

In atherosclerosis, cholesterol, fat, and other molecules have gotten stuck in the arteries and gone rancid (oxidized). The immune system has locked on to this and is trying to remove or neutralize it. Helper T-cells are summoning macrophages to try to engulf the mess. HDL will attempt to clear some of the load from the macrophages. If the HDL cannot keep up, atherosclerosis results.

In cancer, a sequence of DNA mutations has caused a cell, usually a stem or progenitor type, to act abnormally. The immune system is the first line of defense here. The natural killer cells in the innate system will destroy a cell that does not display a correct MHC complex. Further, the adaptive T and B cells may recognize the effects of the cancer and ramp up the attack.

People mainly assume the immune system is all about fighting bacteria and viruses, but its role is much broader.

THE AMAZING ROLE OF HDL

HDL isn't a cell, and it isn't generated by any of the immune system cells. It's sometimes called "good cholesterol," which is only a small piece of the story. One of its many jobs is to rescue the overloaded macrophages in the arterial system by unloading their cholesterol and fat and transporting it to the liver for safe disposal. In spite of its hepatic origins, HDL should probably be considered to be part of the immune system.

How Does HDL Work?

HDL is amazing. If you do whatever it takes to get your HDL level up and functional (no drugs allowed here), you probably won't get sick. It is about as close as the body comes to having a molecular fairy godmother that can fix everything. It alone is that powerful.

HDL is built by the liver and attaches to various cells, where it engulfs certain cellular junk. When "full," it returns to the liver for recycling. HDL is very small and can get in and out of almost any nook or cranny. It has certain cell-like features. It has receptors that bind to various substances, rancid cholesterol being one of the more notable. Its receptor is combined with a transporter that is used to unload toxins from overloaded cells. Quite a handy particle.

There is considerably more to HDL's repertoire. Besides removing cholesterol, HDL enhances blood vessel flexibility, and attempts to down-regulate swollen macrophages' inflammation activity and block their programmed destruction. It's almost as if it is correcting the mistakes of an overly ambitious innate immune system. It comes as no surprise that high HDL translates to a markedly reduced risk of heart disease.

HDL is in some sense programmable. Its specific makeup tends to match the problem. In people with atherosclerosis, it is programmed to go after plaque. If cancer is present, HDL will attack those cells. How this happens and how it is controlled is probably worth a future Nobel Prize.

HDL has at least two cancer-fighting properties. First, its appetite for rancid fat or cholesterol is not limited to the macrophages. It will quite cheerfully help out a normal cell that has gotten in trouble, directly offloading the cell's internal toxic junk. Such stressed cells would be prime candidates for carcinogenic mutations, so this places HDL in the role of a cancer blocker. Second, for a tumor to grow larger than a couple of millimeters, it needs a blood supply. This is called angiogenesis. With the right mutation, it can get one generated, but HDL can block this crucial step too. These steps, and no doubt others, account for HDL's strong anti-cancer properties.

There are some rare diseases where HDL doesn't function properly, and people so afflicted are at high risk for atherosclerosis and cancer.

THE LIVER

Prometheus, a Greek titan (sort of a junior god), ran afoul of the head honcho, Zeus, and was punished in a most imaginative way. He was chained to a rock, and every day, an eagle would arrive and eat his liver. At night, though, his liver would completely regrow, so the punishment was eternal.

Among various questions raised is this one: "Did the ancient Greeks know that the liver could regenerate itself?" And assuming that this punishment wasn't part of their standard penal code, *how*?

As organs go, for vertebrates at least, the liver alone has this unique property; none of the other organs can regenerate. A human liver can regenerate to full function from as little as 30-40%. For all the other organs, we are stuck with the ones we are born with. This regeneration of key bodily items appears to be a pre-vertebrate specialty. Limbs, eyes, livers, even hearts can be regrown in these lesser animals.

The liver is an ancient organ that performs much the same function in humans as it does in lobsters. The liver can be viewed as a food processing factory. The food you eat, arriving via blood vessels coming directly from the intestines, is converted into food your cells can use. It performs dozens of other functions as well.

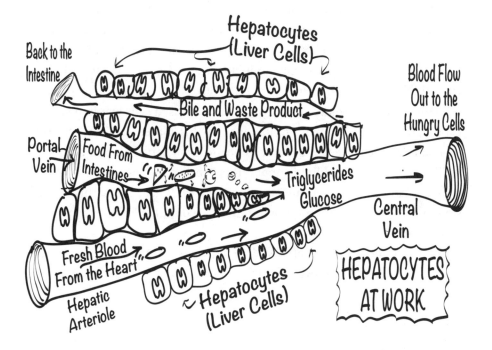

Dozens? Make that hundreds. And the most amazing part is that each cell appears to be its own little tiny factory. There aren't regions that deal with glucose and other regions that deal with fat. Each cell can do it all—all 500 known liver functions—as well as hundreds more yet to be discovered. These magic cells, called hepatocytes, have another handy trick: they can divide. So this, coupled with the lack of compartmentalization and specialization, mean a liver can be regenerated.

The inner workings of hepatocytes is a murky area. They are in most respects a normal cell, but have a much larger protein-making region, which comes as no surprise, given the huge amount of chemical and nutrient processing that is going on.

Generally speaking, much of the food from the stomach and intestines is carried directly to the liver by the portal vein. Unlike the usual arrangement, this vein is bringing stuff in, not providing an exit. A normal artery also feeds into the liver. These two branch down to capillary-sized vessels, and run alongside the hepatocytes, eventually joining up and exiting via a major liver vein. As they flow along the row of hepatocytes, the various types of hepatic magic take place.

Using receptors and transporters, hepatocytes shuffle stuff in and out of the blood, thus maintaining the desired levels of things such as glucose, LDL cholesterol, HDL cholesterol, triglycerides, and hundreds of others. If some items are lacking, the liver cells can probably manufacture them. Fat from sugar, sugar from fat, and many other possibilities: the liver cells are amazingly versatile. The liver also stores a large amount of sugar to use between meals. Here are are some of the more notable liver cell functions:

- **Storing sugar as glycogen.** Up to 30,000 glucose molecules are compacted into huge molecules called glycogen.
- **Dispensing that sugar as needed later.** The glycogen is disassembled back into individual glucose molecules and dumped back into the bloodstream as necessary.
- **Making triglycerides (fat) from sugars.** This is one of the conversions that turn sugar and starches into fat.
- **Packaging lipoproteins.** HDL, VLDL, and LDL are all made up in hepatocytes.
- **Producing bile for digestion**. The hepatocyte assembly line has bile ducts running alongside it and manufactures bile to aid in digestion. The hepatocytes will also dump some waste into the bile.
- **Breaking down many toxins such as alcohol.** Toxins are broken down. Many are converted to urea or marked in some other way for elimination by the kidneys.
- **Storing various vitamins.**
- **Producing blood plasma.** The red and white cells that make up half of the blood come from the bones. The clear part of blood, called plasma, is made by the hepatocytes.
- **Assorted biochemicals.** The liver generates a vast array of various needed chemicals.
- **Blood purification.** Many toxins in the blood are removed and sent into the bile.

- **Immune system assistance.** The liver removes bacteria and other pathogens that have been marked by the immune system.
- And several hundred more that are known, and likely there are as many again that are unknown.

The hypothalamus controls a lot of liver function, or rather tweaks it. Absent the hypothalamus, the liver will trundle along doing its usual routine, but probably not that optimally. It comes as no surprise the liver can operate this way, as it evolved first: many invertebrates have livers, but none are blessed with a hypothalamus.

Given all this complexity, and so little knowledge of how it works, we probably would best consider the liver function to be magical, but a magic that should be well protected and preserved. We cannot survive without the liver, and transplants do not have a high success rate.

KIDNEYS

Kidneys clean the blood, and in many ways, take up where the liver left off. Items in the blood that the liver has marked for destruction, along with other waste, will be diverted into the urine by the kidneys.

The kidneys are usually billed as a filter, but what they are required to do is a tall order for any sort of filter we are familiar with. Since we are building a human from scratch, let's try our hand at kidney design. First the problem: There is a variety of waste product circulating in the blood. Some of it is known, such as urea coming from the liver, and some is unknown, such as snipped-up pieces of a failed bacterial invasion. The size of the trash varies from quite small molecules to fairly large stuff, though most of it is smaller than the circulating red and white blood cells.

So how to go about this? Something like a coffee filter isn't going to work at all. First, it only lets small stuff through, and second, it clogs up and has to be replaced.

Another idea: why not have a bunch of transporters that would latch on to the trash and pull it out of the blood and into the urine? This is not a bad approach, but the problem is that *all* the trash has to be gotten rid of, both the known and the unknown. Since transporters are specific to a certain type of molecule, the kidney would have to have a complete list of every possible sort of trash. Not really feasible. (Note that cells expressing inbound transporters know in advance exactly what they want.)

So it would seem we are stymied. We give up, as the solution is so clever, it would take an Einstein to come up with it. Or someone with a very cluttered desk. Did you ever have such a mess that you didn't know where to start, so you shoved it all into a grand heap, dumped it into the trash, and then picked through it to recover the things you actually wanted to keep? This is how the kidneys work.

Step one: the kidneys squeeze a lot of the blood fluid (plasma) out of the capillaries and into the urine. Think of squeezing a sponge. Only the red and white cells and some plasma would be left in the blood. Now obviously there has to be a step two, or we would be running to the bathroom every 90 seconds and would rapidly dehydrate. We shouldn't even call the squeezed stuff urine, because it's not going to be the real thing until after step two. So then: "pre-urine."

Step two: After step one has squeezed some of the blood into the pre-urine, a downstream process *recaptures everything that should be retained*. This would include most of the water, various electrolytes like calcium, sodium and potassium, and small molecules like amino acids, glucose, etc., and anything else of use. In fact, the recapture is picky. If the blood already has enough salt, the kidneys will just let it go. Hundreds of things are recaptured, at little or no energy cost, and regulated to ideal levels. Anything not taken back goes on to the bladder. Whatever we might notice about urine—color, amount, etc.—directly reflects what the kidneys decided *not* to keep in step two.

So here the body has killed two birds with one stone. It's gotten rid of the waste and performed a regulation operation at the same time. This clever two-step kidney contraption is called a nephron, and is depicted below.

The blood arrives in the cup at the top left and is squeezed out of a tangle of capillaries that are kept under pressure by the two tiny arteries on either side. The blood product that got squeezed out then makes a pass through the "loop of Henlie," where water and various minerals are recovered. In the drawing, the loop of Henlie is way out of scale. It could be a half-inch long. The rest is tiny. We have one and a half million of these nephrons. The biochemical recovery process itself is quite elaborate, and the nephrons play assorted clever tricks, running the pre-urine through different gradients of chemicals in order to pull off the recovery. When everything that interested the nephrons has been extracted, what remains, the "real" urine, continues on to the bladder and further destinations.

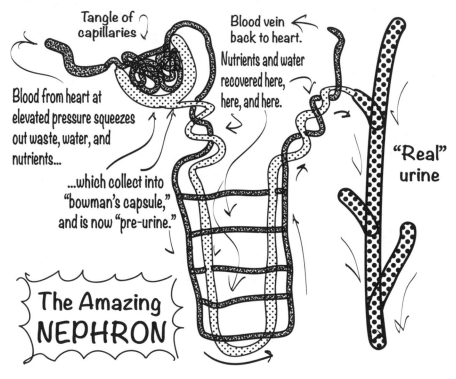

Tangle of capillaries

Blood vein back to heart.

Nutrients and water recovered here, here, and here.

Blood from heart at elevated pressure squeezes out waste, water, and nutrients...

...which collect into "bowman's capsule," and is now "pre-urine."

"Real" urine

The Amazing
NEPHRON

The kidneys also have a few hormone-generating functions, notably:

- Renin. This hormone regulates blood pressure. It is a general signal to constrict blood vessels.
- Calcitriol. This is vitamin D.

And finally, is the hypothalamus sticking its nose into things? As usual, the answer is yes. Is seems that the control is exerted primarily via hormones secreted by the pituitary gland, the hypothalamus's personal hormone factory.

Kidneys, at least a healthy pair of them, represent a tremendous overkill. It seems that we can get by fine on a single kidney, and could probably survive on half of that—at least if it were a healthy one. This is unusually extravagant for our parsimonious body, so there must be some very good historical reason for it. We could ponder what our ancient ancestors were up to. Why did they need so much kidney function? Water retention? Lots of toxins to get rid of?

You have no doubt noticed that there are a lot of small blood vessels involved in the kidney function. If there is artery disease, these are likely to become impaired (clogged) and kidney disease is virtually certain to follow.

ADRENAL GLANDS

The adrenal glands perch atop the kidneys, but have no particular connection with them. They are steroid factories. They are famous for producing adrenalin, the fight-or-flight hormone, but also produce cortisol, the stress hormone, as well as androgen, one of the sex hormones. They generally respond to signals from the hypothalamus, and respond quite quickly.

PANCREAS

The pancreas produces several important hormones, notably insulin, glucagon, and somatostatin. It also aids in digestion.

THE HYPOTHALAMUS AND OTHER TINY BRAINS

We have already sung the praises of the hypothalamus. This little brain appears to have arrived with the vertebrates.

Simpler creatures with nerves seem to use them in "reflex-arcs," which is exactly what it sounds like. This is usually built in rather than learned or trainable in any way. Some learning is possible in some of these animals. Lobsters appear to have a vague knack for this, recognizing the presence of a trainer as a source of food, or maybe making a special move. This seems to be about the top trick they can master. Any vertebrate, no matter how primitive, can easily beat this.

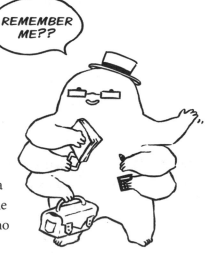

The hypothalamus actually does have a huge store of reflex-arc sorts of solutions—if this, excrete that, etc.—but it's also capable of adapting to new situations. It has the well-tuned regulatory system we are already familiar with. There doesn't seem to be any direct motor control located in the hypothalamus. That function resides in the cerebellum.

The hypothalamus also controls fear level, stress level, and sex drive, but for these sorts of things, it has partners. The hypothalamus is but one member of a tiny brain trust. Several other specialized "brains" also have a say in things. The amygdala and hippocampus are very involved. There are a pair of amygdalae, which deal with emotions. Apparently each amygdala specializes in certain ones. They are also involved in consolidation of emotional memory, and help direct emotional responses, signaling the hypothalamus to turn on the correct hormones: adrenalin for fear, pheromones for other things.

Sometimes, amygdalae are removed as a treatment for violent seizures, and the patient typically experiences major changes in fear and empathy responses.

The hippocampus comes in pairs as well. These are concerned with memory storage and spatial memory. Taxi drivers have significantly larger ones. One young man, Henry Molaison, had his removed at age 27 as a treatment for seizures. It ended the seizures, and he behaved seemingly normally, but from then on, he could never form new memories. The hippocampus appears to be the gateway for that.

The hypothalamus will continue to be the star of the show, though, garnering a bit more attention than it perhaps deserves, as it usually is controlling many, if not most, of the various hormonal and circulating biochemicals that we are undertaking to optimize. In its ancestral view, the neocortex ought to be doing the sorts of things hunter-gatherers have always done. The hypothalamus knows what should be happening in the way of energy and food signals, and knows if things aren't "right." However, it doesn't have an efficient way to communicate that back to the neocortex. Likewise, the neocortex doesn't know what the hypothalamus is expecting. In fact, most neocortices don't even know they have a hypothalamus, much less that they are out of sync with it. You could argue, though, that the conscious self, the neocortex, is actually in control in a larger sense, as it can decide what gets eaten, and what energy gets expended. Would it be possible to facilitate a link between the hypothalamus and the neocortex? Sounds like it would be a health win-win. Perhaps meditation accomplishes this.

The actual functioning of the hypothalamus-amygdala-hippocampus brain trust is almost a complete unknown. To investigate, they stick a knife in it somewhere and observe what breaks. No joke—this is actually what they do. This is like figuring out how a laptop works by drilling holes in it.

The hypothalamus has a billion neurons, which sounds like a lot, but the neocortex has 50-100 times that. The hypothalamus has sensor neurons all over the body gathering information on all sorts of things, and so has a very detailed picture of the general state of things. It has outbound nerves connecting to various organs for fast, specific stimulation. It also controls the pituitary gland, a little hormone factory that will, on command, squirt them into the bloodstream. And the hypothalamus is tiny: the size of an almond.

The pair of amygdalae have around 12 million neurons between them, the pair of hippocampi, 100 million. These decline with age. The hypothalamus, hippocampi, and amygdalae are very interconnected.

These "brains" have a pedigree of note. There are a hypothalamus, amygdala, and hippocampus, doing more or less the same sorts of things, in every vertebrate from our ancient hagfish ancestor on down. Most of these ancient ancestors had no neocortex at all. That type of brain is a relatively recent invention.

When it comes to hormone regulation, all roads seem to lead to the hypothalamus. Many bodily functions once thought to be managed independently by various organs (the liver, for instance) turn out to be controlled and regulated by the hypothalamus. These organs are still doing the same things they are known for, but all of them are under the control of the hypothalamus. More accurately, the hypothalamus is trying to control everything, but it isn't always succeeding. The body can become overloaded, and when it is—from too much starch, for instance—the hypothalamus cannot regulate properly. This causes various hormones and other biochemicals to deviate from their ideal levels, and in turn, many problems follow.

Perhaps "under the control of the hypothalamus" is too strong a term. The liver will trundle along, doing its hepatic thing, even if the hypothalamus is totally removed. It just won't do it as precisely. An apt analogy for the role of the hypothalamus would be an orchestra conductor. If you shoot the conductor, the orchestra can play on, but it's likely to be a bit sloppy and out of time.

In any case, the idea of centralized control can only go so far. Many processes are clearly controlled locally, especially if they evolved before the hypothalamus. The immune system would be a good example. In response to a wound, a little army of specialized white blood cells mobilizes to deal with it, and there doesn't appear to be any hypothalamic activity involved here. First things first, perhaps.

A lot of cellular growth and repair is locally controlled as well, although the hypothalamus can curtail things if it is in a mood to conserve. Blood pressure is locally, regionally, and centrally controlled.

LAND AND DIVERSITY

Around 450 million years ago, plants started to appear on an otherwise barren planet. Around 50 million years later, the insects appeared, and 100 million years after that (300 million years ago), we vertebrates decided to go ashore as well. Fins became fingers and feet. Some sorts of lizard-like creatures would undertake colonization of all these new lands.

Insects and plants were there to greet us, and in abundance. This was a windfall for the vertebrates. With pretty much free rein in this new and delicious environment, they could evolve and expand *ad libitum*; all the tools were there. The closed circulation system facilitated growth to enormous sizes, adaptation to various weather extremes, and metabolism of broad varieties of food. The hypothalamus and hippocampus enabled adaptation. Diversity soared as new opportunities became available. The world was warm and wet—a golden age of vertebrates. Thus evolved reptiles of all sorts, birds, and, hiding in the shadows, mammals. We were nocturnal tree creatures, to better avoid being eaten.

The final organ, the lungs, completes the kit needed for terrestrial living. We now have all the pieces we need.

The next step is mammals, and indeed we turned up around 250 million years ago, probably appearing as hairy-looking lizards. The various features that distinguish mammals, hair, warm-bloodedness, live young, and milk production, seem to have arrived in bits and pieces, with some mammals lacking one or more of these functions still around today.

The hair and warm-bloodedness may well have been adaptations to nocturnal life, given the panoply of predators about in the daytime.

In any event, the fates of many of these wondrous creatures were sealed several hundred million years earlier when a chance collision in the asteroid belt sent one large rock flying out of orbit with our name on it.

THE K-T EVENT

Though it probably didn't seem like it at the time, the huge asteroid that slammed into the Gulf of Mexico 66 million years ago was a windfall for us, or rather for our furry little tree-dwelling ancestors. The 75% of life forms that became extinct included 100% of our predators. Things were probably pretty bleak for a decade or so, then recovery began, and the world, as they say, was our oyster.

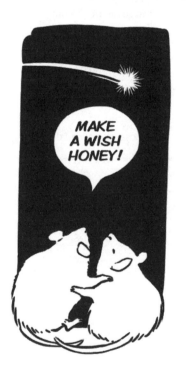
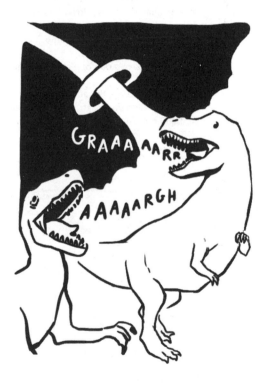

Things moved rapidly ahead. A few million years after the asteroid, lemur-like monkeys had appeared, followed by the real monkeys, the orangutans, the gorillas, and the final fork, seven million years ago, into chimpanzees and humans. We are so genetically similar to the chimps that we can share blood transfusions.

We suppose the human-chimp ancestor was monkey-like. We don't know. No fossils have been found. We have both been evolving, but measured genetically, the chimps have evolved more than us, and have come up with two items we could certainly use: they don't die from AIDS, and they don't get malaria. We, on the other hand, became the most adaptable animal ever known, able to thrive in good health, free of degenerative disease in almost any environment.

We had finally arrived, though we would need several million years to get to our present situation.

Key Points
18 - Vertebrates
- The hagfish is the oldest known vertebrate.
- Vertebrates have an internal skeleton and (usually) a soft exterior.
- Vertebrates have a closed circulation system. Octopus and squid are the only other animals that have this.
- All vertebrates have a hypothalamus, which regulates energy and performs many other control functions.
- All vertebrates have a pair of hippocampi and amygdalae for fear and memory processing.
- With vertebrates came the addition of the adaptive immune system.
- Around 300 million years ago, vertebrates adapted to land.
- Around 250 million years ago, mammals emerged.
- The K-T event, which caused the extinction of the (large) dinosaurs, opened the ecological pathway for mammals.

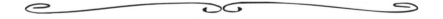

19 - HUNTER-GATHERERS AND THE AGRICULTURAL REVOLUTION

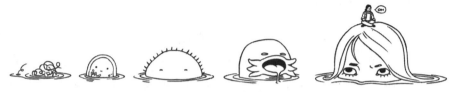

O nly the penguins at the South Pole were safe. Throughout the entire rest of the world, a new predator, of a sort never seen before, had emerged: cunning, ruthless, and able to kill from a distance.

On the eve of the agricultural revolution, hunter-gatherers had spread throughout the planet, were occupying every continent but one, and were thriving in climates both temperate and inhospitable. Everyone today is genetically identical to these people: they are our direct ancestors.

Though degenerative disease was unknown in those ancient times, a myriad of other trials and tribulations typically befell hunter-gatherers. Infectious disease was the primary cause of death, but in some regions, warfare was so endemic that up to 30% died from that. There were further perils from childbirth, accidents, and starvation, but the hunter-gatherers consistently transcended their condition and found ways to adapt, survive, and thrive. The reason is clear: our big brains gave us huge advantages.

BIG BRAINS

As an apex predator, a human being is an unlikely candidate. One needn't search far in the animal kingdom to find abilities that far exceed our own. Virtually every carnivore can outrun us. We can't escape through the air. We foolishly lost our ability to swing through the trees. We have no armor plate or tough leather coat. We are poorly camouflaged. It's amazing that the better equipped creatures haven't already hunted us to extinction.

When we split with the chimps seven million years ago, we took an evolutionary path that favored big brains. The chimps may have as well, but we clearly won the race, as our brain is now about three times the size of theirs. Which path was it that got our brains growing? This is yet another unknown, though one intriguing notion is that there may have been a semiaquatic phase. We like water and are hairless. Chimps don't and aren't.

The ever increasing brain-size trend apparently hasn't continued. Human brains 10,000 years ago were slightly larger than today's models. But what did our ancestors do with those big brains?

Tools and Weaponry

Many animals use tools, but the typical uses are very immediate and primitive, even with chimps. The usual example is termite fishing, wherein a chimp chooses and modifies sticks to extract termites from mounds. But the notion of using tools for somewhat larger game doesn't appear to have occurred to them yet. And why not? How much brain does it take to haul some rocks up a tree and pepper them on predator and prey alike?

To make a meal out of any animal larger than a bug, more serious weaponry would be needed. Sticks and stones were a good start. The domestication of fire gained us a great defense against marauders, and the first spear, a stick with a fire-hardened point, soon became possible. Then a sharp stone tip was added, and finally a slinging sort of device called a spear-thrower, which greatly increased the spear's velocity and range. Already deadly at a distance, someone soon thought of the bow and arrow. This one is a relatively recent development, perhaps 15,000 years ago. Poison-tipped arrows were soon added. There are many other ways to catch animals. One can build traps of various sorts. Ambush is possible if animals migrate along certain vulnerable pathways, or are driven there. No end in sight to this ingenuity.

How good were we at this? Hunter-gatherers today do not live on the most desirable lands; these were taken from them eons ago. They instead survive in remote, inhospitable places that "civilized" man had no use for. We would not expect these to be the most productive habitats. Even so, these modern hunter-gatherers typically spend less than 20 hours a week obtaining their food. This leaves a lot of time to play, sing, tell stories, practice weaponry, invent new and clever gadgetry, and so on.

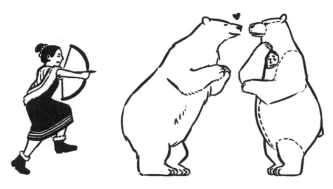

ONE CAN ALSO USE DECEPTION.

Culinary Diversity

Our large brains clearly helped here. For vegetal matter, this would involve a thorough knowledge of what could be eaten. Apparently we are able to eat a huge number of "forest products" that we don't see in grocery stores. Various roots, leaves, mushrooms, etc. Hunter-gatherers would know both the nutritional and medical uses of all these.

From Anthony McMichael, "Typically there is great diversity... Australian Aborigines make use of a total of around 200 different animals . . . 100 different plants. The San and !Kung people 150 plants and 100 animals. With that dietary diversity, micronutrient deficiencies are very unlikely."

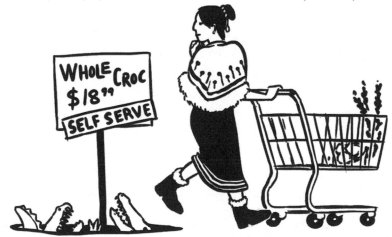

This is indeed variety. Can the local supermarket match it? There are literally thousands of edible and often delicious plants that simply aren't grown commercially. Many are regional, and many don't travel well. And meats? Do you ever eat antelope, bighorn sheep, kangaroo, crocodile, turtle, squirrel, gopher, armadillo, snake, lizard, insects, or larvae?

Despite various claims, there is no evidence that hunter-gatherers were vegans. Why would they be unless it was forced upon them? Animal product is nutritionally denser, richer in micronutrients, and can be better preserved for future lean times.

Flexible Metabolism

We can't eat rock or crude oil like some bacteria, but we can do well with just about any mix of protein, fat, or carbohydrate. These are quite dissimilar and require very specific cellular machinery. Most animals are not omnivores, which greatly restricts their range and diet. Mastery of fire would improve and extend our cuisine as well.

Mindfulness

The notion of existential vacuum is a new one, and there are billion-dollar drug and counseling industries built around the inability of many people to cope with our interconnected, multitasking world. We cannot know what really goes on in Washington, in boardrooms, or in other centers of power, yet these strongly affect our lives, health, and livelihoods. One could easily conclude that anxiety is built right into the system.

Nothing prepared us for such problems. The hunter-gatherers' world was immediate and direct. Everyone knew who they were, where they were going, and what was expected of them. Apparently these societies were quite egalitarian. There must have been alienated or outcast people, but it never seems to have been the norm. By necessity, hunter-gatherers would be connected to their environment, and we suppose had the wisdom to manage its exploitation, at least the bands that survived and thrived. Some Native Americans would apologize to an animal's spirit, explaining that they were sorry to kill it, but had to eat. (Apparently they didn't extend this courtesy to fish.)

This modern view of an enlightened ancient people in harmony with their environment is in sharp contrast with the 19th-century view of ruthless, treacherous savages. We suppose both views are correct in differing times and places. There are many examples of culturally similar people migrating to environmentally similar places and coming to very different ends, some thriving today, and others lasting only a few generations.

Could mindfulness and collective wisdom partly explain human success? Possibly. We would certainly hope so.

ANTHROPOLOGICAL SIDEBAR
Just Who Were the Neanderthals?

These people left Africa 200,000 years ago. They were very similar to modern humans, with a somewhat larger, but differently shaped brain. They thrived all over Europe and Asia until our arrival 50,000 years ago. Within 10,000 years, they were all gone—or were they?

Recent very clever DNA sequencing has concluded that non-African humans share 4% of their DNA with Neanderthals. There is one and only one way to "get" DNA. So somewhere, in some ancient forest, Neanderthal-human offspring were at play. Mitochondrial DNA is only transmitted maternally, and ours differs from the Neanderthal's, which would mean a Neanderthal dad and a human mom. The other possibility might have also produced children, but we find no descendants today.

One of several definitions of species is the ability to conceive fertile offspring. Could we then say that Neanderthals were the same species as us—homo sapiens? We fulfill the fertile offspring requirement, but only partly, so this is up in the air. But in some sense, the Neanderthals clearly do live on. Indeed, 4% DNA is a fair amount. Someone with a Chinese great-great-great grandparent would be at least 3% Asian. What did some of us get from our Neanderthal ancestors? Blond and red hair—and excessive amounts of it—along with blue eyes are strong candidates. In all this genetic investigation, another unknown ancient human turned up as well, which they are calling Denisovans. We are 4% this guy too, though we know practically nothing about him, no fossils having been found.

ELDERLY HUNTER-GATHERERS

Gurven and Kaplan have provided us with an excellent analysis of mortality among extant hunter-gatherer groups. There is, as would be expected, considerable death caused by the harsh nature of the lifestyle. However, those that make it to 50 will probably make it to 75 or more. For these elderly, the causes of death still tend to be illness, accident, or violence. Degenerative disease death rates (cancer and cardiovascular) appear to be around 2%.

This research strongly contradicts the general view we were taught: that hunter-gatherer life was "nasty, brutish, and short." It appears that this more aptly applied to "civilized" society, at least until 150 years ago.

Man lives far longer than animals of similar size. This is no recent development and would have been true 10,000 years ago. There clearly has to be some evolutionary advantage to attaining old age, but no one really knows what it is. One theory, called the Grandmother Hypothesis, holds that a society benefits by freeing the younger women for hunting and gathering while the grandmothers raise the children. While this Paleolithic daycare idea sounds charming, no modern tribes practice it. Longevity may also be due to the uniquely human ability to communicate acquired knowledge and skills. Or maybe not. Chimps live an abnormally long time as well.

HUNTER-GATHERER BLOOD TEST NUMBERS

There is some such data available today for the few remaining tribes. How the data was obtained would be an interesting story in and of itself. In any case, the numbers are almost always pristine even if the specific lifestyles are varied and rugged. Here are some various measurements obtained from a variety of tribes.

Measurement	Ideal value	Americans aged 55	Typical hunter-gatherer value
Blood pressure	110/70	145/85	110/70
Total cholesterol	150	215	125-158 mg/dl
Triglycerides	70	110	73 mg/dl
Glucose	75	103	72 mg/dl

These are quite impressive numbers. It is reasonable to speculate that instances of degenerative disease would be low, which is, of course, confirmed in various skeletal remains that have been discovered as well as in extant tribes.

THE AGRICULTURAL REVOLUTION

Imagine the shock of replacing a life of relative leisure, freedom, and equality, with one of toil and slavery. This is what the agricultural revolution, which began 10,000 years ago, meant to 98% of its participants—the have-nots. A few hours of daily hunting and gathering were replaced by 10-14 hours of repetitive, backbreaking toil; and the varied diet, with its numerous beneficial micronutrients, was likewise replaced by a low-grade starch fare, which was frequently in short supply as well. Further, crowded and unsanitary conditions would prove ideal breeding grounds for new bacterial and viral pathogens.

In the May 1987 issue of *Discover* magazine, noted scientist Jared Diamond called the agricultural revolution "The worst mistake in the history of the human race." This is a rather stark statement when juxtaposed against the standard textbook version that we all grew up on: that the agricultural revolution was a transition from a crude and desperate savage life to an orderly, well-fed agrarian society.

Diamond's premise is that this orderly schoolbook view is simply untrue. People converted to agriculture either out of desperation (perhaps due to diminished resources) or because they were forced to. He mentions that worldwide, hunter-gatherer societies spend little time working and a lot of time sleeping and playing. Further, they are far less affected by famines, as they tend to have dozens of potential foods available rather than one staple crop. This is based on evidence gathered from modern hunter-gatherer societies, who by and large occupy marginal lands of no interest to the agricultural settlers.

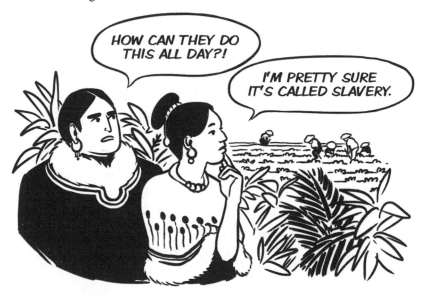

There is a convincing historical record as well. Skeletons of hunter-gatherers and their agricultural peers have been unearthed, and the differences are dramatic. The hunter-gatherer men were 5'9" and the women 5'5". The nearby agriculturists were 5'3" and 5'0". Even as late as the Middle Ages, heights were only beginning to catch up.

Another dig, from an Illinois burial mound, traces a Native American group through their transition from a hunter-gathering lifestyle to corn farming. Numerous skeletal effects, strongly indicative of sharply reduced health, were found. Teeth were bad, and bones had lesions indicating disease and nutritional problems.

The change also brought about class difference. The "haves"—the lucky 2%—tended to be several inches taller and far healthier than the other 98%.

While these notions may be easily dismissed by those of us in today's wealthy West, consider Diamond's challenge: "Would you rather be a subsistence farmer in Ethiopia today, or a Kalahari Bushman?"

The Decline of the Hunter-Gatherers

What caused the decline? In the case of North and South America, hunter-gatherers were wiped out by European infectious disease to which they had no immunity. Deadly disease was the primary Old-World weapon, and went a lot further toward conquering the indigenous peoples than any warfare. In particular, smallpox would often wipe out entire tribes.

Of course, the Old-World invaders were far better equipped and organized as well, though usually less numerous.

By contrast, in Europe and Asia it was always a case of numbers. An army of 500 would always defeat a far healthier hunter-gatherer band of 50.

Agricultural societies could support 10 times the population density, or even a 100. And they indeed did. That was rather the point. But the shift did not happen overnight. Perhaps as recently as 1,000 years ago, half of us were still hunter-gatherers, and given the reality of the transition, who would be in a hurry? Again from Diamond: a Bushman, when asked why his people hadn't adopted agriculture, replied, "Why should we, when there are so many mongongo nuts in the world?"

PROGRESS

Very, very gradually, the lot of the "modern" world peoples improved, punctuated by enormous setbacks such as the Black Death, huge wars, etc. Even in 19th-century Europe, a bad harvest meant starvation for many.

In 1850 England, the life expectancy of urban workers was just under 25 years. Life expectancy averages include everyone, the infants and the elderly alike. The odds were better than 50:50 that you would die before you were 15. If you made it that far, you would probably live another 20 years. Death was almost entirely due to infectious disease, which was rampant. There was no sanitation (sewer systems), few sources of clean water, little medical help, and extremely crowded living conditions.

Significant progress was finally about to be made. One thing missing from our wonderfully evolved immune system is a way to transfer our immunities to our children. Although there is some evidence of immune "memory" via genetics, the explicit immunities recorded by the adaptive immune system seem to die with us, and we don't have a way to directly pass these on to the next generation. But using our big brains, we figured out a way to do something equivalent, and the result was stunning. For the first time in the history of eukaryotic life, the bacteria were no longer going to be winning the arms race.

By the beginning of the 19th century, it was more or less known that smallpox was preventable. A century earlier, the "vaccination" consisted of deliberately infecting people with smallpox, which generally resulted in a less severe case, and conferred lifelong immunity. Smallpox is a killer, with death rates approaching 90% for children under six. Those few who had access to doctors in the 18th century were generally inoculated. It was also known that milkmaids never got smallpox, but they all got cowpox, a related but far less lethal pathogen. Would this be protective?

Edward Jenner decided to explore this possibility. He deliberately infected his gardener's child with cowpox and, once the child had recovered, made repeated efforts to infect him with actual smallpox, all of which were fully resisted. (Imagine a new drug being tested this way today!) Jenner had the political capital needed to promulgate the cowpox solution as well. It was Jenner that coined the word *vaccine*, from the root word *vacca*, latin for cow.

In the 19th century, progress would be made in two major areas: sanitation and the bacterial theory of disease. The former would remove the most common cause of frequent epidemics, especially of cholera and typhoid, and the latter would lead to immunization.

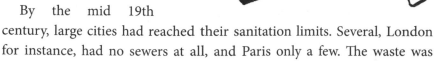

I'M NOT FALLING FOR THAT ONE AGAIN!

By the mid 19th century, large cities had reached their sanitation limits. Several, London for instance, had no sewers at all, and Paris only a few. The waste was collected locally, and removed manually if at all. Water quality was likewise unreliable. Typhoid and cholera epidemics were common, and contaminated water was but one of several possible causes.

In England, Dr. John Snow, who could also be called the father of anesthesia, was convinced that a cholera outbreak in London in 1854 was the result of some sort of bacterial contamination. At first, other theories prevailed, one being that the cause was miasma, or foul odor, which, in sewerless London, was in no short supply. Others blamed the weak constitution of the working classes, and so on. To further convince his peers, Snow sent people out to survey the affected neighborhoods and record the source of their drinking water, eventually narrowing the problem to a single pump. Snow's theory finally carried the day. (The idea of determining disease cause by examining the habits of groups of people is now called epidemiology. Snow could make a reasonable paternity claim there as well.)

Snow's work had a double effect. Cities started installing sewer systems and making efforts to insure a supply of clean water. The bacterial theory of disease would remain a subject of debate, though.

The existence of bacteria had been known for 200 years, having been discovered by the Dutch Leeuwenhoek in 1680, but no one could grasp any way by which these tiny "animalcules," as Leeuwenhoek termed them, could cause any threat to us, creatures so enormously larger. Logical enough, but what was causing all these diseases?

Enter Louis Pasteur. A brilliant scientist, but one who had lost three children to typhoid, Pasteur was convinced that bacteria were responsible for a large number of problems. One major cause was spoilage of liquids by bacteria. It was widely believed that bacteria could "spontaneously generate." (No one at the time had any idea how complex bacteria were.)

This being France, the liquid of primary interest was wine. Pasteur did a series of clever experiments and managed to convince *les savants* of the time that if you killed all the bacteria, they would not regenerate. He killed them by heating the liquid and keeping it sealed. This worked, and the process bears his name to this day: pasteurization.

THEY'RE ONTO US!

Ancient Medicine Sidebar
Medieval Medicine

It is not too hard to pin down when Western medicine began doing more good than harm to the people it served. A safe date would be 1890. The importance of sterility had taken hold, anesthetics had been developed, some vaccines were known, and the microbe theory of disease was safely established.

Prior to this, many serious wounds would result in death, and various sorts of epidemics were commonplace. A very learned 1826 British medical text has material on the cause of almost every known disease, and its appropriate treatment. The causes are almost completely wrong, and the cures are useless when they are not outright harmful.

The late 19th-century advances continued into the 20th. By 1960, most of the scourges of civilization had been conquered, and the medical profession was by all standards deservedly heroic. Its unfortunate segue into the Food Pyramid, high-carb diets, and other medical wild goose chases will hopefully be ultimately rectified and forgotten.

Nonetheless, when it comes to ineffective, misguided, and dangerous medicine, the European Middle Ages are hard to beat. The four humors theory was the central dogma, and most disease was therefore caused by an excess or lack of one of them. The four humors were blood, phlegm, and two types of bile, dark and yellow. An infection would usually produce a fair amount of pus, so clearly this had to be "expelled," typically by making the infection worse with goat dung or the like. This probably led to more amputations than cures, but at least any survivors had a thoroughly robust immune system. Most of these "cures" were presided over by the monasteries. They produced many learned texts, which only they could read, and all of which had almost no basis in fact.

In contrast, surgery of that period was practiced by barbers. This primarily consisted of bloodletting, but sometimes they dealt with wounds, especially if cutting were involved. Some of them followed antiseptic procedures, which would have helped.

The various bizarre procedures commonly practiced are not for the squeamish and will not be expounded upon here, except to say that they were as painful as they were generally useless.

There is one condition today that indeed has a medieval remedy. Excess circulating iron is not good, but is common in menopausal women. The cure for this is bloodletting. Of course, it's no longer called that. It's called therapeutic phlebotomy; less medieval.

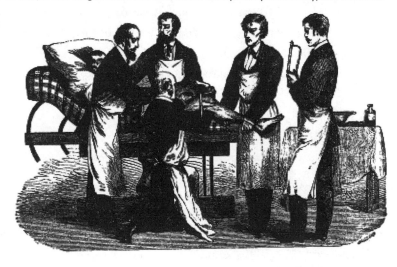

But Pasteur was convinced that the various microbes did a lot more than souring the wine. A key discovery was made via fortuitous accident (not at all rare in science). Pasteur was studying chicken cholera and had inoculated a brood directly with the disease. However, though the chicks got sick, they all recovered. Pasteur then discovered the "problem." His stock of cholera was weak, lacking in virulence. Would this work? Could you produce a weakened version of a dreaded disease and achieve immunity? The answer was yes of course, and Pasteur went on to conquer an impressive list of diseases, notably anthrax and rabies. Blissfully, there are no anecdotes about Pasteur experimenting on his servants' children.

The end was in sight. We now knew the cause, and we also had the potential technology to effect a cure. It remained to identify and conquer the rest of the lethal microbes and devise a means of distribution (still a major problem). One by one they would fall: typhoid - 1896, tetanus - 1897, diphtheria - 1905, whooping cough - 1925, yellow fever - 1937, polio - 1953, hepatitis B - 1980, but the battle never ends. Bacteria and viruses are famous for rapidly evolving, and new pathogens appear like AIDS and Ebola. Nonetheless, we are winning the battle. A century ago, a fever could be nothing, or it could mean a fatal disease, and for half the children of the era, it indeed did. This is clearly no longer the case.

With infectious disease, if not conquered, in full retreat, we should be in the golden age of health. In many ways we are. Life spans have doubled—even tripled—in the last 100 years. However, we didn't arrive where we might have. We aren't living disease-free and we are not living as long as we potentially could.

What went wrong? We have to take a deeper look into the cells to find out.

Key Points

19 - Hunter-Gatherers and the Agricultural Revolution

- Hunter-gatherers became the improbable apex predator.
- Hunter-gatherers seldom got degenerative disease.
- Average brain size 10,000 years ago was slightly larger than today.
- The agricultural revolution had huge negative health impact.
- Civilized health would slowly get better.
- Vaccines were discovered and most infectious disease was conquered.
- In the last 100 years, degenerative disease has replaced infectious disease as the leading cause of death.

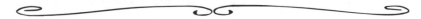

20 - DEGENERATIVE DISEASE
OVERVIEW

Most, if not all, degenerative disease is a direct result of chronic stress, either systemic or cellular or both. The causes of this stress are many, and it almost seems that modern society has conspired to make this so.

We divide lifestyle into four areas. Which choices are made in each contribute significantly to disease cause or cure. Here are the four, along with some of the problems typically associated with them.

Nutrition. Cells are not receiving the micronutrients they need, and at the same time are overloaded with glucose, insulin, and triglycerides.

Exercise. Lack of physical activity directly inhibits the powerful healing properties of HDL, and idle cells tend to load up with toxic trash, free radicals being the best known.

Stress Management. Stress elevates cortisol. High cortisol down-regulates the immune system, increases fat storage, and raises insulin. All of these are promoters of cellular damage. High cortisol undermines the benefits of proper diet and exercise.

Sleep. A lot of the body's extensive cellular repair apparatus works only at night, when energy is not needed for other activities. Poor-quality or interrupted sleep is very detrimental.

Likewise, we focus mainly on the resulting diseases:

Atherosclerosis. This condition, a buildup of plaque in the arteries, leads to heart attacks and strokes. The cause of this buildup is primarily dietary. A correct diet greatly diminishes the proportion of dangerous circulating lipid particles (the main cause of the problem), while the correct exercise greatly elevates the amount and improves the intensity of the repairing mechanisms.

Adult Onset Diabetes. This syndrome, a state of high glucose, insulin, and triglycerides, is a perfect launchpad for all degenerative disease, and is mainly diet driven. It is readily reversed and cured with lifestyle change. Left uncured, multiple serious problems are all but inevitable.

Cancer. This is the unbridled proliferation of damaged cells. Cellular damage is common, but exacerbated by dietary elements, stress, and lack of exercise and sleep. The immune system is entirely capable of blocking cancer if not overloaded with poor lifestyle choices.

Osteoporosis. A sedentary lifestyle will slowly diminish bone strength. This is true for both men and women. Proper resistance exercise can halt osteoporosis and even reverse it.

Our lifestyle choices can also lead to rapid aging, dementia, and osteoarthritis, and these three are preventable as well.

QUANTITATIVE MEDICINE CURES DEGENERATIVE DISEASE

This is a vast statement, and if true, it is the health magic the world has been waiting for, wishing for. And it is completely true—demonstrably so, but the "medicine" part of it requires a lifelong self-discipline that may prove challenging for some, and our use of the word "cure" is not as broad as one could hope. Quantitative Medicine indeed cures degenerative disease, but if that degenerative disease has already taken some toll, perhaps a stroke, then that stroke isn't "cured." Quantitative Medicine cannot reverse that. But the risks one associates with aging are very reversible. That is a clock can be turned back. The sooner one acts, the greater the benefit, and the lesser the risk of any damage that cannot be undone.

Calling Quantitative Medicine "prevention" is to short-change it as well. The health attainable by practicing the Quantitative Medicine protocols is our natural state. It means a long, robust, and energetic life. It is the life we lived for countless millennia. The dietary norms of Western society, with its lack of exercise and chronic stress, are the causes of disease. To be well is simply a matter of knowing the healthy choices and adopting them. This is not disease prevention. This is disease evasion.

Degenerative disease proceeds in tiny steps. One cell mutates and divides. Will it grow into a tumor? Not if the correct life choices were made. Those dividing cells will be spotted and eliminated long before they become anything lethal. However, in their short but virulent life, they were a tiny cancer, a tiny tumor, and the body spotted it, and destroyed it. This is repeated in everyone millions of times. Tiny cancers are cured before modern medicine can even begin to detect them.

Likewise, an army of patrolling HDL particles is continuously removing toxic waste from behind artery walls. That waste is the fuel of atherosclerosis, and the body is curing it long before it can cause a heart attack or stroke.

Clearly a person cannot wait until they are 75 to start worrying about the health effects of their lifestyle. Our modern tragedy is that the choices that offer protection and a lifelong cure aren't practiced in our society, even though they could be. Healthy diets can be eaten. Starch is unhealthy; organic vegetables are healthy. For some reason, the government subsidizes the unhealthy one. Healthy exercises can be performed, but useless ones are preferred. We do have a chance to quiet the mind, integrate our wholeness, and dissociate from the swarm of stress we live in, yet those who seek this are ridiculed.

This brings us to two stark choices. We can either wait for our modern society to enlighten and become aware of what it is doing to itself—what we are doing to ourselves, really—or we can take control now, take matters into our own hands, and thereby choose our own destiny, and perhaps alter the destinies of those around us.

We are about to describe degenerative disease in detail. Our fervent hope is that the additional insight into the diseased state unlocks some doors. Those at risk of atherosclerosis can benefit from knowing exactly which dietary choices are promoting the disease, and which circulating biochemicals are actively involved in clearing it out. Such knowledge engenders a healing focus, a focus that can minimize the dangerous and boost the protective. It is enough to simply do the right thing, and this may be sufficient for many. For the terminally curious, the coming chapters take you a step beyond this into the world of *why*.

As in the preceding chapters, much is still unknown.

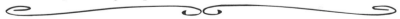

Personal Story Sidebar

My (Charles Davis') Health Measurement Experience

At age 55 we had our last child, a baby girl. I didn't want to drop dead when she was in junior high, so I went to Dr. Nichols and asked if he could order up a battery of tests to find out what I was all about, and hopefully, fix anything that was broken.

Unbeknownst to me, he was about to start a new practice based on this sort of thing and there I was, his initial Human Lab Rat.

I thought my health was pretty OK. I jogged once or twice a week and was trying to keep my weight down. It kept creeping up year by year anyway.

I was sent for a blood draw, which measured about 70 things, and a scan. I saw the scan results before Dr. Nichols and learned that I had calcium on my heart. This freaked me out. The blood tests were incomprehensible to me.

We met when all results were in and I was told the following:

1. You have borderline osteoporosis. (That was a shocker.)
2. The heart calcium is normal for your age and is the body's way to stabilize plaque, but we want to stop it from increasing.
3. Your cholesterol is a bit high, but you are genetically lucky here and don't have the small sized bad cholesterol particles that clog arteries, so we don't care.
4. You are lousy at metabolizing carbs, so a lot of what you eat gets stored as fat.

All this and more from one scan and a blood draw. He then said all this can be fixed, and I was expecting a bunch of pills, but not at all. He said there weren't any that did what I needed.

To stop and reverse the osteoporosis, I needed to stress the big bones. This causes them to gather in calcium, the absence of which is the cause of the disease. This means squats, deadlifts. Heavy lifting. This went fast. I was out of the danger zone within a few months.

To stop the accumulation of heart calcium, I should do exercises that ran my heart up and down. Exercises of an explosive nature. I should give up jogging, which he said was not very useful. So about the same amount of exercise time, but a totally different routine.

If I behaved, heart disease was off the table. This was the really good news.

I needed to get pickier about the carbs, cut out all starches and most fruit, sticking with meats, fish and colored vegetables.

I have doggedly kept this up and the baby girl is in high school. My bone density is in the top 25% now, meaning if I keep at it I am *never* going to have osteoporosis. The heart calcium has crept up a little, but way less than normal. I've got muscles out to there and all my prior chronic back problems are totally gone. My belly is mostly gone too. I built about 10 pounds of new bone and maybe 10 pounds of muscle, but weigh 10 pounds less than I did 14 years ago, so that's 30 pounds of blubber gone. "Now and then" photos show this clearly.

I am not particularly enamored with exercise, but love the results. No real problems sticking to the diet despite some occasional backsliding. I get a blood draw quarterly and a scan every couple of years. That is probably overkill.

With heart disease not an issue, my main health risk is cancer, and I have already had some problems with that. I am trying to modify my lifestyle to turn up cancer prevention. Time will tell; it's a work in progress.

21 - ATHEROSCLEROSIS - CAUSE AND CURE

Atherosclerosis is the buildup of fatty material and other undesirable detritus within the artery wall. It is an inevitable process, beginning in the womb. However, there are counter-processes at work to manage and reduce this load. Like most degenerative disease, progression is a question of which predominates.

Because of this tipping point property, atherosclerosis can be attacked by reducing the processes that build it up, by augmenting the processes that clear it, or preferably both. Diet, exercise, and stress level affect atherosclerosis in a variety of ways.

Atherosclerosis is, in most cases, reversible, but consequent damage, such as a heart attack, stroke, or embolism, is usually not. Nonetheless, further damage can be prevented.

INSIDE THE ARTERY

Recall that the artery has four layers: a tough outer layer, a layer of muscle, an intermediate fibrous layer, and finally an inner layer, the endothelium, which is in direct contact with the blood flow (lumen).

The endothelium is very complex. Its primary functions are nutrient delivery and waste disposal to and from the body's cells. The various ways that the endothelium accomplishes this were discussed in THE VASCULAR SYSTEM in chapter 18.

The endothelial cells seem to be set up to last forever, with life spans varying from a bit over a month to well over half a century. Why do we care about cell lifespan? There is a very important reason: when endothelial cells are being replaced, the artery leaks. This leakage is by far major cause of atherosclerosis, and tends to occur in certain areas where cell life is short. Why certain areas are vulnerable and how to counteract that will soon be covered in detail. (Veins don't leak—or at least not much—because unlike arteries, they are not under pressure.)

There is no regularly scheduled replacement program for endothelial cells of the sort we find for the intestinal or skin cells. Endothelial cells are only replaced when they become damaged beyond repair. Such a cell, terminally damaged, could potentially let quite a lot of material—good and bad—leak through. Very quickly, though, the leak will be plastered over with platelets, which will form a partial patch. Platelets are mini-cells, and their best known function is stopping a wound from bleeding. That's exactly what they are doing here, albeit on a very tiny scale. The platelet patches are temporary, and somewhat leaky.

Besides quickly constructing a patch, the platelets also emit SOS chemicals toward circulating replacement cells. (Although the endothelial cells can replicate in place, new cells usually come from individual cells circulating in the blood.) The platelets send out various chemical signals that act like a sci-fi movie tractor beam and pull the replacement cell into place. The replacement stitches itself to the adjacent cells, and the immune system cleans up and carts away the remains.

This all takes around 30 minutes. Fast, but not fast enough. Some stuff does leak through, and in particular, some toxic particles get through that the endothelium would otherwise have blocked had it been intact. Likewise, bacteria, even those which may have already been captured by circulating immune cells, might also manage to get through.

Why are there toxic particles around? Most cells dump their bodily junk back into the bloodstream or else spill it to the surrounding medium. The spills get mopped up by the lymph system, which eventually drains into the circulatory system anyway. So, any toxic junk will circulate until it is removed by the liver or kidneys.

This buildup of toxic trash behind the cell wall is the atherosclerosis. It only happens in arteries, and most of the time, only in certain places. The veins tend to stay out of trouble because they are not under pressure. Arterial pressure can be fairly forceful. The 120/80 sort of blood pressure number refers to the arteries only, and is quite enough pressure to force blood material through any small holes. Of course, higher blood pressures only make the situation worse. Of more interest, though, is why atherosclerosis seems to set up shop at certain sites. The reasons for this will give us some very useful tools for effectively combating this life-threatening disease.

A Very Short Course in Fluid Mechanics

Fluid mechanics is a branch of civil engineering, and studies how fluids flow. If a fluid flows slowly across a flat surface, it is well behaved, all the fluid goes in the same direction, and all is predictable.

To visualize this, draw a bath, and run your hand slowly through the water. The water is hardly disturbed and flows gently around your hand. Now repeat this, but with rapid motions. Things are no longer well behaved. A wake will form behind your hand and little eddy currents will set up on the sides. This is non-uniform or turbulent flow. Flow is rapid in some areas, but is very slow or may even stop or reverse in others.

Fluid in any pipe, an artery being a pertinent example here, has a tendency to be poorly behaved and turbulent. That is simply the nature of fluid flowing in pipes, and there is nothing to be done about that. Whenever the flow turbulent and non-uniform, there will be areas where the flow is slow, stationary, or even reversed, and it is in these spots that problems arise. The most problematic flows are found at bends or branches, and the arteries are full of these.

Areas of slow, no, or reverse flow are the common sites for atherosclerosis. There are several reasons for this. First, in order to deliver nutrients to hungry cells, blood must be flowing. If, due to non-uniform flow, the blood is just sitting still, or moving slowly, the cells will not get enough food and oxygen. They will become weak and die more frequently, and when they do, they will leak badly. Second, stress on the cell will be exacerbated by circulating toxins, which are likely to stick on regions of the endothelium where there is minimal blood flow. A regular or rapid blood flow will wash such toxins off the endothelial wall. Finally, the repairing platelets and replacement cells will be slower to arrive, since they are carried in the blood. These three problems, all of which occur at regions where arterial blood flow is low, are the root causes of atherosclerosis.

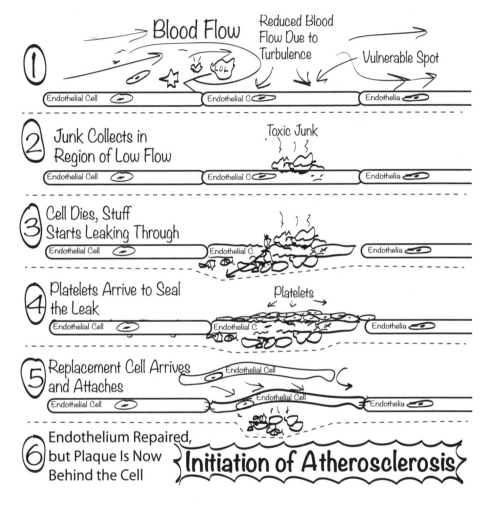

We aren't stuck with this unfortunate state of affairs, though. We can't rewrite the laws of fluid mechanics, but we can do plenty to alter and vary the flow. We can also change the amount of circulating toxins. We can even force some of the toxins toward larger sizes so that they can't slip through the temporary platelet patches. If all these are done and done correctly, atherosclerosis will reverse.

Some of these remedies are dietary, and others are driven by exercise.

Exercise and Endothelial Health

Exercise of the right sort causes blood to rush along the endothelium and literally scrubs it clean. Any unwelcome junk that may have gotten attached will be washed off. This is just what we want. Further, this rushing flow will also alter the flow patterns, and the areas that suffer from slow or no blood flow will temporarily adopt new briskly flowing patterns. If the heart rate is varied, up to the max and back down repeatedly, the entire endothelium will spend at least some time enjoying the benefits of rapid blood flow. This alone will prevent heart disease. Finally, a lot of fresh blood was made available, thus helping out any cells in nutritional need. Hence, exercise which features large changes in heart rate accomplishes quite a lot, especially in the slow-flowing danger zones. The mitochondria benefit as well. The cells become more capable of taking up and using oxygen.

Note that aerobic exercise, where the heart rate is elevated to some fixed level and held there, will not accomplish all of these benefits. Because the elevated rate of blood flow is uniform, the variety of flow patterns does not occur, and some of the slow-flow regions will not receive the rapid flow benefits. This is definitely better than nothing at all (unless carried to extremes), but significantly less effective than intense exercise.

Diet and Endothelial Health

Other than fiber, almost everything eaten ends up in the bloodstream, whether needed or not. A lot of processes, several of which have already been discussed, cooperate to deal with potential overloads. Excess glucose tends to be converted to triglycerides and stored as fat. Excess fat is usually burned unless accompanied by excess sugar, in which case it is stored as fat as well. Toxins such as pesticides may be removed by the liver, the kidneys, or even neutralized by immune system cells. However, all this doesn't happen at once, and while all the dietary excesses and toxins are still circulating, they can cause problems. Besides getting behind cells, or sticking to them and damaging them, they might also trigger other processes that are rough on the cells, such as inflammation.

LDL

What about LDL? The cardiac arch-criminal, accused for years of causing all the atherosclerotic woes, can be a problem, but only if it gets oxidized.

For decades, the "solution" has been to lower LDL, usually with statins, and sometimes with other drugs. This has in large part failed. No drug, including statins, has shown an overall reduction of mortality, and several have made things worse. Cholesterol is essential to life, and lowering it is not the solution. There is mounting evidence that attempting to do so is causing problems. The hypothalamus has set cholesterol to a quite specific level for some good reason, and we shouldn't be second-guessing that.

Rather than rolling the dice with statins, or otherwise meddling with a regulated bodily system, there are several things that will diminish the oxidized LDL threat in far healthier ways. The first line of defense is keeping the size of the LDL particles large. The platelets covering the dying endothelial cells form a pretty tight mesh. Circulating cells don't get in at all, and neither do the larger molecules, and this includes larger LDL particles. In fact, a predominance of large LDL particles will reduce cardiac events two to threefold.

But how can LDL size be controlled? This is pretty easy, but the reason it works is rather counterintuitive. LDL particle size tracks inversely with triglycerides. High triglycerides (circulating fat) means small particles and vice versa. This is an important relationship. More in a bit.

But how is the triglyceride level controlled? Triglycerides are fat. For a long time, the official dogma was "don't eat fat, especially saturated fat." In fact, this is still the official dogma. But it's wrong, and here's the paradox. Eating fat is not what makes triglycerides soar. It is instead high glucose levels, and the subsequent insulin burst, that pushes triglycerides to high levels. There are two reasons for this. First, high insulin tells the cells to use glucose for energy and ignore circulating fat (the preferred energy source for most cells), and second, the liver will convert excess circulating glucose to—you probably guessed it—yet more triglycerides.

So the solution to high triglycerides is simple: cutting down on glucose (primarily starches, sugars, and fruits) will reduce triglycerides and raise the LDL particle size up. Predominance of the larger size is called Pattern A. The necessary triglyceride reduction needed to achieve this pattern varies, but the threshold tends to be somewhere near 100 mg/dl.

Even if excess fat is eaten, so long as it is eaten in the absence of carbs, triglycerides will not increase and will typically fall, especially if coming from high-carb, low-fat regimes. Triglycerides do rise momentarily, but the cells will take the fat out of circulation very quickly. Cells love fat.

SCIENTIFIC DETAIL SIDEBAR

The Endothelium

The endothelium is a lot more than just a simple lining. It could be considered an organ in its own right, albeit an oddly shaped one.

Before we get into its many interesting functions, let's consider how you might repair a damaged endothelium. Most renewable cells have stem or progenitor cells nearby, ready to generate new material should the need arise. Not the case with the endothelium, but it is so important there are two renewal methods. First, unlike most replaceable cells, it can divide. But this apparently isn't good enough. The body also circulates progenitor cells in the blood that can differentiate into endothelial cells if needed. These particular cells come from the bone marrow, which makes sense since the other circulating red and white blood cells also originated there.

So besides providing a slippery lining, what else does the endothelium do? Here is part of the repertoire:

Selective Barrier. When the arteries branch down to capillaries, the two outer layers disappear, leaving only the endothelium and the basement membrane. Oxygen and nutrients need to escape to the nearby cells, and waste product, CO_2 for instance, needs to be transported out. The passage of these various nutrients and biochemicals is controlled by the endothelium.

Nitric Oxide. This important molecule is generated by the endothelium and is involved in vasodilation by relaxing the nearby muscles that form the outer part of the artery or vein. In fact, one cause of high blood pressure is insufficient nitric oxide. Of the numerous things affecting blood pressure, nitric oxide is one of the most local.

Angiogenesis. This is the growing of new blood vessels. This might occur as part of the healing process following a wound. In a clogged area, the body will try to grow new blood vessels around the clog. There are also implications in cancer, as tumors cannot grow much larger than a grain of rice without a blood supply.

Prevention of Clotting. Blood clots quickly so that you don't bleed to death from a wound. But circulating blood that clotted could kill you. A clot needs some surface to stick to in order to get started. However, the endothelium has a very slippery coating that prevents this. If the endothelium is missing or damaged, the underlying material may initiate a clot, especially if it breaks off and escapes into the bloodstream.

A damaged endothelium is always associated with heart disease. Arterial health is largely synonymous with endothelial health. Endothelial damage can come from the toxicity of plaque deposits in the cell wall, from mechanical stresses, and from disease.

Note that soaring triglycerides have another sinister consequence. If triglycerides are high, they remain in circulation as LDL particles longer, and this gives more time for something to go wrong. Oxidized LDL particles are indeed bad news. They can kill any cells that they manage to stick to and will set off a chain reaction of havoc if they manage to get behind cell walls. So keeping triglyceride levels down and their lifetimes short has doubly beneficial consequences. This is primarily diet driven.

High Chronic Stress Will Cause Atherosclerosis

High chronic stress will raise cortisol, which in turn raises insulin which raises triglycerides, which then decreases LDL particle size, which increases the risk of atherosclerosis. Additionally, chronic stress will increase inflammation, increase potential clotting, and reduce endothelial repair. High chronic stress can cause atherosclerosis as effectively as bad diet, perhaps more so.

Triglycerides, Insulin, Sugar, and Starch

Triglycerides are fat. Cells run on them. There are two sources: our last meal and our liver. Triglycerides aren't soluble in blood, so as an additional step, triglycerides are packaged in water-soluble particles called lipoproteins.

The triglycerides from our last meal are packaged into chylomicron lipoproteins by our intestines, which send them, via the lymph system, directly into the bloodstream. Chylomicrons have only a small amount of cholesterol.

The triglycerides made by the liver are packaged into VLDL particles. Viewed from the outside, these are very similar to chylomicrons. Both have an outer layer of water-soluble proteins, then a thick layer of triglycerides. The VLDL particle, however, has a center composed of cholesterol.

As these VLDL and chylomicron particles circulate, hungry cells pluck off the triglycerides. The chylomicrons are gone in minutes, and within a few hours, most of the VLDL particles are picked down to their cholesterol core. These particles, now a lot smaller, are renamed LDL, and are essentially a little ball of 50% cholesterol, 30% fat. If a cell needs cholesterol, it will engulf this entire particle. Otherwise it continues to circulate. Various other processes will eventually take the particle out of circulation, or it may manage to get itself stuck behind an artery wall.

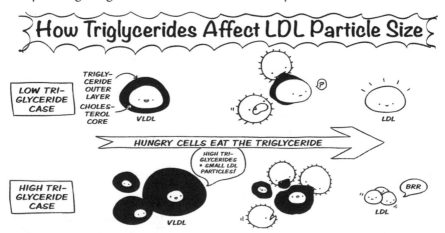

If triglyceride levels are high, the liver makes larger VLDL particles, and crucially, makes more of them. What is crucial about this? The amount of cholesterol the liver allows in circulation is regulated, and stays constant. If the liver makes *more* VLDL particles, then each particle is going to get a smaller ration of cholesterol. Later on, when most of the triglycerides have been picked off, the result is a much smaller LDL particle—just what we do not want.

Oddly, it has been known since the '50s that high carbohydrate consumption causes high triglycerides, and that high triglycerides, in turn, cause heart disease has been known almost as long. Makes you wonder how the high-carb dietary fad of the last several decades ever met medical muster. It's done enormous harm.

Eating a high-fat-diet low-carb diet doesn't increase triglycerides. If triglycerides were elevated due to a high-carb diet, a high-fat diet will usually cause them to drop, and drop fairly quickly. There will be weight loss as well.

Adult onset diabetics can have fasting triglyceride levels of 500 mg/dl or more. Over 150 is considered borderline high by most doctors. Actually, a lower target is preferable, something under 100, or even less. To get there, sugar, starch, and alcohol would have to be cut. Getting triglycerides below 75 will almost always increase the size of the LDL particles to Pattern A, and thus reduce the amount getting behind the artery wall.

Triglycerides and LDL Pattern Size

If triglycerides are below a certain "tipping-point" level, LDL particle size will switch to highly desirable, large Pattern A. A preponderance of smaller, more dangerous LDL particles is called Pattern B and is associated with higher levels of triglycerides. The tipping-point triglyceride level varies from person to person. Usually those with triglyceride levels below 100 mg/dl will have Pattern A, and if below 75, it is almost a certainty. Most people who give up sugar and starch will have triglycerides this low. For a more nuanced view, measurements of pattern size can be made and "calibrated" with a person's triglycerides. The tests that determine Pattern A and B are called lipid subfractions. Unfortunately, this test isn't standardized and there are three competing methods: Ion Mobility (IM), Nuclear Magnetic Resonance (NMR), and Vertical Auto Profile (VAP). We prefer them in that order. They don't yield identical results, but are close.

SCIENTIFIC SIDEBAR
Mitochondria and Vascular Health

Mitochondrial health is important everywhere, and the vascular system is no exception. If the endothelium is in good shape, actively repairing itself (damage is continuous and frequent), and responsive to its various other duties, all will be well. However, if this is not the case, there is ample opportunity for atherosclerosis to develop and prosper.

The endothelium has several crucial functions, and of course, they all need energy, and this in turn requires a plentiful supply of healthy mitochondria.

How can this be attained? It turns out that cell wall shear stress tends to trigger this. Simply put, cell wall shear stress is the force of the blood rushing by. More blood flow—more mitochondria. More mitochondria—better endothelial health—less heart disease. And, of course, an increase in blood flow is best brought about by exercise.

Here is an example of energy management at a very localized level. Exercise for us, as hunter-gatherers, would usually mean food. Hunting was going on, and we were so good at it that an increase in the available food supply was a near certainty.

Of course, rushing blood could also mean conflict or flight.

ATHEROSCLEROSIS - PROGRESSION AND CURE

A few particles of stray LDL leaking behind the endothelium aren't really going to be much of a problem. In fact, cells in need of cholesterol might happily gobble them up, and that would be the end of it. But if these LDL particles become oxidized, or they were already that way when they arrived, the cells won't take them, and so they sit, possibly corroding adjacent cells and molecules. Unfortunately, this is the fate of much of the material that builds up behind the endothelium: it sooner or later goes bad (oxidizes). And as it builds up, it will present a fairly serious threat.

But the nearby threatened cells don't take this lying down. They secrete various chemicals that call for help. These chemicals are called interleukins. Interleukins are mainly used by immune system cells (white cells or leukocytes) to communicate with one another—hence their name—but endothelial cells can generate these chemical SOS signals as well. There are a couple of dozen different ones. They are stringy proteins made (like everything else) from amino acids. These ones are a couple of hundred amino acids long, and curled up like the ribbons on a birthday present. Typically, there are various innate immune system leukocyte cells patrolling any area. If they get the SOS signal, or if they notice some bad LDL or other detritus, they will spring into action: first, they will engulf the rancid particles, and second, they will call for reinforcements—more leukocytes—using the interleukin "hotline."

Small circulating leukocytes respond, squeezing through the junctions at the ends of the endothelial cells—a tight squeeze indeed—and entering into the area behind the endothelium. Once at the "scene of the crime" they also begin engulfing the junk, and if necessary, call for yet more leukocytes. As the leukocytes consume more and more material, they grow and soon are too large to escape back out into the bloodstream. If more rancid LDL piles up, then the process continues and more and more stuck leukocytes get fatter and fatter, eventually forming a significant bulge in the artery.

These fattened-up leukocytes now have a whitened fluffy appearance and are called foam cells. If the process continues, more and more foam cells will form, and the lump in the artery wall will become thicker and thicker. However, the plot is about to take an interesting turn.

HDL

HDL particles soon make their appearance. The HDL particles are going to attempt to stabilize the growing mess behind the artery wall:

- They offload the overloaded white cells by sucking the rancid material from the swollen cells into their own interior. This will cause the HDL particles to swell up.
- They attempt to prevent the white blood cells from undergoing programmed cell death. A dead leukocyte that is full of gunk is yet another mess to be dealt with. The HDL particles carry specific chemicals that are "injected" into the white cells, preventing this death.
- They further try to reduce the inflammatory response, by attempting to curtail the amount of interleukin SOS calls that the on-the-scene leukocytes are making.

If there is enough HDL, and the atherosclerotic buildup isn't overwhelming, the situation can be reversed—a true cure.

So just who are these little superheroes, soaring in to sort out the situation? HDL particles are much smaller than any LDL particle. They are also made by the liver and function as a very clever garbage collection fleet, much like immune system cells. In a just world, they would have full membership in the immune system society, and not merely be known as "good cholesterol." They start out as small, flat, dish-like little particles. Although they aren't cells at all, they have some of the same skill set, including cell-like gadgetry aptly named "scavenger receptors," which entirely describes their function. These HDL particles will scavenge about in the bloodstream, and one of their favorite targets is circulating, oxidized LDL cholesterol. They will directly remove this unwelcome trash.

HDL will also remove junk directly from cells. They will dock on just about any cell needing attention and offload some of the cell's garbage. For this reason, HDL is a cancer fighter as well.

Of great interest here, though, is HDL's ability to remove oxidized LDL and other detritus from behind the endothelium. This one is a puzzler: How does the HDL know where to go? How does it get behind the endothelium? And why doesn't it get stuck, like the bloated leukocytes? In fact, the endothelial cell itself, being in direct contact withthe plaque, knows where the HDL is needed. The endothelial cell will then express an appropriate transporter, grab a circulating HDL particle, and carry the particle through *itself* to the atherosclerotic mess. The endothelial cell actually engulfs the HDL particle and ferries it through in a little bubble called a vesicle, depositing it on the other side. When fully gorged on LDL, the HDL escapes back to the bloodstream via the same route, and then on to the liver, where its toxic contents are safely disposed of. Once emptied, it is ready for another mission.

Of course, HDL will easily get behind the endothelium (along with everything else) when a cell is being replaced.

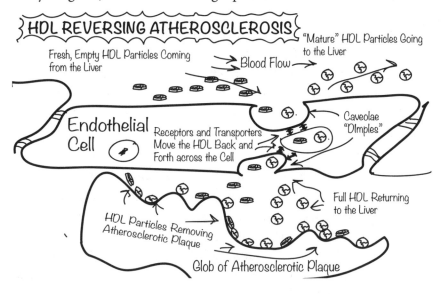

HDL REVERSING ATHEROSCLEROSIS

"Mature" HDL Particles Going to the Liver

Fresh, Empty HDL Particles Coming from the Liver

Blood Flow →

Endothelial Cell

Receptors and Transporters Move the HDL Back and Forth across the Cell

Caveolae "Dimples"

Full HDL Returning to the Liver

HDL Particles Removing Atherosclerotic Plaque

Glob of Atherosclerotic Plaque

HDL's methods are elaborate and varied, and there is still much to learn. However, there is copious evidence that high HDL levels are beneficial. In one study, an increase in HDL by 10 mg/dl not only halved the risk of heart attacks, but decreased cancer incidence by 36% as well. A sedentary person embarking on a new career as a gym rat will increase his HDL by 10 mg/dl or even more, if he does the correct exercises. Of course, the exercise itself will lower the risk in other ways—endothelial scrubbing, for instance. But with reductions of 50% and 36%, we won't quibble over who gets the credit.

It is as if HDL "evolved" for the purpose of cleaning up the mess the leukocytes made—getting stuck behind the endothelium, swelling up, and sending out inflammatory calls for help—but this cannot be. HDL evolved before animals even had circulatory systems. Perhaps HDL particles had rather different adventures in, say, a lobster. Or maybe not. The lobster has a heart and arteries, just no capillaries and veins: an open system. So it may be subject to some of the same sorts of perils we are.

Cells have many proteins that can "bind" to HDL. Some of these sit on the cell surface, acting as receptors. A cell that is overloaded with fat, like our poor bloated leukocyte, is likely freckled with these.

Atherosclerosis Tipping Point

HDL, along with the immune system, is trying to reverse the atherosclerosis. It will do so easily if, first, there is plenty of HDL available to clean up behind the artery wall, second, the buildup of rancid junk isn't overwhelming, and finally, the endothelium gets a periodic exercise-driven scrubbing.

But if these three factors are amiss, the atherosclerotic load increases and increases. The artery actually "remodels" itself, trying to maintain the original opening so that blood can flow unimpeded. The inner diameter of the artery stays the same, and a bulge develops on the outer wall. The blood can flow as before, but the artery begins to look as though an egg were stuck in it. This lump is called an atheroma.

Bulging out to maintain the blood flow is a quite clever trick. A person can (and many do) have a very high atherosclerotic load without a rise in blood pressure. Thus a normal blood pressure doesn't necessarily mean absence of heart disease. High blood pressure, though, usually indicates its presence.

The artery can't remodel itself forever. As the plaque builds up, several things may eventually happen—all of them bad.

Blood Pressure and Attempts to Control It

What controls blood pressure? Short answer: A lot of things. At rest, and in the absence of disease, it is regulated to around 120/80 or lower, and, as important as this is, all the mechanisms that affect blood pressure are not fully understood. Blood pressure control is both centralized and distributed regionally and locally—we don't have a tidy "unified theory."

Let's consider the problem from a logistical point of view. All the cells need to receive oxygen and nutrients, and get rid of wastes like CO_2. The energy demand for any group of cells can vary a lot—a hundredfold or more—and vary quickly as well. So besides delivering the goods, the circulatory system needs to be able to quickly step up the deliveries to the needier cells. People get sleepy after a meal. This is because the digestive system got allocated a lot more blood, and consequently, flow to other areas, the brain for instance, got cut. This is regional control. Another example would be the allocation of more blood flow to muscles during exercise.

The kidneys filter the blood and may require a boost or cut in the flow rate to do their job. Further, there may be a pending emergency, and in anticipation of this, blood flow and blood pressure are going to rise to prepare for the proverbial fight-or-flight.

There are dozens more items that affect blood pressure. How they are all coordinated, if indeed they are coordinated at all, is not known, but that hardly stops modern medicine from tampering with them. Let's consider the arsenal of pills and procedures frequently thrown at high blood pressure:

- Cut nerves to the kidney.
- Ablate certain areas in the limbic system regions of the brain.
- Cut nerves to the adrenals due to their role in the sympathetic system.
- Block calcium channels to decrease tone in the muscle walls of the arteries.
- Block kidney and/or lung-based angiotensin.
- Force sodium from the kidneys.
- Force water from the kidneys.
- Beta-blockers.

None of these are causes of high blood pressure. They are simply areas that can be fiddled with in a futile attempt to compensate for the root cause: poor lifestyle.

Bear in mind, though, high blood pressure is not a problem in and of itself. In intense exercise, blood pressure soars to levels so high that they would be morbidly dangerous if they were to remain there. High all the time—chronic—is the real issue. The body adapts to the chronic condition, but this can be undone, remodeled, relearned, and so on (but outside of Quantitative Medicine, this rarely happens).

The first has to do with the artery opening, which will eventually begin to get squeezed smaller. Blood pressure is raised to try to compensate for this. Even so, there still may not be enough blood flow. This situation is called ischemia, and may result in angina, a painful and dangerous heart condition. Plus the elevated blood pressure has its own issues.

A potentially more serious problem is the integrity of the atheroma itself. As it grows, the endothelial cells separating it from the blood flow are largely destroyed. To try to seal the atheroma shut, the immune system forms a sort of scab, called a fibrous cap. This cap is flimsy, and can break, spewing all sorts of junk directly into the artery, where it immediately clots. This is the nightmare scenario. Now something is loose in the artery that is going to get stuck somewhere downstream as the artery narrows down toward the capillaries. Once it clogs an artery, the downstream cells will be partially or totally cut off, resulting in a stroke, heart attack, or other such problem. The clotting is quite fast. However, for people with high amounts of Lp(a), an LDL variant, the clotting is significantly faster, and they are at higher risk.

Further, the swollen leukocytes cannot live forever. Eventually, they die and spill their remaining toxic contents into the atheroma and the surrounding area. The immune system then tries to mop this up, either by sending in new leukocytes to again engulf it, or by building a larger and larger wall around the mess. The swollen outermost layer of the artery is also weakened and vulnerable. This is the spot where a hemorrhage or aneurism could occur.

After some period of time, some of the atheroma calcifies, which tends to stabilize it, while at the same time making the artery stiffer.

Heart disease is unknown among hunter-gatherers. Evidently, their arterial plaque buildup is more than compensated for by their circulating HDL. Non-hunter-gatherers can achieve this too.

The best non-invasive measurement is the cardiac calcium scoring done in a full-body scan. This measures the amount of calcified material, which in turn gives an accurate assessment of the underlying atherosclerotic load. A measurement of the calcified area is computed. It is known as the Agatston score. A score of 0 means no calcium, and therefore a light atherosclerotic load. A typical 60-year-old man or 70-year-old woman might have a score of 30, which is not a particularly high value, though it could be quite a lot higher. In the absence of exercise and dietary control, the Agatston score will double every two or three years, indicating significant buildup. The score is soon into the hundreds and can go on up into the thousands.

High blood pressure may also indicate atherosclerosis, although there could be other reasons. Likewise, a high level of C-reactive protein could be the result of atherosclerosis or due to other factors.

Reversing Atherosclerosis - Controlling LDL Particle Size

Simply put, ameliorating the causes of the disorder and augmenting the repair processes will reverse atherosclerosis, and both are needed. One involves mainly diet and stress management, while the other mainly exercise. By diet, we mean eating the right food in the right amounts, not "dieting." The exercise must be of the "right" type as well.

However even with proper diet and exercise, high chronic stress will accelerate atherosclerosis, as will poor sleep patterns.

When is LDL dangerous? A high concentration of very small LDL particles, Pattern "B," is a high-risk condition for plaque buildup. It is the smaller particles that get behind the endothelium when cell replacements are taking place. Smoking cessation and trans fat avoidance are two obvious direct steps, and, as previously discussed, reducing triglycerides to below 100 mg/dl will likely insure the desirable Pattern "A."

Reversing Atherosclerosis - Exercise, HDL, and HDL2b

The other side of the equation consists of increasing the amount of HDL and maximizing the percentage of "mature" cholesterol, also called HDL2b. This is HDL which has done a thorough job of collecting bodily junk. A typical number might be 25%, meaning that 25% of the HDL observed was this fattened-up variety. If the percentage is high, then the HDL garbage system is working well. Unfortunately, the HDL2b measurement is a little hard to find. Both HDL and HDL2b increase in response to exercise. Exercise should have these attributes to be effective:

- Varying the heart rate up to its (safe) maximum and back.
- Explosive, a sudden burst of activity.
- Concentric, meaning muscle should be shortening.

In sedentary people, HDL tends to be low and inactive. A typical HDL level for non-exercisers might be 30 mg/dl, with an HDL2b of 15%. Not a lot.

On the other hand, a person doing the right concentric and explosive exercises will probably have an HDL closer to 60 mg/dl, and an HDL2b above 35%. This represents a large increase in cellular garbage collection. The HDL system here is cleaning up three to four times more bodily junk than the sedentary individual. The benefits are huge. There is a substantial reduction in atherosclerosis, and cancer as well, and all from exercise alone. When such exercise is combined with proper diet, atherosclerosis clearly has little chance to develop.

Why does exercise raise HDL so much? There is a combination of factors at work here. The concentric, explosive, intense exercise has the direct effect of running the heart rate up and down, and washing clean the endothelium, but there is also an indirect effect. Overall HDL level is controlled by the hypothalamus, and if the exercise is concentric and explosive, the HDL level will be increased, along with numerous other healing and repair functions.

Exercises that could be interpreted as migration, like jogging, do not raise HDL and HDL2b very much. Here the hypothalamus thinks a food shortage is coming and conserves. Plus the physical movement and blood flow variation of the arteries is not as intense.

There are certain rare diseases where HDL will not clean up the arterial mess, and these unfortunate people have a very difficult time.

LIPOPROTEIN(a)

Elevated levels of lipoprotein(a), also called Lp(a), can be a risk factor for atherosclerosis and for clotting as well. Lp(a) is a slightly modified form of LDL lipoprotein particles. The modification involves the attachment of an additional protein string called apo(a). The apo(a) string sticks tightly to the LDL particle at one spot, and tends to cling to the LDL particle, covering it. If the particle is flowing rapidly, during exercise, for instance, the apo(a) string unfurls like a streamer. These streamers come in a large variety of lengths. Some people have mostly short ones, and others mostly long. The increased risk is with the shorter lengths.

About 10% of the Caucasian and Asian population has high levels of Lp(a). High usually means above 15 mg/dl. Such people have double the risk of heart and clotting problems. The Black population has an even higher rate of elevated Lp(a), around 20%, but is not at increased risk of heart problems, as this group has predominantly longer apo(a) strings.

There is no cure for Lp(a), nor is there a known reason for its existence, as people with little or no Lp(a) appear to do fine. Despite the increased heart and clotting risks, there seem to be a couple of benefits. First, the cancer rate is lower in those with high Lp(a), and second, there may be a longevity benefit, as a disproportionately higher percentage of centenarians have elevated Lp(a). (Note that is not the same thing as saying that people with high Lp(a) are more likely to become centenarians.) Also, some research has reported a lower incidence of adult onset diabetes in those with high levels of Lp(a)

Lp(A) Has Several Properties That Cause It to Be Dangerous.

First, the apo(a) protein string closely resembles plasminogen and interferes with its action. Plasminogen causes clots to dissolve. With its function partially disabled, clotting risk increases. Heart attacks and strokes are both caused by clots. The risk for heart attack is close to doubled for those with levels above 30 mg/dl. Stroke risk is also increased.

Second, high Lp(a) levels accelerate atherosclerosis. There could be several reasons for this. Circulating LDL particles are frequently engulfed by cells that need cholesterol. However, these cells will not take the LDL particles that have the apo(a) string attached. Hence these particles stay in circulation longer, have a tendency to oxidize, and also have a tendency to stick to the endothelial wall, which will promote cell death and repair. Further, if the particles are abundant, they are more likely to get behind the endothelium during repair activities.

Combating Lp(a)

To avoid the cardiac consequences, the Quantitative Medicine protocols are a must. However, if strictly done, not only will heart problems be prevented, but most others as well. Lp(a) has its "vulnerabilities," from which a strategy can be developed.

First, consider how Lp(a) is formed. The apo(a) string generation happens in the liver, but the attachment to LDL particles happens outside the liver, in the bloodstream. So one defense is to keep the LDL particle size large. These larger particles will have a harder time getting behind the endothelium. The strategy then is to push the LDL size up by pushing triglycerides lower, as explained earlier in this chapter.

Second, stop the Lp(a) particle from sticking to the endothelium. This means varying your blood flow with frequent vigorous, but brief, exercise. Barrel up stairs two or three steps at a time. Trot up hills. Keep things stirred up.

Another benefit of exercise is speculative. The rushing blood may cause the apo(a) strings to unfurl. As such, it may be exposed to various circulating enzymes that can snip it up.

We did not intend to preach in this chapter, but, readers with high Lp(a): you must combat it. Otherwise cardiac problems are very likely, and often at an early age (forties). Atherosclerosis is much easier to prevent than reverse, so a life-long commitment is called for. However, a person with high Lp(a) who undertakes this will probably avoid all other degenerative disease too. This is no small reward for all that effort.

The Lp(a) Measurement Is Problematic

Low means there is no danger regardless of the measurement technique. However, the measurement is not standardized, and there are several techniques that, unfortunately, do not yield comparable results. Further, it is very difficult to figure out how a specific lab did the analysis. At this point, anything over 20 mg/dl should be considered dangerous. It is hoped that a more definitive measurement will be developed in the future.

To actually pin down the risk, we probably need to know how many of the LDL particles have the apo(a) string stuck to them, and the length of the strings. The measurement situation is in a very bad state. The usual measurement is volume amount of Lp(a).

Therapies and Possible Breakthroughs

Aspirin and niacin are frequently proposed, though neither have been properly studied in a way that would determine long-term effects. Until such time, these should probably be avoided.

One promising new development is called antisense therapy. This drug is a complement of the messenger RNA that encodes the apo(a) protein string (hence the term "antisense"). The drug attaches to the messenger RNA, thus inactivating apo(a) production. The drug is quite new (2015) and may have numerous problems or side effects. However, so far, in very early trials, it managed to lower Lp(a) up to 80%. So stay tuned.

REVERSING ATHEROSCLEROSIS - A RECAP

If the triglyceride level is safely below the tipping point, Pattern A will result and there will not be many of the very small LDL particles. This reduces the supply of potentially atherosclerotic material. Exercise that varies the pulse rate will tend to keep the endothelium healthy, reducing turnover. Such exercise will also reduce the amount of toxic junk that can get behind an artery. If, through exercise, HDL is elevated, any existing plaque will be removed. It's largely that direct. The balance between the factors causing atherosclerosis and those curing it has been favorably altered. The body is more than capable of controlling atherosclerosis. Any deposited calcium will persist a long time, but this is not dangerous.

If these dietary and exercise patterns are maintained throughout one's life, heart disease is never going to develop at all. This is the case with virtually all hunter-gatherers. However, it's never too late. A lifestyle change that promotes these protective elements will immediately start reversing heart disease regardless of prior damage.

Key Points

21 - Atherosclerosis - Cause and Cure

- Atherosclerosis is a buildup of fatty material behind the endothelium.
- Small LDL particles are caused by excess glucose: big LDL particles pose little danger.
- Small LDL particles get behind the endothelium when dead cells reproduce.
- Particles become oxidized (rancid) and are attacked by immune system cells.
- Immune system cells engulf oxidized material and become fat.
- Bloated immune system cells become a foam-like mass.
- HDL is raised by exercise.
- HDL migrates behind the endothelium and can reverse the situation.
- Exercise with rapidly varying heart rates cleans the endothelium.
- Atherosclerosis progresses or reverses depending on which process is dominant.
- Proper diet and correct exercise will prevent and reverse atherosclerosis.

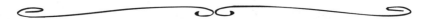

22 - CANCER

Like several other degenerative diseases, cancer can be prevented, and at the earlier stages, reversed. In fact, almost all cancer is eradicated by the immune system long before it forms a tumor large enough to be detected or cause damage.

A cancerous cell is one that is damaged at the DNA level and is then replicating that damage. These cells must be killed or otherwise immobilized, either via the immune system or by medical intervention such as surgery or chemotherapy. Repair isn't really possible at this point.

Many people are unaware that the immune system can fight cancer. In fact, it is the first line of defense and prevents almost all damaged cells from going very far awry. Natural killer cells are specifically searching for cancerous cells, and for such cells to proliferate into a tumor, the natural killer function has to be thwarted, along with quite a few other things.

One might think that DNA, redundant, protected, and tucked away in the cell nucleus, is pristine and reliable. This is not the case. Damage to the DNA is common. Something like 60,000 repairs are made to a single cell's DNA daily. Multiply this by the 100 trillion cells and you get some idea of the astronomical level of DNA repair that is continually going on.

CANCER INITIATION

Heart disease and adult onset diabetes are mainly caused by inappropriate lifestyle choices. However, cancer has a variety of causes and many of them are not under our control:

- Smoke from cigarettes or other sources
- Ultraviolet light from the sun
- Toxic materials in the food chain
- Air and water pollution
- Radiation from radioactive materials or the cosmos
- X-rays
- Infections: e.g., gastric lymphoma due to H. pylori

Cancer and DNA damage can also be initiated by several factors within our control. A diet lacking in nutrients could weaken cells, as could an imbalance of various cellular biochemicals, or an overabundance of free radicals. Chronic stress levels and poor sleep patterns also diminish the immune system's natural cancer-fighting ability.

SPECIFIC CANCER SIDEBAR
Colorectal Cancer

Colon cells are short-lived, turning over about every six days. This means very active replacement is going on, and hence a cancer risk. The stem cells reside in "crypts," small protected pouches found throughout the small intestine, colon, and rectum.

Should these cells become pre-cancerous, they will fill the crypt and erupt out of it. At this point it is called an adenoma and resembles a small bump. The bump can grow larger into a mushroom-like structure called a polyp. It is not necessarily cancerous at this time. In a colonoscopy, these are usually snipped off and examined. Less than 10% of polyps become cancerous, but virtually all colorectal cancer starts out as a polyp. Hence, in a colonoscopy, all of them are removed.

A cancerous polyp will initially be contained within the intestine (and easily treated), but may grow through the intestinal wall or spread into the circulatory system (metastasize).

Screening for colon cancer means having a colonoscopy. Officially, this isn't recommended for people under 50, but this is a mistake. A full 20% of people between 40 and 50 have some sort of abnormality that may become cancerous. This fact is known, but the medical reasoning is that it will be caught when these people have a colonoscopy at age 50. The seminal paper that found the 20% abnormalities in the 40-50 group concluded that it was OK to wait. This idea was not wholly subscribed to and developed into quite a kerfuffle. Waiting seems foolhardy to us. It does save money presumably, but even this is debatable. Treatment of anything caught early is always far cheaper.

Does red meat cause colon cancer? This is widely believed to be the case, but it is definitely not true. The contorted history of this association follows that of saturated fat and heart disease. People who did not have health as their top priority, who smoked, who drank, got a disproportionate share of colon cancer (and heart disease and just about everything else). Red meat was blamed. More recent trials have completely upended this. Red meat per se is not harmful at all, and causes less inflammation than many vegetables.

Quality of meat is important. If it is loaded with chemicals, it is not going to be healthy. It is best to vary meats: some red, some fowl, some fish. Reasonable consumption is not going to increase the risk of colorectal cancer.

Does whole grain wheat prevent colon cancer? Compared to refined grain product, the answer is slightly, maybe. Compared to not eating grain at all, the answer is no. Grain, whole or not, causes high insulin. High insulin causes cancer.

Repairing Cellular DNA Damage

Regardless of the source of the damage, the cell has considerable machinery available to attempt repairs. As with any other cellular function, cellular health is a prerequisite for efficient performance of any such repairs. The following sorts of damage are usually repairable:

- Direct damage. In this case, the DNA nucleotides have sustained specific damage—maybe some molecule got stuck to one of them. There are several cellular mechanisms that can set this straight.

- DNA single-strand break. There are a couple of mechanisms that remove the bad stretch and manufacture and install a correct one. The intact piece provides a pattern for the repair.

- Mismatched complements in the DNA. Recall that A pairs with T and C pairs with G. There are cellular proofreaders that look for violations of this rule. This raises the question: which strand is the correct one? Somehow, the cells seem to be able to get this right.

On the other hand, a double-strand break is usually not repairable and this is the dangerous one. The blueprint for possible reconstruction—the complementary strand—has also been obliterated. The typical repair consists of tossing out the broken section and rejoining the broken strands. This isn't so much a repair as a cellular kludge, and clearly, that "repair" might cause problems. Almost always, the cell won't make it through the next cell division, but if it does, we now have two new maverick cells, with unknown intent, that can replicate—so this again is a candidate for tumor generation. Note that some double-strand breaks, particularly those in regions of repeated patterns, can be effectively repaired.

The "standard procedure" for these unrepairable cases is that the cell commit suicide, which is called apoptosis, or else the cell may just sort of fizzle out, which is called senescence. Of course, the cell has to be functioning well enough to do this, which is an obvious weak spot. Broken cells that don't follow the "rules" are also tumor candidates.

What about the mitochondrial DNA? Mitochondria, being essentially enslaved bacteria, aren't blessed with the elaborate DNA repair machinery available to the host cell. However, mitochondria do have one trick that the host cell lacks. Mitochondria have multiple copies of the same DNA, typically hundreds. So a dividing mitochondrion could "choose" to replicate only the intact DNA, purging the broken ones. The jury is still out on this one, but the evidence is strong that this winnowing process does take place. In any case, mitochondrial mutations don't directly cause cancer, although they can certainly be an indirect cause by reducing available cellular energy. Another piece of evidence for the purge route of repair is that it is known that exercise sharply reduces cancer risk. At the same time, exercise sharply increases mitochondrial health and turnover.

Most Cancers Begin in Stem or Progenitor Cells

A single damaged cell may do goofy things, but is unlikely to cause any harm unless it can divide. After all, it's only one of a hundred trillion. Normally, only stem and progenitor cells have the ability to divide. As cells differentiate down toward their working everyday versions, the ability to divide is lost. Likewise, some cell types are around for life, and there is little or no division going on there either.

Thus, where you find cancers is where you find the stem and progenitor cells, and you find these associated with tissues that renew, like skin, intestines, colon, lungs, throat, and so on. Cancer is far less common in the permanent cells, like the brain, heart, muscle, etc.

(Actually, brain cancer almost always involves a cancer that started somewhere else and then took up residence in the brain—metastasized—or else a cancer originating in the glia cells, the brain cells that provide structural support for the neurons. Unlike neurons, these glia cells do divide.)

Stem and progenitor cells are usually as protected as they reasonably can be. The ones that make skin are under several skin layers. Those for the intestine are in little intestinal cubbyholes called "crypts," safely tucked away from the caustic intestinal lumen. The white and red blood cells are generated in the middle of bones—hard to get more protected than that.

A Sequence of Mutations Is Needed to Launch and Sustain a Cancer

Given how many things have to go wrong to get a life-threatening tumor, you would think it could never happen. Of course, we know otherwise, but consider the sequence of events required:

1. A mutation in a cell's DNA needs to happen. We have already discussed numerous causes for this.

2. This mutation has to cause uncontrolled division. Most mutations are completely unrelated to division.

3. Various cellular mechanisms specifically designed to block unregulated proliferation must somehow be disabled.

4. Another mutation must also thwart the cellular mechanisms that cause programmed cell death.

5. Senescence must similarly be blocked.

6. Yet another mutation has to deceive the meandering white cells that are looking for cell abnormalities. Specifically, the mutated cell has to display an MHC complex indicating that it is intact and normal, when, in fact, it is not.

7. Angiogenesis. The cells may begin proliferating, but they need nutrients. Without a blood supply, tumor growth is limited to about the size of this "O." Further cell division and growth will stall out from lack of nourishment. At this point, another mutation is needed that will start producing an enzyme that causes new blood vessels to grow, a process called angiogenesis.

8. With a blood supply, the tumor can grow, possibly fairly large, but it may not yet be life threatening. In fact, a tumor bigger than a raisin can be spotted with an MRI—provided one is done, but people aren't routinely scanned. If there is a symptom—some pain for instance—and a scan detects a contained tumor, successful removal is usually possible. For the tumor to evade this type of detection, it will need to maintain a stealthy symptom-free profile.

9. To continue its lethal course, the tumor must now metastasize, and for this, a mutation is needed that will allow tiny pieces of the tumor to detach and enter the bloodstream or the lymph system. Note that this step would be an easy one for any sort of cell that normally circulates in either system. This is the situation with leukemia, where the leukocytes (white blood cells) have become cancerous.

10. The bloodstream and lymph system are fairly loaded with immune cells, so the cancer will have to have a way to evade detection there.

11. Still another mutation is needed to enable the tumorous material to burrow back out of the bloodstream or lymph system and inflict itself on some other organ.

12. Depending on where the metastatic tumor material landed, additional mutation may be needed in order for it to thrive further.

With so many hoops to jump through, why do we ever get cancer? The odds are small, but the number of cells is so large that rare sequences do happen. In a sense, we always have cancer. In anyone's body, numerous cancers are at various stages of development. How far any of them get depends a lot on cellular health, mitochondrial health, and an active immune system, and all of these are strongly influenced by lifestyle choices.

Many anti-cancer therapies attempt to block one of these steps. For example, if angiogenesis—the production of new blood vessels—can be blocked, the cancers are stuck at a small non-lethal size.

Staging of Cancer

Staging varies from cancer to cancer, and roughly reflects how far into the above sequence of mutations the cancer has traveled. A system in general use is the TNM system (also known as the UICC or AJCC system). TNM stands, respectively, for **T**umor, lymph **N**ode, and **M**etastasis.

The T score identifies the size of the primary tumor. A following number indicates tumor size. T0 means no tumor found, with T1 through T4 indicating larger sizes. N0 means no spread to the nearby lymph nodes, and numbers N1-N3 indicate the extent of the spread. Finally, M0 indicates no metastases, and M1 indicates that some were found.

Many specific cancers use variants of this system, and some cancers use completely different systems. Breast cancer uses TMN and a I, II, III, & IV system as well. Colon cancer has an ABCD system as well as TMN.

CURING DETECTABLE CANCER REQUIRES MEDICAL INTERVENTION

A cancer that has gotten far enough to be detectable is not likely to go away on its own. It is possible, but bear in mind that a tumor large enough to be detected on a scan has probably gotten past the angiogenesis stage. This is a tumor on the march, and medical intervention is required. This can mean removal of the tumor by surgery or killing it in place with chemotherapy or radiation. If a tumor is spotted early, these therapies are very effective, and are becoming far more precise, with less destruction to surrounding tissue.

Cancers That Can Be Detected

These cancers are detectable at stages where they are still curable:

Colorectal Cancer. These are screened with a colonoscopy, either a real one or a virtual one, which is slightly less unpleasant. This should start at 40. Forty-year-olds do not typically get colon cancer, but a full 20% have something pre-cancerous that ought to be closely watched.

Carcinoembryonic Antigen (CEA), normally present only during a pregnancy, could also indicate colorectal cancer. Change is important, so a history of this measurement should be maintained. CEA could also be present in people with breast, pancreatic, or lung cancer.

Breast Cancer. This is detectable by self-examination. Most breast cancers, 70% to 80% in fact, are initially detected this way.

Standard practice calls for mammograms. However, these have a "false alarm" issue in that they detect "Ductal Carcinoma in Situ" (DCIS), which is really a pre-cancerous condition, and usually goes away of its own accord.

After any initial indication of a problem, the usual procedure is to follow up with MRIs, ultrasounds, biopsies, and other tests.

As a preventive measure, insulin, IGF-1, and estradiol can be monitored. If these are in normal ranges, breast cancer risk is significantly reduced.

Prostate Cancer. This can be detected with a PSA measurement, a simple blood test. There are several other detection methods, including ultrasound, MRIs, and biopsies. PSA alone is not a very good indicator. A trend, determined from a series of measurements is needed.

Squamous Cell Skin Cancer. This is spotted as an abnormal skin growth.

Malignant Melanoma. Any dark or mole-like spot anywhere needs to be checked by a doctor.

Liver Cancer. AFP, normally present only in pregnancy, could indicate liver or pancreatic cancer. AFP can be measured by a blood test. Change is important, so a history of the measurement should be maintained. AFP could also be present in people with ovarian or testicular cancer.

Ovarian Cancer. CA125 may indicate ovarian cancer. Again, trend is more important than level, so it is important to have a series of measurements. High AFP may also indicate ovarian cancer.

Except the skin cancers, all of these could show up on a full-body scan. The resolution of such a scan is 3-4 millimeters—pea sized. A tumor that size may or may not have accomplished the angiogenesis step (growing a new blood supply). It's right on the edge. If angiogenesis hasn't occurred, the tumor is, for the time being, stuck at that size.

Catching a tumor early requires looking for it, and there is currently an unfortunate trend away from screening.

Here are the odds of five-year survival for several common cancers:

Cancer Type	Odds If Localized	If Spread to Lymph Nodes	Odds If Metastatic	Chance of Getting It	Chance of Dying From It
Malignant Melanoma	90%		10%	2.5%	0.5%
Squamous Cell Skin Cancer	~100%		10%	7.5%	0.01%
Bladder Cancer	88%	55%	15%	2.5%	0.6%
Breast Cancer	~100%	72%	22%	12%	3%
Prostate Cancer	~100%	~100%	28%	15%	2.6%
Colorectal Cancer	92%	65%	11%	4.6%	1.9%
Esophageal Cancer	40%	21%	4%	0.9%	0.7%
Lung Cancer	31%	15%	2%	6.8%	5.8%
Pancreatic Cancer	14%	7%	1%	1.5%	1.35%
Liver Cancer	28%	7%	2%		
Leukemia	Varies	Varies	Varies	1.4%	0.8%

Cancers that are rare, or that are rarely fatal, aren't listed here.

Now even with a "war on cancer" that began 50 years ago, there is no clear evidence we are winning. Certainly there are breakthroughs, but people live longer and can then get more cancer, plus heart disease is down and adult onset diabetes is up, both of which tend to skew the disease statistics toward cancer. In fact, cancer is now the leading cause of death in America, the UK and France.

The Trend Away from Screening

From the above chart, we see that melanoma, breast, prostate, colorectal, and bladder cancer are essentially curable if caught early. Nonetheless, they account for half the cancer deaths. Are a full 50% of cancer victims today dying needlessly? Shouldn't this sound the alarm: prevention—prevention—prevention? Yet the trend is clearly away from screening. Endless excuses are offered: not cost effective, stressful, over-treated, etc. This cut in the screening is a death sentence for a huge number of people.

If you have the ear of anyone influential, for the sake of all of us, bend it. We don't need less detection. We need better processing of the results. Why isn't this obvious?

This trend away from screening is thoroughly disturbing. Prostate cancer is typical of the reasoning. Most men will get prostate cancer and most will not die from it, but when an elevated PSA is detected, many men panic and opt for surgery. So we should stop detecting it? Instead, perhaps we could persuade the eager surgeons and radiologists to refrain from rushing terrified patients into lucrative surgeries or other pricey procedures. Frequently treatment is not necessary, at least not immediately, and the cancer can be closely monitored with additional PSA measurements. (This is called "watchful waiting.") Ignoring the presence of prostate cancer solves nothing and sentences many to death. The other cancers seem to have similar screening stories. The trend away from screening has financial roots as well.

Miracle Cures Are Rare

Miracle cures very rarely happen. Otherwise, they wouldn't be considered miracles. Something like 1 in 50,000 terminal cancers simply go away. This makes for good press, but not for good medicine. By far the best shot is with the medical experts. There has been considerable progress and there will be more. Treatment procedures are getting more and more targeted, with less consequential damage to non-cancerous tissue.

LIFESTYLE CHOICES FOR CANCER PREVENTION

Diet, exercise, meditation, and sleep all have significant effects on cancer. Optimizing these using the Quantitative Medicine protocols affords the strongest cancer prevention possible. Of course, sensible avoidance of known carcinogens is important as well. We suppose health-conscious people will do this as far as practicable.

As to the controllable aspects, we break up lifestyle into the usual main categories:

- **Stress**. Stress causes high cortisol, which increases insulin and down-regulates the immune system. This is practically a formula for cancer. Stress can be reduced through meditation or other spiritual disciplines.
- **Diet**. The biggest dietary risk element is elevated insulin and glucose, both of which directly encourage cancer. High insulin goes hand in hand with elevated glucose.
- **Exercise**. Exercise fights cancer in a variety of ways. HDL is elevated, which improves cellular health. Exercise improves mitochondrial health, which further reduces cellular stress.
- **Sleep**. A lot of bodily repair occurs during sleep. People whose work inherently disrupts their sleep pattern have a significantly higher incidence of cancer.

STRESS AND HIGH CORTISOL CAN CAUSE CANCER

Any stress event raises cortisol. This is normal. Cortisol is the stress hormone, after all. However, cortisol sets in motion a variety of alterations to basic bodily functions which compromise long-term health in return for a short-term improvement in survival likelihood. This makes sense if you are a hunter-gatherer or in a combat situation, but is otherwise out of date.

A short burst of stress and its consequent cortisol elevation aren't particularly harmful, provided that things return to normal.

Chronic stress causes chronically elevated cortisol. This may be external—a difficult partner or working relationship—or internal—a chronic infection or overloaded metabolism. This elevated cortisol triggers several changes: much of the immune system is disabled, insulin is raised, and blood glucose is raised as well. Each one of these is carcinogenic. Hence, chronic high cortisol greatly increases cancer risk.

Reducing *average* cortisol to a safe level, say under 15 µg/dl, is very important. Unfortunately, there is no convenient way to measure average cortisol, so fasting levels are used. Cortisol is a very fast-acting hormone, and any minor stress prior to a blood draw, such as an argument over billing, could run it up. So unless you are in a normal relaxed state, the measurement should be taken with a grain of salt, or ideally, taken again.

Ten minutes a day of some sort of meditation or other spiritual discipline appears to work wonders, and the wonders worked are primarily stress and cortisol reduction and their consequences.

Chronic Inflammation Causes Cancer

Chronic inflammation could result from chronic stress, or from any number of other things. Inflammation indicates cells in distress and is an immune system response. If the immune system cannot solve the problem and the cellular stress continues, various sorts of cellular damage will occur. Cellular stress due to nutrient overload or a lack of essential micronutrients would indicate a need for a dietary change. Likewise, inactivity causes mitochondria to shut down and increases the presence of reactive oxygen species. In small amounts, these aid in cell regulation, but in high amounts, they can wreak cellular havoc. High glucose and high insulin are also causes of cellular stress.

EXERCISE AND HIGH HDL PREVENT CANCER

According to one study, for every 10 mg/dl higher HDL, a 36% reduction in cancer was observed, a very impressive result. This rise in HDL can be brought about by proper exercise and diet. There are some drugs, niacin in particular, that also raise HDL, but raising HDL this way increases mortality, an unexpected and, of course, very undesirable result, so it seems it has to be exercise. It doesn't take a lot of additional exercise to raise HLD 10 mg/dl.

Was it the increase in HDL that actually reduced cancer, or was it some other benefit associated with exercise? In a way, the answer is moot. We want that 36% reduction no matter what. Truth is, we really don't know the answer. Probably both. Things are too entangled.

HDL is very directly implicated in the reduction of heart disease, and that same exercise-driven HDL increase will reduce heart risk 50%, an even more impressive result. In this case we know what is going on. HDL is cleaning the arteries.

Prostate Cancer

Prostate cancer is the second most common cancer in men, after skin cancer. Annually, in America, 230,000 are diagnosed with it and 30,000 will die from it—largely unnecessarily. Current guidelines are tending to suppress screening, so the number of men dying unnecessarily is destined to increase. It should be perfectly clear from the numbers—230,000 diagnosed, 30,000 die—that this is a survivable cancer. The travesty is twofold. First, 30,000 die needlessly; and second, unnecessary (but expensive and lucrative) life-altering procedures are performed on hundreds of thousands of men annually. The medical profession has realized that the disease is over-treated, so to solve this, they have decided to reduce the amount of disease by reducing the amount of screening. Sound absurdly Orwellian? You are not alone if you think so.

Let's do a reality check on prostate cancer:

1. Prostate cancer is the tortoise of cancers. It takes decades to develop.
2. Almost all men eventually will get it. The odds a man has it are approximately equal to his age.
3. Most men aren't screened. If all men were screened, the number of new cases would be more like two million a year. Very few of these men will die because of prostate cancer. Perhaps 1%.
4. The low rate of death from undiagnosed or untreated prostate cancer, plus the high incidence of unnecessary and aggressive treatment has resulted in a policy decision to stop screening. Makes some sense in the grand scheme of things, but this will kill in excess of 30,000 men per year.

There really should be some way to stop practitioners from rushing their frightened clientele into unnecessary procedures while at the same time treating men who actually need it—at least you would think. Some people look at the big cost picture and say don't screen, don't treat. Others look at their six-figure incomes derived from treatment and form other opinions. Altogether this is medicine at its worst.

The prostate's sole function is to manufacture and ejaculate semen. Making semen is a glandular function, and propelling it is a muscular one. For most post-adolescents, this occurs once a day or less, so metabolically, little is going on, things run slowly, and a cancer is usually very slow to develop.

The prostate lives in one of the more inaccessible locations, nestled between the penis and the rectum. The urethra, the duct for urine, runs through it, as well as the nerves controlling erections. Therefore its removal or destruction by radiation will frequently affect these functions, as well as the "quality of life" associated with them.

The prostate is a hormone-driven gland. It "runs" on dihydrotestosterone, a very "high-octane" version of ordinary testosterone. Cancer is but one of several possible defects in the prostate that will cause it to spill some of its internal stuff, called Prostate Specific Antigen, or PSA, into the bloodstream. Not much is spilled, though, as it's measured in nanograms/milliliter. The rule of thumb has been to suspect prostate cancer if PSA is over 4. This is the wrong rule. To detect prostate cancer, change is needed, and the rate of change. A person with a PSA of 1 that went to 2 in six months probably needs treatment. On the other hand, a person with a PSA of 4 that hasn't changed much in a decade may have prostate cancer, but it is stable, and no immediate treatment is needed.

In an ideal world, at least how Quantitative Medicine imagines it, all men's PSA would be measured when they are young, say 40. At this point, twice-a-year measurements would begin. Any sudden lurch would be investigated, and if necessary, treated. Non-aggressive prostate cancers would be left alone, or possibly treated with dihydrotestosterone-blocking drugs, which starve the prostate and slow things down even more. Practitioners would not be allowed to bully frightened patients into meaningless treatments that degrade the quality of life while providing little benefit.

In the artery wall, HDL performs its magic by draining excess fat from immune system cells, decreasing inflammation, and extending cell life. It turns out that HDL is willing to perform these good deeds for just about any needy cell. Unloading excess fat and reducing inflammation are anti-cancer activities, though extending cell life wouldn't necessarily be.

Exercise that increases mitochondrial health will also have anti-cancer activity. So exactly apportioning individual contributions will remain a bit blurred, but the net effect of exercise is a significant overall reduction in cancer risk.

The right exercise is strongly anti-cancer. The right sorts are explosive and concentric. They increase mitochondrial health, reduce cortisol, increase HDL, and place growth factors at optimal levels. We have already covered this form of exercise in PART II, chapter 10 - STEP III - LIFESTYLE CHANGE GUIDELINES - EXERCISE, and will cover it more deeply in chapter 28 - EXERCISE.

Exercise of a continuous nature, such as jogging or brisk walking, will have much less effect, and if carried to extremes, such as in a marathon, can actually be detrimental.

Overexercising can also be detrimental. The effect of overexercising is to raise cortisol, which triggers several cancer-promoting processes.

Exercise Prevents Cancer by Increasing Cellular Health

Anything that improves cellular health will decrease cancer risk. Cellular health, in turn, is optimized by improvement in all four lifestyle choice categories—diet, exercise, spiritual discipline, and sleep. Specifically, exercise helps by increasing metabolic throughput. Idle cells are not healthy cells. Nutrients will accumulate, and underutilized mitochondria will spew free radicals into the cell, which will react and oxidize the accumulated nutrients, making them toxic.

The Effect of Exercise on Growth Factors

Exercise will increase growth factors such as testosterone (both male and female) and IGF-1, which in turn cause cellular repair and turnover. As mentioned above, there are optimum levels set by the body for these powerful hormones and at these optimum levels, they are cancer preventive. At elevated levels (from supplementation) they may cause cancer.

CANCER SIDEBAR
UV, Skin Cancer, and Malignant Melanoma

The relation of exposure to ultraviolet light, normal skin cancer, and the risk of malignant melanoma is a source of grand confusion. Currently, parents are slathering their children with sunscreen, which in cases of normal sun exposure is a bad idea and actually increases cancer risk.

Examining first ordinary skin cancer, also called basal cell cancer and squamous cell cancer, we find that these two cancers are almost never fatal, easily removed, and caused by exposure to the sun. They occur mostly on the face and later in life. Presuming they are treated, such are little more than a nuisance.

Melanoma, on the other hand, will usually be fatal if untreated. Melanoma may be connected to sun exposure, or perhaps not. Factors associated with melanoma tend to be conflicting. Melanomas often occur in areas that get little or no sun. Melanomas occur more frequently in fair-skinned people, and more frequently in the Nordic countries, which is also odd, as the sun is less intense in northern locations. It may be that repeated sunburn is a risk factor.

Some sun, though, may be protective of melanoma. From *The Lancet*, we have: "Sunlight is the main environmental cause of most cutaneous melanomas. Exposure to intense bursts of ultraviolet radiation, especially in childhood, starts the transformation of benign melanocytes into a malignant phenotype. Paradoxically, outdoor workers have a decreased risk of melanoma compared with indoor workers, suggesting that chronic sunlight exposure can have a protective effect. Further, some melanomas form on sun-exposed regions; others do not."

Now, staying out of the sun or using sunscreen will prevent vitamin D generation. Low vitamin D may cause a 20% increase in other cancers. Of course, you can, and probably should, take vitamin D supplements. However, this is not equivalent to sunshine.

Our recommendation:
- Avoid sunburn. Use sunscreen for this.
- Otherwise, don't use sunscreen and be sure to get some sunshine.
- Keep up with the latest findings on melanoma. It is a work in progress.

Bodybuilding Supplements Can Cause Cancer

Bodybuilders supplement with all sorts of things: testosterone, insulin, IGF-1, cortisol, to name a few. For the most part, the body regulates hormones to the healthiest (for you) level. Any attempt to artificially change this will cause problems. Specifically, since cancer is out-of-control growth, it should be fairly clear that taking a "growth" hormone has the potential to make things worse.

EXCESS GLUCOSE AND INSULIN CAN CAUSE CANCER

Several dietary attributes can contribute to cancer. First and foremost, high levels of circulating insulin significantly increase cancer risk. A close second would be the presence of excess fat and glucose in a cell. A 2007 Swedish study found strong associations between high levels of fasting glucose and cancer. Overall, the highest quartile had 25% more cancer than the lowest for women and 8% for men. This is significant, but what particularly stands out is that some cancers were strongly affected while others were hardly affected at all. For instance, ovarian and breast cancer in women under 50 more than doubled with the high glucose conditions. Kidney and pancreatic cancer doubled as well. Melanoma and bladder cancer were up 70%. Several other cancers were unaffected by sugar levels. Prostate cancer was actually slightly lower. Oddly, the study did not measure insulin, which may have been the principal cause of the cancers. Clearly, it can be concluded that certain cancers are strongly associated with high glucose levels.

An Austrian study found a fourfold increase in liver cancer in people with high glucose levels.

Insulin May Be the Primary Culprit

Insulin in particular seems suspect. How do we conclude this? A very misguided approach to adult onset diabetes is administration of additional insulin. This lowers glucose, but raises insulin. Instances of cancer increased by 50% in those receiving additional insulin. If glucose were the primary culprit, we would expect a decrease in cancer with increases in insulin, but this is not the case.

In fact, adult onset diabetics, most of whom have chronically high insulin, have a much higher cancer rate even without adding extra insulin.

Though high insulin is clearly implicated in increased cancer risk, chronically high insulin is primarily found in those with chronically high glucose levels, so whatever may be said of one applies to the other.

Low-carb Diets

A low-carb diet fights cancer by reducing available glucose and lowering insulin. Given what we know about high glucose, high insulin, and cancer, this low-carb benefit is rather obvious. Low carbs means lower glucose and lower insulin. This will clearly work.

Sometimes you will see vegan diets promoted as anti-cancer, with the implication that meat somehow caused the cancer. This is completely untrue. Meat, at least clean meat, doesn't cause cancer. It is protective. The best way to fight cancer is to get the various blood markers into healthy zones as rapidly as possible, and a vegan diet isn't going to accomplish that at all.

CANCER SIDEBAR
Breast Cancer

The breasts consist of a system of milk-producing lobules, which deliver the milk to the nipples via ducts. Usually breast cancer develops in either the ducts (ductal carcinoma) or lobules (lobular carcinoma). Is there a cancerous stem cell behind all this? It is generally thought so, but this has apparently been hard to pin down.

The standard screening currently is the mammogram. This is controversial because of both false positives and false negatives. A positive reading will usually be followed by additional diagnosis, encompassing one or more of: a more focused mammogram, ultrasound, an MRI, or a biopsy.

Treatment can consist of surgery, radiation, and chemotherapy.

The most commonly occurring cancer is Ductal Carcinoma In Situ (in place) (DCIS). Most of these are precancerous conditions and never cause a problem. However, treatment is often applied anyway, as it is hard to tell which DCIS will remain passive or disappear, and which will invade. Ductal arcinoma, both the _in situ_ and Invasive variants tend to show up on a mammogram.

Lobular carcinoma is more serious. It also has an _in situ_ variant. Lobular carcinoma is not usually detected with a mammogram.

It has been the experience of Quantitative Medicine that women with low insulin, normal IGF-1, and normal estradiol are at low risk for breast cancer. This is also supported in the literature. Adopting a lifestyle that tends to manage these three markers accordingly would be a good prevention strategy.

Phytochemicals Might Prevent Cancer

Colored fruit and vegetables have a variety of chemicals that protect them against various predators: bacteria, fungi, bugs, and so on. While we may share a vulnerability to bacteria, other plant predators pose little risk. It is then somewhat odd that on the whole, these assorted chemicals are quite beneficial for us, especially considering that the plant had no such altruistic notions in mind when it decided to evolve them.

These phytochemicals have, or may have, cancer-fighting properties. This would be good news were it true, and it most likely is, but most studies haven't found anything particularly strong. In any case, the colorful vegetables are by far the healthiest plant-based food you can eat. The only thing wrong with the fruits is their sugar content. Those with glucose issues should avoid these. If not, enjoy them too. (All the phytochemicals can be obtained from eating vegetables alone, though.) Owing to their high phytochemical content, the berries are especially healthy.

Poor Sleep Patterns Cause Cancer

Shift workers, nurses for instance, and people with irregular schedules, such as airline employees, appear to have a 50% higher rate of cancer.

There seems to be no general awareness of this, but it should be an area of significant concern. The principal cause may be the disruption of the melatonin cycle. Melatonin is a hormone that is triggered by darkness and mediates sleep timing, and is thought to have anti-cancer properties as well. Shift work is known to disrupt or even eliminate the melatonin cycle.

Poor-quality sleep is also a risk factor for cancer, apparently interfering with the immune system as well as disrupting the melatonin cycle.

QUANTITATIVE MEDICINE AND CANCER

The general principles of Quantitative Medicine afford the strongest possible resistance to cancer. Likewise, recovery is also significantly enhanced. If cellular stress is kept to a minimum, repair mechanisms enhanced, and immune system surveillance boosted, most cancers will be contained and eliminated before they become dangerous.

Unlike the case with atherosclerosis and adult onset diabetes, we do not have a tidy set of blood markers that predict cancer risk. We have mainly cortisol as a direct measure of stress, and some idea of mitochondrial health from the exercise-related markers. However, given the sharp increase in cancer found in adult onset diabetics, glucose and insulin levels are reasonably included as cancer promoters too. So then, the Quantitative Medicine formula for avoiding cancer consists of:

1. Minimizing environmental stress. Give up smoking, avoid pollution. Try to eat organic, especially berries and root vegetables. Get some sun, but avoid getting sunburned.
2. Modifying diet to bring insulin down. This essentially means cutting glucose intake—sugar and starch. Make sure to eat a variety of natural animal and vegetable product.
3. Reducing cortisol. More than any other measurement, cortisol is predictive of cancer. Meditation, contemplation, prayer, yoga, and Taijiquan activities reduce cortisol.
4. Sleeping well. Cellular repair occurs during sleep. Cellular damage causes cancer.
5. Exercising. Exercise fights cancer in several ways, increasing both HDL and HDL2b. Likewise, exercise improves mitochondrial function. Finally, exercise signals higher levels of hormonal

growth and repair activities both systemically and locally, all of these reduce cellular stress. QM exercise also modulates and improves cortisol levels directly.

There is scant evidence that hunter-gatherers get cancer.

Besides appropriate lifestyle choices, effective screening is also key. There is a large amount of research and development currently (2016) ongoing aimed at finding better and less intrusive cancer detection methods. A fair amount of this is based on emulating the cancer-sniffing ability of various trained dogs. Everyone should keep their eye open for new developments in this fast-moving area.

Key Points
22 - Cancer

- The immune system fights cancer.
- Millions of tiny cancers form and are blocked by the immune system. Only a very few go on to become larger tumors.
- Cancer is caused by damage to cellular DNA.
- Besides lifestyle, DNA damage can come from many things: UV light, pollution, etc.
- The cell can repair a lot of DNA damage.
- Cells that cannot repair DNA damage are supposed to commit suicide, aka apoptosis.
- Colorectal, breast, bladder, prostate, squamous cell, and malignant melanoma are usually curable if caught early.
- There is a disturbing trend away from screening.
- Most breast cancer is detected by self examination.
- Colorectal cancer is detected with a colonoscopy.
- People should get a colonoscopy at age 40.
- Prostate cancer is detected with a PSA blood test.
- Full-body scan may detect cancers as small as 3-4 mm.
- Lifestyle choices can cause cancer.
- Chronic stress causes cancer.
- Chronically high glucose or high insulin causes cancer.
- Exercise reduces cancer risk by raising HDL level and for other reasons.
- Poor sleep patterns can cause cancer.
- Colored vegetables have anti-cancer properties.

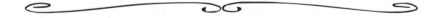

23 - ADULT ONSET DIABETES

Adult onset diabetes is not genetic and is curable. Many in the medical profession would disagree with both claims. Quantitative Medicine clinical practice has cured adult onset diabetes consistently and repeatedly.

Logical proof that adult onset diabetes is not genetic is simple: A lot more people have it now than 50 or 100 years ago. Genetics simply cannot change that fast. Our body manages sugar and starches as it has for tens of thousands of years, as though we were still hunter-gatherers. That's how fast genetics works.

Genetics may make a person more susceptible to adult onset diabetes, but does not mean that he or she will inevitably get it. Genetic disposition to this disease is a survival skill. The ability to store large amounts of nutrients would mean life or death in situations where food supplies were disrupted for long periods, such as ice age winters. The people that could store excess food survived and went on to reproduce. Thus that genetic trait was selected and passed down to some of us. Of course, food shortage is no longer the human circumstance, at least in the Western world, and the genetic ability to store large amounts of nutrients for a bleak or uncertain future is no longer a healthy attribute.

Reversal of adult onset diabetes can be difficult, but judge the alternative: Left to its own devices, adult onset diabetes kills the eyes, the kidneys, the fingertips and toes, the brain, and the heart. It lowers testosterone, impairs memory, and speeds the loss of bone mineral density. It causes heart attacks, strokes, and cancer. It causes aging at very high speed. It is effectively all degenerative diseases packaged as one.

Adult onset diabetes is also called Adult Onset Diabetes Mellitus, Type 2 Diabetes, and non-insulin dependent diabetes. For the rest of the chapter, we'll use its most common acronym: AODM.

AODM is usually defined as a failure to properly manage glucose. Since it is the "job" of insulin to get rid of glucose, AODM got categorized as diabetes, i.e. not enough insulin. Although it is possible to have an impairment in insulin production, by far the principal cause of AODM is not a lack of insulin, but instead, way too much glucose.

DIAGNOSIS AND INSULIN RESISTANCE

AODM is usually diagnosed from glucose levels alone, and it is odd that insulin is not part of the diagnosis. There are three glucose measurements that are usually considered.

- Two-hour glucose. This is meant to simulate the body's response to a meal: 75 mg of straight glucose is administered intravenously, and the glucose level measured after 2 hours.
- Fasting glucose. This is blood glucose concentration after a 12 to 14-hour fast.
- Average glucose, also known as Hemoglobin A1C, or simply A1C, is a surrogate measurement, meaning that the percentage of blood hemoglobin that is "glycated" (has a sugar molecule attached to it) is measured. This is normally given as a percentage of total hemoglobin. Often an equivalent blood glucose concentration is presented. A 5% A1C means an average glucose level of 97 mg/dl, 6% means 126 mg/dl.

Here are the levels that usually define AODM.

	Healthy Level	"Normal" Upper Limit	AODM Lower Limit
Two-hour Glucose	120 mg/dl	140 mg/dl	200 mg/dl
Fasting Glucose	<80 mg/dl	110 mg/dl	125 mg/dl
Average Glucose (A1C percentage)	<100 mg/dl (5.1%)	125 mg/dl (5.9%)	140 mg/dl (6.5%)

However, people with AODM can have glucose levels significantly higher. Above 250 is considered dangerous.

Three Important Points

1. It is possible for a type 1 diabetic to be an adult onset diabetic as well. This is probably the case if significantly increased amounts of additional insulin are needed to maintain good glucose levels.
2. Note that the AODM diagnosis is only about glucose. However, chronically high insulin is dangerous too. A type 1 or 2 diabetic may drive their glucose down to a safe level. However, if doing this requires chronically high insulin levels, the purpose is defeated. To be healthy, both glucose and insulin need to be at safe levels.
3. AODM and obesity are not the same thing. It is possible to be obese and not have AODM. Think sumo wrestler. It is also possible to have AODM and not be overweight.

HOW DOES AODM START?

As chronic diseases go, AODM is something of a con game. The victim is lured in with sugar and starch. Then hormones and cellular metabolism change and make him dependent on it—in effect locking him in. It becomes difficult to roll this back.

Insulin Resistance

The mechanism that powers this trap is called , and the trap itself works like this:

Fat in the form of triglycerides circulates in the blood, packaged in lipoprotein particles: chylomicrons and VLDL particles. Any cell needing a meal can snatch a triglyceride molecule from the passing particle parade. This is the "fuel" we are evolved to use, at least in all areas but the brain.

Glucose is different. All carbohydrate food that is digested is converted to glucose, and enters the bloodstream as such, but muscle and fat cells don't grab passing glucose particles unless there is elevated insulin in the blood as well. The insulin acts as a switch. If the insulin level is up, the cell must grab that passing glucose. If not, ignore it. Cells that consume primarily, like neurons, don't do this little dance with the insulin. Neurons will grab what they need.

This insulin switch is an odd complication. Why not just let the muscle and fat cells grab the glucose if they want to?

This glucose control is in place so that the brain won't starve. The brain cells won't eat circulating fat. Actually, they probably would if they could, but blood that is available to the brain has to cross a fine mesh filter called the blood-brain barrier. And it's really fine. Even though fat molecules are pretty small, most can't get across this barrier. Bacteria and viruses are far too large. Glucose, though, is a very tiny molecule and easily makes it across. So the brain runs primarily on glucose. The brain has top priority. Therefore, the other cells, muscle and fat, are not going to be allowed to hog the glucose. Hence the insulin on-off switch.

However, after a meal that includes a lot of starch or sugar, there's a surplus. The non-brain cells can now have some glucose. The body raises the insulin level, which circulates, attaches to cell receptors, and effectively rings a dinner bell. The cells then activate transporters that can pull in the glucose. But the insulin does a bit more than just start a glucose feeding frenzy. It also signals the cells to *stop* eating fat. If circulating glucose is high, a storage molecule called glycogen, which is found in the liver and muscle (but not in the fat cells) is topped up. Once these are full, the rest of the glucose is converted to fat and stored in the fat cells. The body clearly does not want high levels of circulating glucose. High levels foul up cellular functionality in a variety of ways.

At least this is how it is supposed to all work: the body will secrete enough insulin to bring the circulating glucose back down to the homeostatic level: around 80 mg/dl.

The Topsy-Turvy World of Insulin Resistance

Suppose glucose levels get high. We aren't "designed," as it were, to run on glucose. Our hunter-gatherer ancestors normally got little. Our body treats excess glucose like a windfall and tends to store it, but it really doesn't handle excess amounts very well. (Fat is a different story: the body deals quite efficiently with excess fat.)

Suppose the cells refuse to take up any more glucose. The glucose is high, insulin is high, but the cells turn up their noses. Both levels remain high, and are essentially stuck there. This is a very unhealthy situation. This cellular refusal to take in the glucose is at the core of insulin resistance. The cell is "resisting" the insulin's orders to use the glucose. This insulin resistance trap was, in the past, called Syndrome-X.

Now why would cells refuse glucose? This isn't fully known, but here are some possible reasons. Reason #1 we have already mentioned: they're full. This could certainly apply to muscle cells. They maintain little local glycogen storage depots to store excess glucose, but once these are full, they've got no place to store more glucose. But fat cells don't get full so easily. They stretch and expand to make room for more. Reason #2: The cells have aged. They just don't respond to insulin like they used to. Reason #3: Fat cells appear to have their limits too. Once a fat cell is reaching its limits, it gets inflamed and won't store more.

This does make some sense. High insulin is an attempt at force-feeding. The cells just aren't going for it. Actually, the body's ability to produce insulin tends to become impaired in a high-glucose environment as well, further adding to the problem. High glucose tends to kill insulin-producing beta cells. Carried to the extreme, this can result in type 1 diabetes on top of the type 2 version.

Why Does Insulin Shut Down Fat Metabolism?

There may be several reasons, but one is that high insulin and glucose are significantly more dangerous than high fat. So insulin-glucose clearance gets a priority.

On a more anthropological level, let's take it as a given that, metabolically speaking, we handle food the same way as our hunter-gatherer ancestors. What did those guys eat? Animals they could hunt and plants they could gather. Animals year round, vegetables for a portion of the year, and fruit in the summer.

Food shortages were a way of life for many hunter-gatherers. Those living in the north would also have to contend with ice age winters. So when that summertime fruit was available, why not store it all as fat for the impending ice age winter? That's what bears do. That's what we did (and still do). We don't hibernate, but we have a lot of the skill set. High insulin? Store everything.

The Effects of High Glucose and High Insulin

A consequence of chronically high glucose is high triglycerides—circulating fat. It might seem odd that levels of fat would be high in conditions of glucose overload, but there are two reasons for this. First, as mentioned, high insulin inhibits the cells from burning fat for energy, so circulating fat naturally piles up, and second, the liver makes *more* fat particles.

Why would the liver do that? The liver makes those fat particles from the circulating glucose. The liver, it seems, is also joining the effort to reduce glucose levels. The body can safely tolerate a much broader range of circulating of fat. Triglyceride levels from 20 to 500 would not cause any immediate problems, whereas glucose at either of those extremes would be quite dangerous, even fatal.

High Fat Intake and AODM

High fat is a bit of a red herring. Because of the excess circulating fat (triglycerides) that is invariably found in those with AODM, advice is frequently given to minimize it, especially saturated fat—medicine's standard boogeyman. It is widely believed that saturated fat *causes* insulin resistance, and numerous studies have elicited various mechanisms tending to revolve around fat cell impairment due to inflammation, with saturated fat the leading culprit.

But, in fact, this "it's the fat" hypothesis does not hold up at all. There are so many interconnected metabolic pathways in AODM that it is very difficult to figure out which factors affect what. That is one reason why, after all these many years, there is no clear consensus. Sadly, the most common diet recommendations, high-carb low-fat, do not appear to work at all, and will usually exacerbate the disease.

One problem is that much of the experimental work is done on mice; perhaps as many as 15,000 studies. (A Hamelin of mice studies?) It seems that the dietary recommendations for diabetic mice do not translate well to humans. There are even several papers that examine this. Extrapolation to humans is a general problem with mice studies. Mice are available for research, and sometimes the results carry over to humans, but other times not.

To cut this medical Gordian knot, as it were, we can simply look at the effect of high-fat and high-saturated-fat diets on people that have AODM. The results here are starkly clear. A variety of well-done studies simply do not implicate fat. Quite the opposite. High-fat, low-carb diets are curative—high-carb diets are not. Virtually every study shows dramatic improvement with high-fat, low-carb diets. This could hardly be the case if fat were promoting insulin resistance, but that is almost beside the point. Low-carb diets are curing people, and curing with immediate results. In fact, it is quite difficult to find any study, well done or otherwise, where a high-fat, low-carb diet did not significantly improve AODM symptoms.

With results this dramatic and strong, you would think that all AODM diet recommendations would be immediately revised. Sadly this is not the case. As of 2016, it's still lots of carbs and low-fat.

CONSEQUENCES OF AODM

AODM is a perfect metabolic storm: high glucose, high insulin, and high triglycerides. And with the high triglycerides, we have the consequent Pattern B LDL particles, which were discussed in detail as heart attack risks in ATHEROSCLEROSIS, Chapter 21. The cellular stress of all this produces a general, overall inflammation (high levels of C-reactive protein). Cortisol tends to be high as well, and the immune system function is curtailed.

This is a very unhealthy environment, and it should come as no surprise that adult onset diabetics, who represent 35% of the population in the U.S., have 80% of the health problems.

The AODM condition is a launchpad for a variety of degenerative diseases. The top four risk areas are:

1. Impairment of micro-vascular health. There is little public awareness of micro-vascular health. In this scenario, the blood circulation is impaired, and tissue starts to die. This could occur in the eyes, the kidneys, the fingers and toes, or any other extremity. Erectile dysfunction could be a consequence.
2. Impairment of macro-vascular health. We refer here to atherosclerosis. AODM conditions cause atherosclerosis. This leads to high blood pressure, ischemia, heart attack, embolisms, and stroke.
3. Cancer. Due to cellular stress, AODM substantially elevates cancer risk. The immune system tends to be suppressed along with HDL levels, aggravating the problem.
4. Dementia. The same markers that define AODM are high-risk factors for dementias, particularly Alzheimer's.

VIRTUALLY ALL ADULT ONSET DIABETES CAN BE CURED BY LIFESTYLE CHANGE

Further, virtually all patients that have been treated for AODM with Quantitative Medicine lifestyle changes *have* been cured. It is largely a matter of getting the body out of its glucose dependence and AODM-induced torpor.

DIETARY

If it's all about glucose rising to high levels because the cells don't want it, isn't there a solution just screaming at us: CUT THE GLUCOSE?

And if study after study shows substantial improvement with low-carb diets, isn't the message clearly: CUT THE GLUCOSE?

We do not know what could be a plainer truth. Obvious, logical, verifiable, and repeatable, but adding to the absurdity, this was once common knowledge.

Here is an excerpt from a 1917 book, easily available online, called *The Diabetic Cookbook*. It has this list of strictly forbidden food.

This book goes on to allow freely: all meats, fish, poultry, dairy, all sorts of fat, most colored vegetables.

This was the right diet. It worked then, and it still does. Now this book was written for type 1 diabetics, but dietary needs are identical for AODM. This diet is very pointedly trying to minimize glucose.

At some point in the '60s, this cookbook and its sage

DIABETIC COOKERY		13
TABLE IV		
Foods Strictly Forbidden		
1. Sugars	15.	Beets (on doctor's
2. All Farinaceous Foods		order)
and Starches	16.	Large Onions
3. Pies	17.	All Sweet and Dried
4. Puddings		Fruits
5. Flour	18.	Honey
6. Bread	19.	Levulose
7. Biscuits	20.	All Sweet Wines
8. Rice (by permission only)	21.	Liqueurs
9. Sago	22.	Cordials
10. Arrowroot	23.	Syrups
11. Barley	24.	Beer
12. Oatmeal (by permission	25.	Ale
only)	26.	Stout
13. Tapioca	27.	Porter
14. Macaroni	28.	Chocolate
29. Condensed Milk		

advice were tossed out the window. The medical authorities today have extensive advice about proper AODM diet, and though some of it is good, there are invariably certain recommendations that completely derail the healing process. Here are some examples:

American Diabetes Association

- "Starchy foods can be part of a healthy meal plan, but portion size is key. Whole grain breads, cereals, pasta, rice and starchy vegetables like potatoes, yams, peas and corn can be included in your meals and snacks." "Wondering how much carbohydrate you can have? A place to start is about 45-60 grams of carbohydrate per meal."
- "A healthy meal plan for people with diabetes is generally the same as a healthy diet for anyone—low in saturated fat"

British National Health Service

- "Increasing the amount of fibre in your diet and reducing your fat intake, particularly saturated fat"
- "Increase your consumption of high fibre foods, such as wholegrain bread and cereals, beans and lentils, and fruit and vegetables"
- "Choose foods that are low in fat – replace butter, ghee and coconut oil with low-fat spreads and vegetable oil"

U.S. National Institute of Health

- "Eating a variety of whole-grain foods, fruits and vegetables every day"
- "Eating less fat"
- "Using less salt"

We are in total disagreement with these specifics, but why should you believe us? We seem to be enamored with a 1917 cookbook. Are we hopelessly out of date?

Wake up institutional medicine! If the problem is an inability to metabolize glucose, what is the obvious solution? We don't give alcoholics more alcohol. We don't give addicts more drugs. Why is AODM any different? Due to the mechanism of insulin resistance, sugar/starch has become an addiction. Fat is not the problem. Glucose is the problem. Why complicate things? Cut out sugar and starch and get well. Sugar and starch exacerbate the problem. Fats reverse it, and this includes saturated fat. Without exception, cutting glucose has reversed AODM for every Quantitative Medicine patient that presented with it and followed the protocols.

Why the Huge Disconnect?

The 1917 cookbook shows that we once had it right, but things changed. There are political agendas and history at work here. Baby boomers and beyond will remember the dietary advice that preceded the Food Pyramid. There was the idea of a balanced diet, represented by a plate, divided in thirds, with a meat, vegetable, fruit portion, and, interestingly, no bread. Sounds sensible, and it more or less was. Then along came the demonization of cholesterol, the demonization of saturated fat, and the demonization of red meat. These three dietary witches were simultaneously burnt at the stake with the introduction of the Food Pyramid. At the base were breads and cereals, then came fruits and vegetables. Over half the pyramid was now starches and sugary fruits. Dairy, beans, nuts, meats, eggs, and oils then competed for the tiny space at the top. Whole grain got promoted to the level of wonder drug.

This was shock treatment. A huge change in recommended food consumption patterns. The high priests of nutrition were absolutely, positively sure this would cure all health problems past, present, and future.

So 40 years later, what have we to show for this? An adult onset diabetes epidemic. The food pyramid did nothing to cure this. It caused it. Make no mistake about that.

What were they thinking? Hunter-gatherers, who never get AODM (as long as they stay away from us), wouldn't even recognize the bottom bread and cereal layer as food. But so confident are the gurus that all this sage advice lives on. There are rebellions brewing here and there, but high-starch, low-fat is still the mainstream advice. We suppose they intend to keep it going until it works—or we're all dead.

We Do Not Need Any Sugar or Starch

There is some general notion that dietary glucose is essential, the basic fuel of life, or essential for the brain, or something along those lines. It is true that the brain runs mainly on glucose, but it can also run on the smaller fat molecules and on ketones. The liver will *always* supply enough nutrients for the brain no matter what you eat. It can and does synthesize glucose as needed, and can also synthesize ketones, which are a backup fuel for the brain, and a perfectly satisfactory one. In fact, it may run better on ketones. Several studies have indicated that a ketogenic diet has significant benefits for dementia sufferers.

None of the other cells in the body need glucose. In fact, they run cleaner and better on fat.

How can we be so sure that we don't need dietary glucose? Again, back to our hunter-gatherers. Not a lot of vegetal matter grows in winter, especially an ice age one. For arctic hunter-gatherers, there is little available year round. But these people thrived on a diet of protein and fat. They were (and are) very healthy. Starch and sugar were typically a windfall, and invariably stored as fat. As their descendants, we have the same dietary tendencies.

It's Quite Hard to Cut the Glucose

AODM locks you in. After a period of time in a high-glucose environment, the cells are thoroughly "programmed" to run exclusively on glucose. They are literally programmed. The cellular mechanisms that metabolize fats are suppressed and inactive, while those metabolizing sugar are fully engaged. This has the attributes of addiction: a need for more, and cutting is painful.

Suppose glucose is cut dramatically—no sugar, no starch. Circulating glucose and insulin will immediately start to come down. This is disease reversal, plain and simple. However, the cells aren't quite ready for this and do not utilize the available circulating fat—at least not at first. The cells get hungry, and their owner gets hungry—for sugar and starch. Resisting this phase takes substantial willpower, but there is no danger here. Eventually, the cells will respond and start using the fat. Insulin will drop. Glucose will drop and the craving for sugar and starch will completely cease. This could take a couple of weeks or several months, but it will definitely happen.

Once the transition is made:

- No more craving.
- Weight will tend toward the ideal homeostatic level.
- Lipid profile will improve dramatically.
- Well-being and focus will improve dramatically.
- Sugar and starch will taste a little weird.
- If this is coupled with an exercise and spiritual discipline program, cancer and atherosclerosis will reverse.

To its general discredit, the medical profession assumes no one has the willpower to pull this off. However, in the Quantitative Medicine practice, cutting the starch/sugar, along with an intense exercise program, has been successful almost every time, and compliance has been high.

Why does the medical profession assume that no one has willpower? Simple. The ones that had the willpower got cured and didn't come back. The repeat customers are those that couldn't successfully change their diet—but that's not entirely their fault. Successful treatment is usually dependent on patient awareness of these three key components:

1. Knowledge of the real consequences of AODM. Many view AODM as a weight issue, but it is far worse than that.

2. Certainty that the Quantitative Medicine protocols work: why they work, what they consist of, and how long they take.

3. A means to track the progress. The periodic Quantitative Medicine measurements provide this information.

Is This Really a Cure?

High glucose, high insulin, and high triglycerides will subside to healthy levels fairly quickly. Other key numbers will likewise improve, though up to a year many be needed. When all the numbers are in their ideal zones, the health risks associated with AODM will be completely gone. It is hard to argue that this is not a cure.

However, if the dietary discipline is broken, the AODM will return, and likely fairly quickly. In this sense, there is no cure.

Frequently doctors and others will toss around terms like "incurable," implying that AODM is out of your control. This is absolutely untrue.

Two AODM Therapies to Absolutely Avoid

It seems completely obvious that supplementary booze is not a cure for alcoholism. Why, then, is it not also completely obvious that additional glucose is not a cure for AODM, or that additional insulin is not a cure for AODM? Yet a high-starch diet is often recommended, and additional insulin frequently prescribed. High starch makes no sense at all, yet as late as 2016, the British National Health Service and other health authorities are recommending *increasing* consumption of breads and cereals (whole grain of course). To be fair, this recommendation is controversial in many spheres beyond our own.

Administration of extra insulin is a widespread practice. High insulin causes cancer. Higher insulin causes more cancer. In fact, there are numerous studies that indicate increased cancer rates of more than 50%

for adult onset diabetics receiving insulin therapy, though simultaneously taking metformin may somewhat mitigate the cancer risk.

Could the increased cancer risk be from high glucose instead? There are two strikes against this one. First, insulin is a known growth factor and cell division promoter in several cancers. Second, insulin therapy does indeed reduce glucose levels, at the expense of increased circulating insulin levels. If glucose were the culprit, cancer would go down in this case, not up.

EXERCISE

Exercise may be more important than diet. In one small study, eight AODM men performed six sessions of high-intensity training over a two-week period. The training consisted of stationary bike riding at 90% of their maximum heart rate, specifically one minute of pedaling, one minute of rest, repeated 10 times. Painfully hard, but blissfully short. This program amounted to a grand total of 60 minutes of bike riding. Their bodies responded by lowering average glucose from 170 mg/dl to 143 mg/dl. Now this is an astonishing result, halfway to a cure. It is even more amazing given the short duration of the exercise program.

A more program would be the exercise protocols described elsewhere in the book: two intense 45-minute sessions per week, with a third "easy" session added for balance and joint health. However, there can be many other routines that work and embody the ideal elements.

SPIRITUAL DISCIPLINE OR MEDITATION

High circulating cortisol can literally cause AODM. High cortisol causes fat storage and blocks fat metabolism. Why? This is another case of the stingy body. Conserving energy in a stressful situation probably made survival sense for a hunter-gatherer.

DO ALL THREE

The Quantitative Medicine protocol is all of the above. Switch to a sensible diet free of starches and sugars. Undertake twice weekly intense exercise sessions. Practice a spiritual discipline 10 minutes each day. Some raw commitment will be needed the first few weeks, but reversal will begin immediately.

TWO INTERESTING CASE STUDIES

The first case, "Jones," is unusual in that insulin resistance is absent. The second case, "Wilson," represents a strong insulin resistance situation, but one that would go unnoticed without Quantitative Medicine measurements.

Dr. Mike Case Study
Curing Adult Onset Diabetes

"Mr. Jones" was an identical twin. When he got diabetes, his brother did too.

"Mr. Jones" was 39 years old when I met him. He came into my office with a copy of his last set of blood tests. Across the face of the copy his doc had written, "Eat better and exercise more." His doc had tried several medications and offered standard advice on diet and exercise, and had done as much as office time would normally allow. Yet the young man I met was clearly motivated and wanted very specific and detailed advice and guidance and was willing to follow such direction if it worked. His identical twin brother was not interested.

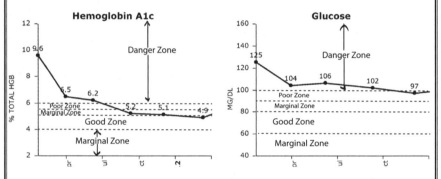

As I was going to ask "Mr. Jones" to undertake intense exercise, and given the severity of his diabetes (an A1C of 9.6, which represents an average blood sugar of 264), I had him undertake a nuclear stress heart test to make sure it was safe for him to exercise so intensely. His stress test was positive. In other words, he had coronary artery blockages, which put him at risk of a future heart attack. His ischemia, a sign of blockage, occurred at a high enough heart rate and work load that we were able to begin his training, without a stent, by carefully monitoring his heart rate to peak at just above his ischemic heart rate. This is called ischemic heart rate training. Never (!) do this on your own. Following my training protocols, carefully monitored by an accomplished personal trainer, and dietary guidelines, outlined in the book, he lowered his A1C to 5.2, an average blood sugar of 108—well below diabetes level—and eventually he had a negative nuclear stress test. He had reversed his coronary artery disease.

"Mr. Jones" was an exceptionally motivated patient and was meticulous in following guidance and by any standard did an amazing job of fixing his diabetes and heart disease. He is also unusual in that his diabetes is not from your typical insulin resistance syndrome; his diabetes is not driven by high insulin, his is driven by a liver that dumps and stores out of sync with his insulin. Still he cured his diabetes.

His brother did not make the changes and remains a diabetic and obese. The fact that they are maternal twins (identical) proves the main point that a person's will can overcome their genetics to a remarkable degree.

This story illustrates that while genetics plays an important role in illness, choices—character if you will—are even more important.

Dr. Mike Case Study

Curing Adult Onset Diabetes

"Mr. Wilson's" case illustrates a very common problem that can be missed unless you look a little deeper. Notice on his graph that his fasting glucose is 100mg/dl. This level has the formal name "impaired fasting glucose." Note too that his HDL is low at 39. His A1C is 5.6, which is less than the pre-diabetes number of 5.7. At 47 he is at very real risk of developing diabetes.

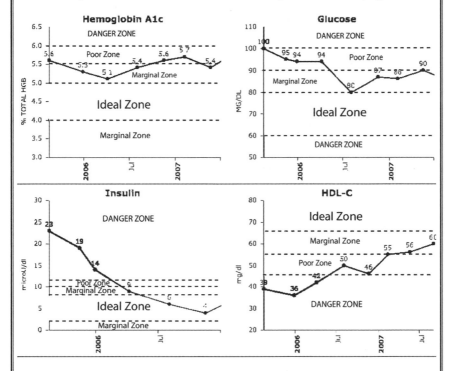

Often overlooked is fasting insulin. Note Wilson's initial level of 23. His diet at that time was high in starch and so tended to cause a high level of insulin. Upon switching to the QM diet, his insulin decreased to 10, yet his glucose dropped as well. This means the QM diet is making insulin more effective, and hence the QM diet "cured" insulin resistance.

Contrast this with the example of "Mr. Jones," who had full-blown diabetes but low insulin. I don't want to sketch out all of the possible scenarios, including some stages of insulin resistance syndrome (IRS) that can look like "Mr. Jones" without being just non-IRS diabetes but keep in mind that "Mr. Jones" did not have a fasting glucose level near as high as his average of 265, whereas "Mr. Wilson" has a fasting glucose of 100 and an average glucose of 122 (A1C of 5.6). So "Mr. Jones" had wildly variant fasting and average glucose numbers with low insulin and "Mr. Wilson" had similar fasting and average glucose numbers with much, much higher insulin. These are differences that matter and that become important when giving dietary advice. "Mr. Jones" needs to be careful to eat every three hours, including a bedtime snack to help stabilize his liver's response to insulin, and "Mr. Wilson" needs to mostly focus on eliminating anything that stimulates insulin. Clearly there are overlaps in the dietary advice each should get but the focus and guidance and ability to comply differ by personality. And this is where the external and objective guidance of numbers needs to work with the internal and subjective character of each of us. This is, after all, a human enterprise.

SOME OTHER TYPES OF DIABETES

Gestational Diabetes

In about 7% of pregnancies, glucose will increase to diabetic levels, typically in the third trimester. Normally this goes away, but this is known to be a risk factor for AODM, so it should be followed.

Type 1 Diabetes

This is also known as juvenile diabetes or insulin-dependent diabetes. In this version of the disease, the body cannot make insulin at all and it must be obtained externally. Type 1 diabetes is beyond the purview of Quantitative Medicine, but we mention it because a type 1 diabetic can become a type 2 diabetic as well. Insulin resistance is a risk for either one. Should insulin resistance begin to occur, a type 1 diabetic will require more and more insulin to maintain proper glucose levels. This high level of circulating insulin is dangerous. A type 1 diabetic who has become a type 2 diabetic should also cut the dietary glucose.

Key Points

23 - Adult Onset Diabetes (AODM)

- AODM is not genetic. A population's genetics cannot change as rapidly as this disease has appeared.
- AODM is defined as chronically high glucose levels.
- AODM is curable with lifestyle change.
- Overweight people do not necessarily have AODM and vice versa.
- The body tries to regulate glucose downward by raising insulin levels. Hence insulin levels become chronically high as well.
- Both chronically high insulin and glucose cause cancer.
- High glucose levels are due to excess dietary sugar and starch.
- High glucose levels cause high triglyceride (circulating fat) levels.
- High triglyceride levels cause small LDL particle size, which causes atherosclerosis.
- Cutting sugar and starches, perhaps completely, will reverse and cure AODM.
- Exercise greatly speeds up the process. For a cure, both are needed.
- It will be difficult to cut down sugar and starch and may take up to six weeks to adapt.
- Much advice recommends high carbohydrates and low saturated fat. This advice is dangerous and completely wrong, and will worsen the disease.
- Successful treatment depends on patient awareness and means to monitor progress.

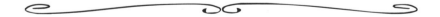

24 - OSTEOPOROSIS

O steoporosis is widely thought to be an affliction of elderly women, but it frequently strikes both men and the non-elderly as well. It is also widely thought to be incurable and irreversible. These too are both wrong. Osteoporotic bones lead to the reduction of stature and the hunched-over appearance that everyone is familiar with. This is tragic, but made even more so by the fact that it is 100% preventable.

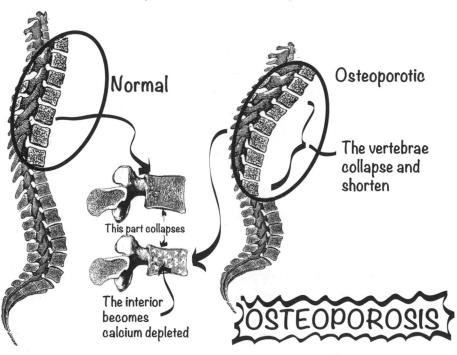

Normal

Osteoporotic

The vertebrae collapse and shorten

This part collapses

The interior becomes calcium depleted

OSTEOPOROSIS

Osteoporosis is caused by a lack of calcium in the bones. This causes them to weaken, eventually to the point of not being able to support the weight their owners place on them. At this point, they start to crush in on themselves. This is called the "fracture threshold." Bones in this weakened state are also much more likely to break in a fall.

How Is Bone Built?

Most people's knowledge of bones comes from the remains of a meal, or from those that amuse their dogs. They are seen as hard, rock-like, hollow, and inert. They look like they will last hundreds of years. These are dead bones. If they have been outside for a while, all that's left is the calcium deposits that made them so hard. This is deceiving. A bone is quite complex, and is often considered an organ. Besides providing structural support, it also acts as a mineral depot and houses the cellular factory that manufactures red and white blood cells. It has an elaborate blood supply and is continually tearing itself down and rebuilding itself.

A live bone is a lot stronger than Rover's plaything. A bone is constructed rather like a steel-reinforced concrete pillar. Concrete is immensely strong under compression, but not strong at all if pulled apart: a tension-type stress. For this reason, reinforcing steel bars, called rebar, are embedded in the concrete pillars to provide the needed tension strength. Civil engineering copied this from bones. The hard mineral part of a bone is quite strong for compressive forces. It's built around a cellular-generated matrix made of collagen, which has enormous tension strength, just like the rebar. Ligaments and tendons are also made of collagen. Collagen is made of fibrous strands, and for its weight, is actually stronger than steel.

This structure is maintained by a busy construction crew of bone cells. The three types of interest are osteoblasts, osteocytes, and osteoclasts.

The first two of these are differentiated from mesenchymal stem cells, which are plentiful both inside bones and in the surrounding sheath.

To build new bone, the osteoblasts tightly align themselves in a rectangular formation. They then secrete collagen, forming a very strong scaffolding-like matrix. To this they attach mineral crystals made mainly from calcium. This is the bone material. As they build layer upon layer of this, they effectively wall themselves in. At this point they are renamed osteocytes. However, they do not die. They live on, and still have several functions. Thus bone is living tissue, even the "bony" part.

How we get bone in the first place is quite complicated. A baby has mainly cartilage. This is replaced by bone via an elaborate process that we won't go into, assuming here that you are already grown-up, and have a full set. Let's consider the part we normally think of as bone, the hard stuff. It is a bunch of layers of osteocytes, which are alive, but imprisoned by the hard calcium wall they themselves built. Surrounding this is a tough layer called the periosteum. It is loaded with mesenchymal stem cells, and will, if conditions are right, lay down another layer of osteoblasts, which will form a collagen matrix, already strong, and then coat that with the mineral bone material, making new bone. The periosteum also has a very strong outer sheath that will tend to hold the bone in place in case of a fracture, basically acting as a cast.

Inside the bone is a spongy layer, called the cancellous, and inside that, the marrow. The marrow is a factory for red and white blood cells.

New bone tends to be made where it is needed. A weight lifter will build new bone in his or her back and legs. A jogger may develop new bone in his or her feet. These are easily seen on X-rays as striations of calcium.

The body knows *where* to build bone because of an amazing property of collagen. It is piezoelectric. Remember piezoelectricity from high school physics? If you put pressure on a piezoelectric crystal, an electric field results. Bone is built over a scaffolding of piezoelectric collagen. Where bone is weak, the collagen scaffold gets pushed and twisted and creates an electric field that attracts new calcium and other minerals.

However, as usual, there is more to it. A variety of growth factors need to be present as well, notably IGF-1, the general "OK-to-build" signal. Of course, that same exercise that stressed the bones in the first place will cause these growth factors to increase as well. So it's a combination: Do the exercises. The growth factors will say, "Build new bone," and the local piezoelectric fields will say, "Build it here."

The collagen piezoelectric effect is important in large fractures as well, where new bone must be built quickly. Clearly there is little strength at the fractured mineral scaffolding, so the collagen there is getting deformed quite a bit. This is why fractures will heal much more quickly if they are not put in a cast, but instead worked a bit.

The bones also play a major role in calcium regulation. Very precise regulation of calcium is important, and the body uses the bones as a storage depot. To reduce circulating calcium, the thyroid secretes calcitonin, which also stimulates bone building, effectively moving calcium from the bloodstream to the bone.

Bone Is Also Torn Down

Bone is torn down for two reasons. First is repair. Although fractures are rare, micro-fractures are common and inevitable. They are just what they sound like. Second, if the body needs calcium, it will tear down bone to get it.

The cells that tear down bone, called osteoclasts, are odd indeed. They have multiple nuclei (five of them typically) and are huge: about five times wider than a normal cell. They look a bit like leeches. It appears these form by fusing multiple white cells together, meaning that they are effectively part of the immune system. However, instead of gobbling bacteria or other invaders, they go after bone. But which bone? The huge cell-leeches are looking for micro-fractures. Micro-fractures occur wherever a rigid structure is used over and over. Remember the walled-in osteocytes? If the micro-fractures involve bone that they made, they secrete a chemical that attracts the osteoclasts. The osteoclasts arrive, attach, and dissolve the bone and collagen matrix. The grand plan is that osteoblasts will come along right after this and build new bone.

The osteoclasts are also involved in calcium regulation. They are responsive to the parathyroid hormone PTH, which regulates calcium by increasing the amount of bone that is torn down, which in turn increases the amount of calcium in the blood supply.

So again, we have an overall signal that says, "Tear down bone," and the micro-fractures say, "Take it from here."

How Is Bone Renewal Regulated?

About 10% of bone is renewed per year. Bone density peaks at about age 21 at around 200 mg/cc. These are strong bones. Beyond this point, the body starts tearing down more bone than it is building, losing bone at a rate of about 2% per year. At first this has little effect, but eventually, bone mineral density is down to around half, at 105 mg/cc. This is the fracture threshold.

The bones can no longer support the weight required of them, and start to crush in on themselves. This is osteoporosis and can happen to both men and women. It can be stopped and reversed by putting more demand on the body's large bones through exercise.

But why the decline? In a large sense, it is almost surely caused by lack of exercise, since hunter-gatherers don't get osteoporosis. To see what is specifically going on, we have to look at the parathyroid hormone, which tears down bone, and thyroid-generated calcitonin, which builds it back up. This tear-down/rebuild process, charmingly called remodeling, prevents the micro-fractures from accumulating.

Now clearly, the thyroid and parathyroid need to cooperate. The levels need to track. We can get a lot of remodeling (tearing down and rebuilding) done by pushing PTH and calcitonin to higher levels. Exercise does this. Likewise, a sedentary lifestyle regulates both of these downward.

We are most interested in altering the tear-down/build-up ratio, so that we get more build-up and avoid osteoporosis. Exercise does just this. It tilts the ratio in a positive direction and thus grows and protects our bones. In fact, it can swing that ratio quite quickly. A three-month resistance exercise program will build bone and have significant, measurable effects.

We do not have a clear picture of exactly how the tear-down, build-back-up process is regulated, but the growth hormones that accompany exercise probably help push it over the threshold so that more new bone is built than destroyed. Whatever the causes, for virtually everyone, building exceeds tear down if proper resistance exercise is undertaken, and since more new bone is being built than is being torn down, osteoporosis is being reversed.

MEASURING OSTEOPOROSIS

The presence or potential risk of osteoporosis is determined by measuring bone mineral density using X-rays. A full-body scan in either an EBT or 256-slice CT machine normally measures the density of three vertebrae. For most people, 105 mg/cc is the fracture threshold, but this is not a firm line. A person is already in trouble at 135.

It is important to catch this before any collapse has occurred. It can then be reversed and avoided for life, with no loss of stature.

Celiac Disease

Low bone density is an expected side effect of celiac disease. Hence, if there is suspicion of osteoporosis, it would be a good idea to test for celiac disease as well, and vice versa.

"STANDARD TREATMENT" FOR OSTEOPOROSIS

The standard therapy is calcium supplementation, possibly with added vitamin D. These are administered ostensibly to correct a calcium deficiency, or to increase the available calcium. From the above bone building descriptions, and the knowledge that calcium is tightly regulated, it is pretty easy to predict what is going to happen:

1. The circulating calcium is tightly regulated and will remain constant. (This tight regulation is critical for proper functioning of neurons and muscles.) Thus the osteoblasts will have no additional calcium, and will not particularly build more bone.
2. PTH will be down-regulated since more circulating calcium is available, which will curtail the activity of the osteoclasts. Thus less bone will be torn down.

This has the effect of slowing down osteoporosis, but doesn't cause new bone to be built, kind of a mixed benefit. The bones basically aren't really any stronger either. All this would probably be mildly beneficial, but in fact, calcium supplementation increased heart attacks 17% in one study.

At low vitamin D levels, calcium supplements no longer work, so vitamin D supplementation is often prescribed as well. Vitamin D may cancel out the negative cardiac effects of calcium supplementation alone.

Rather than playing dangerous games with calcium in hopes of retarding bone loss, a far better strategy is to grow new bone by up-regulating the entire remodeling process with exercise. It doesn't take enormous amounts of exercise to accomplish this, just exercise of the proper sort—resistance exercise that stresses the big bones. With such an approach, the disease is reversed rather than merely retarded, and no risky meddling with a critical bodily regulation system is needed.

If vitamin D levels are low, supplementation would still be a good idea, but without the calcium. Or better still, get more sunshine. Sunshine has many benefits beside vitamin D.

EXERCISES THAT REVERSE OSTEOPOROSIS

Bone can be built by stressing the big bones: the spine, legs and hips. This means weight bearing exercise. This will turn on the growth hormones and up-regulate bone remodeling, building new bone, reversing and curing osteoporosis.

The best exercises for this are squats and deadlifts. Doing three sets of ten each, once a week, correctly and with whatever weight represents a safe challenge, will effectively stop and reverse osteoporosis. Both men and women should do this.

OSTEOPOROSIS CASE STUDIES

The Quantitative Medicine approach is to refrain from taking calcium and instead do big bone resistance exercise—squats, deadlifts, and the like. We have a lot of data on Dr. Mike's cohort. Bone density was increased an average of 20% for those below the fracture threshold. This is reversal and cure for most.

And of course, if other recommended exercises are done as well, heart attacks are reduced 50% or more. This is a considerable improvement over the calcium pill "standard practice," to put it mildly.

Study Detail

In Dr. Nichols's cohort, around 400 of 2,000 patients obtained a bone density measurement. Of those, 92 got a second one, so for these, we can determine a change in bone density. Now of those 92, 51 were in trouble. Their bone density was less than 135. They were all told to stop taking calcium and do the recommended exercises. We do not know how many actually did. Compliance is always hard to discern. However, the average increase in for the 51 people with dangerously low bone density was 14%. This is dramatically better than the calcium "standard-treatment" number of 1% or so, and of course, rather than increasing the risk of heart attacks, the exercise reduced it.

Now of the 52, a smaller group, 19, were in serious trouble with bone density below 105. This is below the fracture threshold, so these people were already experiencing the effects. The average bone density improvement for this group was 20%. All but 3 of the 19 gained bone density, thereby reversing the disease. Two of those three showed no change and one lost more bone. Eight of these people managed to pull themselves above the fracture threshold and are therefore no longer osteoporotic. This is disease cure. Most doctors will tell you this is impossible. Yet here it is.

The worst three, with densities below 60, managed to increase their bone density 45%. That's a huge amount of new bone and certainly put the brakes on osteoporosis.

The typical time between the bone density measurements was one year.

The time between bone density measurements for the calcium supplementation research (which reported a paltry ~1% improvement) was three years.

We conclude from the cohort data that osteoporosis can be reversed and cured for more than 90% of people who comply. Of the 19 in serious trouble, 16 grew new bone. We do not know why two did not. One was known to be non-compliant.

These are remarkable results. There is no pharmaceutical protocol that can come anywhere close to this.

Key Points
24 - Osteoporosis
- Osteoporosis can afflict men and the non-elderly, it is not limited to elderly women.
- Osteoporosis is due to calcium loss in the bones.
- Bones are continually torn down and rebuilt to repair micro-fractures.
- Without correct exercise, bone density decreases 2%/year.
- Below a certain density, bones cannot support the weight placed on them and begin to crush in.
- Calcium supplements slow this down, but increase heart attacks. Calcium with vitamin D ameliorates this.
- Resistance exercise, done once a week, will prevent and reverse osteoporosis.
- The resistance exercise should be done with perfect form and be challenging. Large bones, the legs and spine, should be stressed. Squats and deadlifts are ideal.
- In Dr. Mike's cohort, osteoporosis was greatly reduced for most participants.

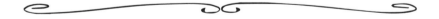

25 - OSTEOARTHRITIS, ALZHEIMER'S, AND AGING

A degenerative disease is one brought about by cellular and mitochondrial degradation. Aging could be considered a degenerative disease, we suppose, though it's not normally thought of that way. Nonetheless, lifestyle choices will have a very noticeable effect on aging. Virtually everyone who has undertaken the protocols has received flattering comments to that effect.

Two other degenerative diseases of note are osteoarthritis and dementia, especially Alzheimer's, the latter said to be a coming epidemic. Osteoarthritis can definitely be prevented and reversed if it hasn't gone too far. The picture is less clear on dementia, although there is strong evidence that exercise is much more preventive than, say, working Sudoku puzzles. Additionally, a very low-carb diet helps markedly, which once again implicates sugar.

OSTEOARTHRITIS

Osteoarthritis is degradation of the joints due to disuse, or, in some cases, trauma. Rheumatoid arthritis is different, and is a deterioration due to inflammation. In osteoarthritis, inflammation is the result, not the cause of the damage. Osteoarthritis is by far the most common sort.

There are several types of joints. The ones that cause problems are the ones that can move a lot, and these are called synovial joints. We'll need to look at these in a bit of detail. Let's dissect the knee joint, since it is a notorious troublemaker.

The ends of the bones that meet to form the knee are covered with a thick, smooth, tough protective layer called the articular cartilage. You have seen this on the ends of chicken bones. It doesn't look like the rest of the bone, being shiny, hard, smooth and white. The articular cartilage is manufactured by a cell type called chondrocytes, which originate within the bone. They are first cousins of the bone-making osteoblasts, both of which descend from the mesenchymal stem cells.

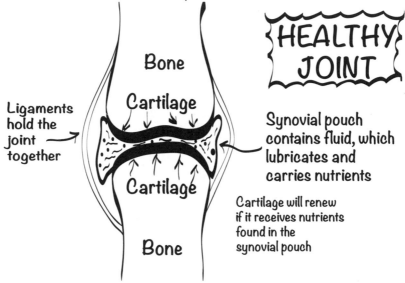

Bone

Cartilage

Ligaments hold the joint together

HEALTHY JOINT

Synovial pouch contains fluid, which lubricates and carries nutrients

Cartilage will renew if it receives nutrients found in the synovial pouch

Cartilage

Bone

The articular cartilage on these bones is around an eighth of an inch thick. The chondrocyte cells that manufacture it migrate from the bone to the surface, building and rebuilding the tough, smooth collagen layer. The cells on the outermost layer are squashed flat by the joint pressure. As they wear, they are replaced by those below. The middle part of the articular cartilage is somewhat rubbery, which absorbs shock and helps spread the load. The layer next to the bone is a tough layer resistant to compression.

The articular cartilages in the knee joints have tough pads inserted between, called the meniscus, which further helps distribute the load. The joint is then enclosed in a flexible sort of pouch called the synovial cavity. The wall of the pouch is made up of two types of cells, one of which secretes thick lubricating fluid, which fills the cavity. The well-lubricated articular cartilages can now slide against one another and the meniscus in the synovial cavity. The synovial cavity is sometimes called the joint cavity.

Surrounding the joint and the joint cavity is a system of ligaments that holds everything together.

The chondrocyte cells in the cartilage, though living, have no blood supply. How is this going to work? The solution is a little strange. It turns out that they get their nutrition straight from the synovial fluid. The cells that make up the synovial pouch wall do get blood, and release nutrients right into the synovial fluid. Making sure this fluid is made available to the cartilage-growing chondrocytes is the key to joint health. The joints get no nutrients from the bone itself.

Even though the synovial fluid provides nutrients, there is no oxygen available, so the chondrocyte cells have to generate energy solely from fermentation. This is a lot less efficient.

Osteoarthritis Initiation

This feeding system for the articular cartilage is a weak link. If the joints are immobile, hardly any of the fluid leaks through, things just sit, and the articular cartilage starts to starve and doesn't repair. This is the initiator of osteoarthritis. Armed with this knowledge, it is easy to devise exercises that will keep the joints in good shape. Two attributes are needed:

- The joint needs to go through its full range of motion. This spreads the synovial fluid all about, and spreads the wear as well. Limited ranges of motion will cause certain points to wear out quickly, while surrounding regions may degenerate from lack of nutrient.
- The thick fluid in the synovial cavity needs to be compressed and released. This forces synovial fluid into the articular cartilage where it can lubricate and nourish. This is akin to squeezing a wet sponge.

Exercises that embody the two of these will generally prevent osteoarthritis. Furthermore, early osteoarthritis, where the synovial pouch is still intact, and the cartilage not worn off, will reverse. In fact, even more serious cases can frequently be reversed. See chapter 10.

It helps to actually visualize the joint that is getting exercised. Is it getting compressed and released? Is it full range? Getting a full range of motion in everyday life is equally important. Walking, standing up, climbing stairs, etc.

Other movable joints are different in configuration, but all have the articular cartilage lubricated with synovial fluid. So compression and full motion are essential.

Unlike other degenerative disease, osteoarthritis does occur in hunter-gatherers, but largely from trauma. However, we do not have to endure their typically punishing physical existence, so we can usually avoid this.

One promising new treatment for osteoarthritis involves injecting mesenchymal stem cells into the knee joint. The cells are harvested from the patient's own bone, thus avoiding any tissue rejection issues, and allowed to reproduce freely in the lab till they are abundant. They are then injected into the joint. No surprise that this would work: mesenchymal cells are "injected" when you do full range motion exercises.

DEMENTIA - ALZHEIMER'S DISEASE

Alzheimer's is the most common dementia. It is sometimes referred to as type 3 diabetes. Diabetes has to do with insulin management, and one would think that type 1 or type 2 diabetes would cover any such issues. A lot of recent research, though, has noted that there tend to be insulin deficiencies and insulin resistance in the brains of those with Alzheimer's. However, type 2 or adult onset diabetics have a much higher incidence of Alzheimer's, so there is a confusing overlap.

Inside the brain of someone with Alzheimer's, neural tangles, plaques, and amyloid beta build-ups are found. This environment is not good: various neural units lose function.

There is a lot of current research pointing to some sort of cerebral version of the metabolic syndrome being a likely cause of Alzheimer's. Specifically, research has centered around the hippocampus and short-term memory. The hippocampus is also involved in memory consolidation—long-term storage. Glucose issues seem to be connected with both.

Normally, the neurons get a relatively steady flow of glucose from the their GLUT-3 glucose transporters. This transporter is not insulin dependent and has a high affinity for glucose. (It draws in more than the other glucose transporters.) It appears that when the hippocampus is dealing with a new memory, it needs a sharp, temporary boost in its glucose supply. To get it, GLUT-4 transporters are expressed. This is just like a "normal" cell, asking for a glucose boost, and here is where the troubles begin.

Recall from chapter 23, ADULT ONSET DIABETES (AODM), that the cells won't express glucose transporters (the GLUT-4 type) unless insulin is present. One would think the hippocampus would be spared this indignity, but that is not the case. So if there is no insulin, or—crucially— if the cells have become insulin resistant, there won't be enough glucose for short-term memory to work. This insulin-memory result is really quite a breakthrough; 15 years ago, no one thought insulin had any role at all in the brain. Insulin's role has been confirmed by several different studies, some associating insulin and insulin resistance with cognition, and others examining improved cognition after insulin administration.

Another body of research that appears to confirm the sugar-insulin hypothesis involves a ketogenic diet. This is a no-carb diet, which, after a week or so, will cause a glucose shortage. The brain must always be fed, so the liver starts generating ketones, the brain's backup fuel. People with memory impairments benefited from this diet. In fact, the higher the ketone level, the better the memory function.

Ketones do not make their way into neurons via the GLUT transporter family; other transporters are used, so there is no insulin effect. In fact, insulin would normally be very low on a ketogenic diet. A very low-carb (or even no-carb) diet can be difficult for some to sustain, but it is possible to do it and it is safe as well. Such a diet reverses a number of other metabolic sins, especially AODM, so this may well become a standard treatment. Or perhaps not. The ketogenic diet, which necessarily involves animal product, is heresy in some influential circles.

So what are we left with? The evidence is mounting for some sort of glucose-insulin problem in Alzheimer's. It would be reasonable to grant it "official" status at this point. In fact, the insulin level in a normal brain is quite high compared to the rest of the body, surprisingly so.

Of course, an insulin-glucose problem, analogous to AODM, would cause the same sort of deleterious cellular conditions. Cells and their mitochondria will lose functionality: brain functionality in this case.

A more advanced model of the process stems from the idea that the brain does its own insulin-glucose regulation and makes its own insulin. This research is state-of-the-art. Researchers haven't pinned down the source of the insulin, but seem to be closing in on it. Various control mechanisms are also being explored. It's a very active and exciting area.

Suffice to say that the brain uses high and variable levels of insulin to meet various dynamic glucose needs. If this system becomes impaired, cerebral function declines in general, but particularly in areas where there is intense glucose dependence, which includes the above-mentioned hippocampus, but also the hypothalamus.

There is no cure for Alzheimer's. The ketogenic diet helps noticeably, but is in no way a cure. Is there reversal there? Perhaps some.

Just to have a working model of the disease, let's suppose that the brain manufactures and regulates its own insulin supply, and that the root cause of Alzheimer's is the deterioration of this system. The big question then becomes: how can this be prevented?

Prevention of Alzheimer's

Prevention of adult onset diabetes (AODM) would be a good place to start. Alzheimer's is twice as prevalent in this group, which tends to indicate that the high glucose levels and insulin resistance characteristic of AODM have, in some way, "spread" to the brain. Perhaps neurons became overloaded with glucose too, or the excess glucose abetted the formation of the characteristic amyloid beta plaques. The exact mechanism isn't known, but high glucose and high insulin are clearly strong risk factors.

Do we have other association clues of this sort? A Canadian study of their indigenous populations found very low rates of dementia. Of course there are many attributes of that lifestyle that could be factors, but very low sugar consumption is certainly one of them.

So primary prevention for Alzheimer's is then the same as everything else: Get the glucose and insulin under control. Measure it and adjust your life accordingly. There is another important component that will be fully elaborated in the SLEEP chapter, and could be called general brain health.

The brain is odd in many ways. It prefers glucose, and is very isolated with its blood-brain barrier. It (probably) has its own glucose-insulin regulation system and so on.

Another way in which the brain is odd is how it disposes of waste. Normally the lymphatic system performs this, but the lymphatic system does not extend to the brain. So where does the waste go?

The brain consists of several types of cells. The neurons get all the attention. After all, they can think! However, there is an extensive network of cells named glia that build the support structures and otherwise act as the neurons' personal handmaidens.

These glia cells also build a drainage system around the outside of the blood vessels, meaning that in our brains, we have a network of inner pipes (the blood vessels) surrounded by outer pipes (drainage). Only the brain has this sort of setup. The key point—and it's an important one—is that this glia cell drainage system, called the glymphatic system, works only while you sleep. When you are awake, your brain doesn't drain! Waste just piles up. It has to be sleep; it won't work if you are unconscious and it won't work if you are resting. This means if you are sleep deprived, you brain is going to fill up with cerebral garbage, and mitochondria will shut down, with the expected loss of function.

Sweet dreams are sweeter than we imagined.

AGING

"Old age ain't no place for sissies," actress Bette Davis informs us. The choices are stark: do all the stuff recommended in this book, which will slow aging down as much as possible, or do nothing and endure its inflictions. One choice means a lot of work, and the other a lot of pain and suffering. Not so easy to put a pretty spin on "the golden years."

There are many theories of aging. As far as Quantitative Medicine is concerned, there are two principal components:

- Mitochondrial damage. Mitochondria reproduce every three weeks or so. Damage to DNA could be replicated. Though the body has numerous defenses against this, the damage slowly accumulates.
- Stem cell damage. Stem cells replicate. Although the stem cells are somewhat hidden out of harm's way, there is some damage, and this too slowly accumulates.

Retard Aging by Protecting Stem Cells and Mitochondria

If cells that are periodically replaced are to remain "youthful," the stem cells that produce them, and the mitochondria that power the operation, need to stay as healthy as possible. The four most damaging situations are:

- High iron
- Sedentary lifestyle
- Adult onset diabetes
- High cortisol

The first one, high iron, could be hereditary, could occur with the onset of menopause, or could occur as a result of various dietary choices. The excess iron is toxic to the cells, and, if untreated, will greatly accelerate aging. The blood marker for this is ferritin. The treatment is periodic bloodletting (therapeutic phlebotomy).

The other three causes are quite familiar to us by now. And once again, Quantitative Medicine is the solution. Interestingly, though, to seriously slow down aging, all four significant lifestyle components, diet, spiritual discipline, sleep, and exercise, are necessary.

It may be a bit of a surprise that a sedentary lifestyle accelerates aging. A principle to bear in mind is that busy cells are healthy cells. If a cell is being challenged, its mitochondria complete their energy production cycles, nutrients are consumed, and all is well. If the cell is idle, the mitochondria are inactive. They will skid to a halt partway through their energy production cycles. If they are in this state very long, they tend to kill themselves, and loose certain oxidizing radicals into the cell. This frequently kills the cell as well. This is a simple catabolic response. The body is removing unnecessary cells.

However, this process is not entirely clean. The oxidizing radicals might damage the host cell, but not kill it. The mitochondria might reproduce, though damaged. Now we don't fall apart if we don't exercise, so it goes almost without saying that the body has numerous mechanisms to block the damaged cells and mitochondria from reproducing. But some damaged ones will reproduce. It may seem odd that rapid cellular turnover translates to slower aging, but that is how we are designed.

Suppose all the cells are stressed for some other cause. An environmental issue, or hormonal or biochemical imbalance could cause this. The two most common causes of chronic imbalance in our society are chronic stress and adult onset diabetes (AODM). Chronic stress causes chronically high cortisol. High cortisol boosts insulin and glucose levels, shuts down the immune system, curtails anabolic cell renewal activity, and interferes with sleep. This alone would be a good launch into AODM, and frequently is.

Adult onset diabetes stresses all cells and their mitochondria. When accompanied by a sedentary lifestyle, the problems are compounded. Given the widespread damage that AODM causes and the numerous diseases it triggers, it comes as no surprise that aging is accelerated as well. AODM is a very unhealthy environment, and accumulating cellular damage would be an expected consequence.

So again, QM to the rescue. Get the numbers right, and get stress under control. This removes chronic stress and reverses AODM. Exercise causes cells to run cleanly again and aging slows.

The Telomere Theory of Aging

This theory is as widespread as it is false, but we suppose it has certain philosophical implications (also false) that keep it going. Here's how it works: When we evolved from bacteria, with their circular DNA, into eukaryotes, with DNA strings, we needed a way to mark and protect the ends. This is the job of telomeres. A telomere is a specific sequence of nucleotides and it is repeated, typically 100 times, rather like wrapping a thread around the end of a rope to keep it from fraying. This part is true.

When a cell divides it loses a telomere. 99, 98, 97 . . . 1, 0, done. So in this theory, lifespan is programmed. However, if you look one level deeper, this falls apart. The intestine replaces itself every four days. By the telomere theory, we would run out of replicable cells in about 400 days. Obviously this doesn't happen, and it turns out that there is cellular gadgetry that will fashion new telomeres and tack them on. This process occurs where it is needed. We are never going to run out of telomeres for the cells that need them. That's pretty much the end of the Telomere Theory of Aging.

However, telomeres do throw a nice monkey wrench into cancer promotion. As a cancer cell replicates, it also loses a telomere. It would run out unless it could also replace the telomeres, so this is another barrier. Not an insurmountable one obviously, but cancer cells are defective, so some can't pull off the new-telomere-construction bit. The more ways cancer cells can run aground, the better off we are.

Bats

An extreme example of retarded aging is the bat. North American bug-eating bats weigh less than a mouse, but outlive it tenfold. The principal reason appears to be that bats have great mitochondria. Or is it that they have a lot of them? Likely both. Flying has such a high metabolic demand that any animal able to do it has to have a huge amount of mitochondria. Bats live 25 years. So do hummingbirds. Some of the larger birds outlive us. These animals do not seem to age. Of course, there are no retirement homes for flying animals (with the possible exception of parrots). When birds and bats can no longer fly, their life is over. So everything has to work in this high-energy mode until the end. That their life should be so greatly extended over their landlubbing cousins attests to the power of busy, healthy mitochondria and the consequent cellular health.

We can't fly, but we can make the choices that will likely get us to 95 or beyond in one piece. Bats have no monopoly on that. Get the numbers in the right place and it all happens. Of course, the changes that must be made, the exercising, and all the rest can seem quite daunting. There are no shortcuts, no fountain of youth, no super-statin pills, but the ability to lead a long and healthy life and reap its benefits is built into all of us.

We hope the book provides this guide. The QM method works. This much is known and thoroughly established.

Key Points
25 - Osteoarthritis, Alzheimer's, and Aging
- Osteoarthritis is the wearing away of the special cartilage used for joints.
- Joint cartilage has cells that will rebuild it, but they only get nourished through movement and pressure.
- By adopting joint exercises, it is possible to prevent osteoarthritis, and reverse it if the cartilage has not been destroyed.
- Alzheimer's is now often called type 3 diabetes.
- People with Alzheimer's have high and unregulated glucose in the brain.
- Alzheimer's may stem from high glucose in the diet, because Alzheimer's is much more prevalent among people with adult onset diabetes.
- The rate of aging can be slowed considerably with correct lifestyle choices.
- Aging is due to slow degeneration of the mitochondria and the stem cells. Slowing the degeneration slows aging.
- The telomere theory of aging is incorrect.
- The four most common causes of rapid aging are excess iron, sedentary lifestyle, adult onset diabetes, and high cortisol.
- Excess iron is resolved by bloodletting, which now goes by a more civilized term: therapeutic phlebotomy.

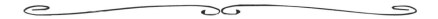

26 - LIFESTYLE OVERVIEW

Various elements of lifestyle have differing effects on degenerative diseases, though the correct choices, properly implemented, prevent them all. This is rather magical, like a single pill that could cure everything. "Just take two QMs and call us in the morning."

For the constitutionally lazy, such a magic pill would certainly be welcome, though it's quite a stretch to conceive of any pill that could supplant the elaborate processes at work to heal degenerative disease. Of course, medical hopes spring eternal, in both the minds of the public and the marketing departments of the pharmaceutical industry.

It's not where we are headed, at least as far as degenerative disease is concerned. There are some pathogen-focused breakthroughs, such as the recent cure for hepatitis C, but the medicines that are promoted as magical cures for degenerative disease either don't work, as is the case of statins, or do net harm, like beta-blockers and ezetimibe. They don't work because these medicines are not treating the disease, they are merely prolonging it or moving its locale.

We will suppose that if you got this far, you probably agree that our modern civilization is the disease in a sense, and the cure is in the amelioration of its worser components. Moreover, how to do this has been elaborated separately and also in the context of specific disease cures.

Why, though? Why are meats and plants good for us? Why are fats better for us than sugars? Why aren't we eating coal instead? Why does short-duration intense exercise work several times better than long sessions of aerobics? Why is the mind so resistant to tranquility? Why sleep at all?

337

Curiosity is itself a curious affliction. Correct exercise will work its wonders without any specific insights into its inner workings, yet somehow the human condition won't quite be appeased by that. We want reason and logic. We want motivators. We want to be able to defend what we do. We want to proselytize.

Like everything else we have talked about, many of the reasons we are the way we are find their roots in evolutionary happenstance. We reinvented little. We kept the lobster's innate immune system and added a new one on top of that. We are as built of layers as any geological formation. Our DNA goes back to bacteria.

We will excavate a few of these layers, but like everything else, far more is unknown than known.

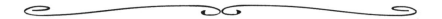

27 - NUTRITION

Metabolism means getting energy we can use from the food we eat. The energy portion of food is called macronutrients. We also need to get relatively small amounts of vitamins, phytochemicals, and minerals. These are called micronutrients. Food contains both, but many dietary items common in the Western diet are woefully lacking in the latter. However, if we are clever about what we eat, we will get enough of both in the same diet, and we need adequate amounts of both.

WHY CAN'T WE EAT COAL?

We can. At least pure coal, which is to say carbon. We just don't have a way to convert it to energy, to metabolize it. We can metabolize something if we can convert it to Acetyl-CoA, which is the input fuel to the Krebs cycle—a very efficient energy converter. The Krebs cycle was discussed in chapter 15.

The two most common macronutrients are glucose (sugars and starches) and fat. Both are small molecules made exclusively of carbon, oxygen, and hydrogen. These two are sliced up into Acetyl-CoA and feed directly into the Krebs cycle.

Proteins can be macronutrients as well. Proteins we eat are broken down into their constituent amino acids and circulated as such. The amino acids are made of carbon, oxygen, and hydrogen atoms and have one or more nitrogen atoms in addition. These also go through various reactions and are then fed into the Krebs cycle.

This is a broad dietary repertoire. In fact, the only abundant living material we can't digest is cellulose. Ruminants (cows, etc.) and termites can. There is cellulose in our diet. It is usually called dietary fiber, and is considered a wondrous thing these days. It is frequently prescribed as a cure-all supplement by gastroenterologists. The medical reality probably dwells somewhere between useless and overrated. Should real benefit be found, though, it would mean that the nutritional content of breakfast cereal could be improved by eating the box it came in.

Though the Krebs cycle can spin along quite merrily on glucose or fat, or even protein, the body manages these fuels quite differently. Stored bodily fat is generally available to the cells, but glucose supplies are hoarded. Energy policy varies enormously from animal to animal according to their ecological niche. Our own niche appears to be hunter-gatherers living in an ice age, and while fat is generally made available to hungry cells, glucose is preserved, both as fuel for our oversized brain, and, after conversion to fat, as a reserve supply for winter.

The Brain Needs Glucose or Some Substitute

The brain cannot use most fat molecules. It can run on the very short ones, but prefers glucose and ketones. The glucose supply is tightly managed. To insure an adequate supply of glucose foe the brain, cells that can run on both fat and glucose will effectively be forced to choose fat. An exception is made if there is excess glucose available.

However, even if glucose runs low, the liver will always supply enough nutrient for the brain. At first, it will synthesize glucose from fat. If this proves inadequate, it will start producing ketones, which are a perfectly satisfactory backup fuel for the brain and some other organs.

The rest of the cells in the body do not need glucose and run cleaner and better on fat.

Cholesterol and Saturated Fat

At some point in the 1970s it was concluded that America's health was deteriorating and that the U.S. Congress should be doing something about it. Thus the federal government officially got into the nutrition business. As is usually the case, a myriad of special interests piled on, attempting to sway things one way or the other, and out of this mire was fashioned the famous Food Pyramid, its base the delight of the cereal industry, and red meat all but abolished. This spread far and wide. Soon low fat and high carbs were all the rage and the obesity epidemic was launched. Many readers will have lived through the entire saga. It is by no means over. Many prepackaged and processed foods still proudly boast "low-fat," and many august organizations still rail against saturated fat.

So let's look at saturated fat and cholesterol themselves. The finding 50 years ago was that saturated fat increased cholesterol, and that heart attack victims had a lot of both in their veins. However, heart attack victims frequently smoked, drank too much, and had a sort of "I don't really care about health" attitude. These studies also lumped trans fats (margarine), processed meat, sausage, bologna, and the like with saturated fats. By stirring this grand mixture together, the conclusion was reached that saturated fat was dangerous and a major cause of disease.

But what about those that don't smoke, don't drink too much, do pay attention to quantity and quality of what they eat, don't eat trans fat, and are picky about processed meat? Further suppose they regularly eat cholesterol-laden eggs or red meat and frequently indulge in clean saturated fats, like butter, cheese and grass-fed meat. The health implications of this kind of behavior are starkly different. In this setting, cholesterol and saturated fat do not cause problems. In fact, quite the opposite: they tend to reduce them. And the evidence for this is, at this point, fairly overwhelming.

Cholesterol - Cell Wall Material

Cholesterol is needed for cell walls and the cells make their own. Without cholesterol, we would collapse into a gooey puddle. In fact, since cells need it so badly, the body has evolved a centrally located cholesterol factory (in the liver) that will make more if necessary and distribute it via the bloodstream. The liver uses any cholesterol it happens to find in the food we eat, and then makes up the rest from scratch. If we eat less cholesterol, it will compensate by making more, and vice versa. The amount in the bloodstream stays constant, regulated to a hypothalamic reference point (yet another feedback control system). The amount of cholesterol eaten doesn't matter. This is no recent discovery, yet many, doctors included, are unaware of it.

Ancel Keys, a famous researcher in the '60s and '70s, led a war against saturated fat, believing that it raised cholesterol and caused heart disease (untrue). However, even Keys pronounced dietary cholesterol (the cholesterol found in the food we eat) innocent, proclaiming in 1997: *"The evidence—both from experiments and from field surveys—indicates that the cholesterol content, per se, of all natural diets has no significant effect on either the serum cholesterol level or the development of atherosclerosis in man."* This is hardly the way the ever-political Keys was hoping things would turn out, needless to say.

This wasn't news in 1997. Keys had said the same thing in 1952. But countless millions have been told to avoid eggs and the like. And still are. Most people who love eggs are enraged to learn that the prohibition that was in effect for the last four decades was completely bogus.

Saturated Fat - The Universal Building Block

But can you have bacon with those eggs? What's "saturated" about saturated fat is that the fat molecule has as many hydrogen atoms as it can hold. It's "saturated" with hydrogen. Saturated fat molecules are straight, and because of this, they pack better. This is the reason saturated fat is solid at room temperature. Monounsaturated fat has a single kink in the molecule, and polyunsaturated fat has several kinks, which usually force it into sort of a curl. The fats come in several lengths as well, so there are a lot of different sorts of fat molecules available to the cells. To build and rebuild cell walls, the cells need various fat molecules with very exact specifications. Rather than wait for the right ones to float by, each cell has a bunch of tools that slice and dice the available fats (the ones you just ate) and convert them into the special ones needed. As it happens, cells can make everything they need from saturated fat. Other types of fat are a bit problematic and can potentially impact the integrity of the cell walls. Trans fat that is man-made is very problematic. Cells don't recognize it as odd, and attempt to use it anyway.

Besides cell wall construction, fats are also used to generate energy. The various sorts of fats are pretty much interchangeable in this regard, though it's a bit more work to extract energy from the unsaturated ones.

YUM!

Some surprising science: A huge study ranked saturated fat consumption among European countries from high to low. France won that one, consuming the most saturated fat of all. Another study ranked countries according to the lowest rates of heart disease. France won that one too. High saturated fat, low heart disease, hmmm. But it's not just a French thing: it's a very reliable trend. Other countries that consumed a lot of saturated fat also had lower heart disease. In fact, they were almost in lockstep. The more saturated fat, the less heart disease. This is nice *raw* data. It hasn't been beaten to death and cherry-picked by well meaning, but possibly biased researchers. More saturated fat, less heart disease. In spite of almost 50 years of vilification, there is really only one possible conclusion: saturated fat is good for you.

Polyunsaturated fat is the one that doesn't keep well. This applies to storage in your pantry, or sitting stuck in your arteries. For this reason, consumers of polyunsaturated fat appear to have a slightly higher mortality rate than those that mostly consume saturated or monounsaturated fat.

Mother's milk is highly saturated. Butter is saturated. Cheese is saturated. There is no need to worry about saturated fat: it's good for us.

Here is a strange fact. The American Heart Association website is still (2016) persecuting saturated fat, lumping it with trans fat, calling it bad fat, even graphically illustrating its vileness with cartoons. Yet, *on the very same website* can be found research *they funded* comparing saturated fat intake to heart disease, and this research reaches quite the opposite conclusion. Research exonerating saturated fat can now be found in most of the blue-chip medical journals. One wonders who reads them.

Why is trans fat bad? We grew up on margarine. This was a great source of trans fat. Our parents bought margarine because butter was too expensive. Butter was too expensive because the federal government guaranteed a price floor and bought up the excess, which kept the price elevated. *They still do this!* Maybe they are trying to protect us from butter. Some trans fat occurs in nature, and this sort causes no health problems whatsoever. Palm oil would be a good example. Man-made trans fat has a different structure that does not occur in nature. It's similar enough to natural fat to fool the body into using it, but the uses the body puts it to tend to have defects and weaknesses. However, no one suspected how serious this could be. In one study, 30,000 premature deaths annually were attributed to trans fat—a number comparable to annual traffic fatalities in the U.S. Fortunately trans fat has all but disappeared.

Practices for raising animals vary widely. Many of these animals are kept in very close, unsanitary conditions and fed antibiotics and other supplements, along with a nutrient-poor diet. As you might expect, this meat, along with its fat, is not the healthiest and, when possible, should be avoided. This is not a condemnation of saturated fat, but rather of industrially produced meat.

How Do Macronutrients Get to the Cells?

Fat. Let's follow a fat molecule from our mouth to a cell. The fat we eat is mostly in the form of triglycerides. A triglyceride is constructed of three fat molecules attached to a glycerol backbone. These enter the upper part of the small intestine and are disassembled into free fatty acids, carried through the intestinal wall, and, once across, reassembled again as triglycerides, which are then packaged into large lipoprotein particles called chylomicrons. These travel via the lymph system, eventually dumping into the bloodstream up near the neck.

Why this? Why doesn't it go through the liver and get sorted like all the other food, instead of bypassing it? And why dump it into the bloodstream at the neck, a seemingly unnecessary additional distance? Quite a puzzler, this.

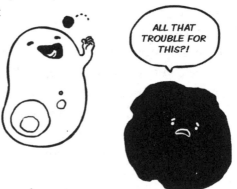

A chylomicron is the largest lipoprotein, significantly larger than VLDL, but it isn't that large, being about a tenth the size of a cell, so it isn't going to get stuck. Once in circulation, hungry cells consume it within minutes. Cells love a chylomicron treat.

A cell interested in a fat snack will indicate this by secreting an enzyme called lipoprotein lipase, and posting it, sticky-notice-like, on the wall of the capillary endothelium. When a chylomicron happens by, lipoprotein lipase does exactly what you might suppose. It grabs off a triglyceride and snips it up into its constituent pieces, specifically two free fatty acids and a third fatty acid with the glycerol attached. These can then diffuse into the cell—or do they need a transporter? This detail is unknown. In any case, once inside the cell, the journey is over. They will either be used for construction purposes—building cell walls for instance—or burned for energy in the Krebs cycle.

Glucose. Starch will be broken down largely to glucose by the small intestine and sent to the liver. Table sugar and fruit are likewise broken down to roughly a 50-50 mix of fructose and glucose. These go to the liver as well. The liver will use these sugars to top up its glycogen reserves. It will use the fructose first, then the glucose. Typically, the liver will store all the fructose you eat. The extra glucose, though, will then be sent into general circulation.

So far, a much simpler journey for the sugars, but that's about to end. The brain has first dibs on the sugar. Its neurons get it by expressing a glucose transporter called GLUT3. The neuron actually has to poke this transporter through the blood-brain barrier. GLUT3 is a strong glucose magnet, and will quickly gather any that is available.

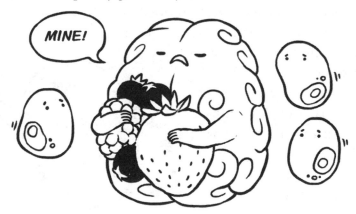

If there's just enough glucose for the brain, say 80 mg/dl, then the rest of the cells, in particular, the heart, muscle, and fat, don't get any. It's not that they don't like sugar. It is *forbidden* unless insulin is high. The body is preserving the glucose for the brain.

However, there's a catch here. High circulating glucose is bad, and after a big starchy meal, glucose could soar very high indeed. To reduce this in a hurry, cells are now forced to use the glucose. The mechanism is interesting. In response to the elevated glucose, the body will secrete additional insulin, thus raising the level. Receptors on the cells monitor this, and if the higher level of insulin is present, the cells express glucose transporters, which are called GLUT4. It's not optional. If they need energy at all, and insulin is high, they have to get it from the circulating glucose. This will usually quickly bring the glucose level down to normal, except, of course, in the case of adult onset diabetes.

The liver gets into the act as well, getting rid of excess glucose by first topping up its glycogen stores and then converting the excess glucose to triglycerides. Better high circulating fat than high circulating glucose it would seem.

Most of the macro-nutrition is via the fat and glucose, but the body has two other ways of creating energy: amino acids and ketones.

Amino Acids. Dietary protein is broken into amino acids in the small intestine, and may or may not be carried across into the bloodstream. Transporters in the intestine determine this. The circulating amino acids can then be picked up by cells expressing the appropriate transporter in the cell walls. Amino acids would normally be used for construction purposes by the clever ribosomes. However, there is a bit of a design flaw in the amino acid transporters. Rather than locking on to a specific amino acid, they tend to collect several roughly similar ones. Hence, to be sure of having the right ones on hand, the cell has to gather more than it actually needs. The excess is then sent over to the Krebs cycle for energy generation.

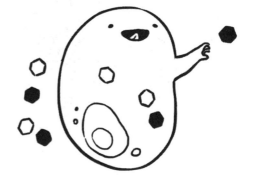

Ketones. Last on the list are the ketones. We don't eat these,

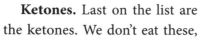

at least not intentionally. It turns out that the brain doesn't have any way to access most fats. The larger fat molecules can't cross the blood-brain barrier, and the neurons don't seem to have any machinery for pulling them in. Normally, there will be glucose available, but if carbohydrate consumption is reduced enough, the glucose will run out. This could be caused by a no-carb diet, which would include the Inuit, at least those still eating the traditional fare, and Atkins dieters. A glucose shortage could also be caused by a prolonged fast or a starvation situation.

If the glucose runs out, it means the liver has used up all its glycogen. So the backup plan for getting nutrients to the brain is to have the liver generate ketones from fat. This includes acetone, the active ingredient in nail polish remover, and two other ketones. The reader may be surprised to learn that acetone, which will remove most paint and dissolve most plastic, is not a deadly poison. In fact, most people can tolerate 6-8 oz. of it with no problem. (Not part of our proposed diet, though.) The circulating ketones are used by the brain, heart, and muscle. The transportation details are unknown.

In insulin-dependent diabetes, a lack of insulin will block glucose from being used. The liver senses this somehow, and starts generating ketones, which may reach a dangerously high level. This is called ketoacidosis, and is very dangerous.

All this metabolic versatility is impressive. Like having a car that could run on gasoline, diesel, junk mail, and lawn clippings.

The Bottom Line on Macronutrients

Excess is not good. Variety is good. A varied diet should be eaten. However, sugar and starches should be avoided if there are any issues metabolizing glucose. Eating whole foods, something our ancestors could have hunted or gathered, is a generally safe strategy. A plate with one-third protein and two-thirds colorful vegetables should provide a healthy spectrum of macronutrients (and micronutrients as well). Foods should be varied, with preference to organic and grass-fed. Industrially packaged food should be avoided. There is no need to worry about red meat, cholesterol content, or saturated fat. Human-made trans fat should be avoided. If a tree, bush, plant, or animal made it, it's probably fine.

PROTEIN AND AMINO ACIDS

We can only make about 12 of the 21 or so amino acids we need. The other 9 must come from the diet. We need around a gram or two of each of these daily.

Most protein sources have all 21 amino acids available, so this is not normally a problem. However, sugar and fat contain no protein at all, and starch only a tiny amount.

Is Eating Excess Protein Dangerous?

Suppose excessive proteins are eaten? This seems to be a bodybuilder favorite. What does the body do with this? Excessive amounts of anything are bad, and protein would be no exception. Currently, articles are published that indict high-protein diets, especially animal protein, as cancerous, hard on the kidneys, and aging accelerators. There is no reason a priori to believe that amino acids from meat are particularly different than those from plants—molecules are molecules. It would probably be harder to consume excessive amounts of protein solely from vegetables, though. We do not think there is any reason to worry about protein. Eat a sensible amount. This isn't rocket science.

Why Can't We Make Those Nine Essential Amino Acids?

Only one explanation. Follow the food chain. Some creature or plant has to be able to generate those missing ones. Somewhere in our evolutionary past, we lost the ability to generate them because we could get them by eating. But losing nine amino acids seems like a lot. One or two could perhaps be excused, but losing nine seems downright careless.

How Do We Make the Twelve Other Amino Acids?

We know that a ribosome makes up proteins by assembling strings of amino acids, which we imagine floating about forming a reliable supply. But shortages occur and each cell synthesizes its own supply. The pathways for each of these are different and, within the cell, are self-regulating. Interestingly, for many of the amino acids, the basic molecule is plucked from one of the eight intermediate steps in the Krebs cycle. Quite handy, the Krebs cycle.

MICRONUTRIENTS

In one experiment, a modern hunter-gatherer led a researcher on a tour through a local forest and emerged with 200 edible plants. Now that's diversity! Are there 200 different vegetables available at the local grocery store? Perhaps at the better ones.

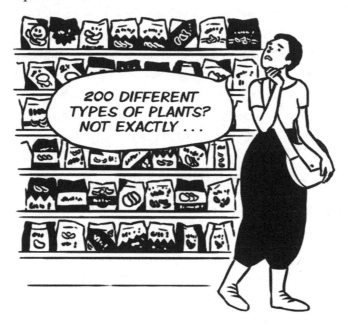

We may become known as the "sound bite" generation. How many times have we heard that something is rich in antioxidants? That has been the "in" vegetable attribute for quite a while. This fad is fading now that there is research confirming that antioxidants are yet another bodily function that shouldn't be tampered with.

The core problem is this: plants and meats have literally thousands of micronutrients. A pomegranate has well over a hundred identified phytochemicals alone. Are these important? Definitely. Which ones? We don't know. Maybe all of them, or a combination, or more likely, the important ones are the ones your body has a current need for, and it will grab these and deliver them where needed. This will be different for different people, and vary from day to day as well.

We would do well here to take a humbler attitude and defer to the body. Provide it with a healthy variety and trust it to do the right thing. Bear in mind that any sensible diet will provide the right amount of micronutrients. The body will take what it needs, and ignore the rest (or burn it for energy). Armed with that admonition, let's look into the world of micronutrients.

Vitamins—Except for Vitamin D

These vitamins are all necessary biochemicals that we used to be able to make, but no longer can. We must obtain these from food. Deficiencies are dangerous, but are rare with any normal diet. Nonetheless, for a good part of the last 75 years, vitamin supplementation has been standard. This does not appear to have been a very good idea. One by one, the alphabet soup of vitamins have shown themselves to be detrimental if used as supplements. In particular, supplementation has not been shown to decrease mortality for any of the vitamins, and for some vitamins, mortality has actually increased. Note that B_{12} is an exception, as it comes only from meat. Vegans and possibly vegetarians should supplement with this.

So What about Vitamin D?

The jury is still out on D, but it's not really a vitamin. Vitamin D is effectively a hormone, and has a variety of important functions. It is needed to build bone, is believed to be protective against cancer, and has a number of other benefits. We can still make vitamin D, and we really don't get much from food. It's made by the skin from sunlight and cholesterol.

Skin color is an adaptation likely driven by vitamin D needs. Dark-skinned people living in northern climates do not make enough vitamin D. The sunscreen-slathering ritual is adding to the problem, and we all spend a lot more time indoors than was traditionally the case.

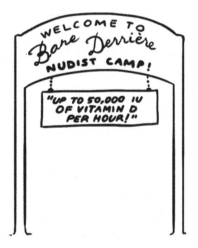

Many authorities recommend taking something like a 1,000 IU pill per day. A hour by a pool in the summer sun would generate 12,000 IU. Excess vitamin D is stored in the muscles, and a lot can be stored, enough in principle to last through a cloudy northern winter. But this does have its limits. Given the current popularity of vitamin D, toxic overdoses are common. A safe dosage should average to no more than 4000 IU daily. If a greater amount is made available by basking in the sun, the body has a way to regulate this and make less: we will get tan.

Vitamin D supplementation is recommended only if levels are low, say below 30 ng/ml, and measurements should be made first. More sunshine may be the fastest and most effective remedy. Failing that, supplementation would be in order. If supplementing, the Quantitative Medicine recommendation is to take 20,000 IU once a week, and remeasure quarterly. Daily pills appear to be rejected rather than being stored.

In some northern European countries, 50,000 to 100,000 IU are administered orally to children once or twice a year.

Phytochemicals

Phytochemicals are found in plants and go by these names:

• Monophenols	• Hydrolyzable tannin
• Polyphenols	• Aromatic acid
• Flavonoids	• Phenolic acids
• Isoflavonoids	• Hydroxycinnamic
• Flavonolignan	acids
• Lignans	• Capsaicin
• Stilbenoids	• Phenylethanoids
• Curcuminoids	• Alkylresorcinols

Several mouthfuls here, and these frequently have health benefits ascribed to them, like cancer-fighting or antioxidant and so on.

The plants "invented" phytochemicals as chemical defenses against predators, so all of them are toxic to something (bugs, bacteria, mold, etc.). What is absolutely amazing is that they should be good for us. Actually, in some cases, we are prey to the same predators as the plants, but in other cases, not. Nonetheless, the phytochemical assortment seems to have significant benefit.

Here is an interesting tale. A Southern California pomegranate company, POM Wonderful, funded a UCLA study to research the effects of their pomegranate juice on men with prostate cancer. The research showed that the cancer slowed quite dramatically. However, when a similar test was done on their dense processed pomegranate extract, the results were fairly good, but substantially less impressive than those obtained by simply drinking the juice. Now industry-funded studies have their own issues, but the point here is that the plain pomegranate juice seemed to work a lot better than the extract. Other things being equal, we would expect the extract to do better as it is low-sugar. However, the process of changing it from juice to an extract appears to have greatly tamed its prostate cancer-fighting properties.

A typical plant has a hundred or more phytochemicals. They tend to be simple and fragile. As soon as a plant is found to be beneficial, the supplement industry mobilizes, isolating a couple of chemicals, and pronouncing them responsible for all the benefit. Soon a new supplement containing the chemicals appears, along with a string of vague claims.

However, in the case of pomegranate or broccoli or green tea or whatever might be beneficial, we have good news: the original vegetables and fruits are still available, complete with all their phytochemicals—exactly like the ones grandma used to eat. There is no need to wait for the supplement industry to do their New Product Rain Dance, and there is precious little point in worrying about which foods have which phytochemicals, and what each phytochemical is good for. If we eat a variety of colored vegetables and fruits (assuming no sugar issues), we will enjoy all the health benefits of the 10,000 or so phytochemicals we will be consuming. The body knows which are which, and what to do with them. No need to lose any sleep trying to figure out which specific are needed. We need them all.

Minerals

Minerals mean elements. Mostly, we are made up of the big four: carbon, oxygen, hydrogen, and nitrogen. C, O, H, and N. They are abundant in food, and we need a lot. We get these from macronutrients, fat, sugar, and, to a lesser extent, protein. But you can't create a human from just C, O, H, and N; a few more ingredients are needed. Specifically, we need, in order, a reliable supply of calcium, phosphorus, potassium, sodium, sulfur, chlorine, magnesium, and in addition, a pinch of boron, chromium, cobalt, copper, fluorine, iodine, iron, manganese, molybdenum, selenium, silicon, tin, vanadium, and zinc. That makes 25 elements total. Calcium through magnesium account for about 4% of us, and the 14 "pinch" elements—properly called trace elements—are less than 1%, but we need these too. If they are lacking, disease results, such as goiter in the case of an iodine deficiency.

Almost all these elements are toxic in their "plain" form. Sodium and chlorine, for instance, are deadly, but when combined into some sort of molecule, table salt in this case, they are rendered harmless. Elements contained in a compound that the body can access and use are said to be bioavailable, and any mineral we need will have to have this attribute. The body knows exactly how to process and distribute these bioavailable minerals, but how can we know if we are getting enough?

Here again is where "real food" comes in. A variety of meats, fish, fowl, and dairy, and vegetables and fruits of all colors, will contain far more than are needed. The body takes what it needs and discards or burns the rest.

Sugar, starch, and fat contain only small amounts of the essential minerals. Hence someone living on starch alone will suffer a variety of deficiencies. This has been made dramatically clear by fortuitous archaeological digs at ancient sites where (likely enslaved) field hands were fed starch only, but the nearby hunter-gatherers had access to the variety a forest could offer. The differences were profound. The hunter-gatherers were six inches taller, had better teeth, no signs of arthritis, and were generally more robust. An extreme but illuminating illustration of lifestyle difference.

Minerals Are Tightly Regulated

It is not possible for the body to predict which load of minerals will be arriving in the next meal-shipment, so all of them are tightly controlled and regulated. This regulation goes on at several levels. At the most local level, a cell needing, say, magnesium, will "express" a transporter that will latch on to the circulating bioavailable magnesium and haul it into the cell. There are literally hundreds of different transporters, one for every occasion. Some cells have transporters that operate in the opposite direction, and insert minerals back into the blood.

The cell has a way to regulate its own needs, but the circulating levels are tightly regulated as well. This is a system-wide function. Calcium is the most studied, as it is used in bones and endless other places. It is regulated by the thyroid, parathyroid, and the "hormone" vitamin D. The hypothalamus may or may not control this. Odds are it does, or at least has a hand on the handlebars.

The other two dozen or so minerals are regulated as well, many of them quite tightly. What organs or mechanisms are doing the regulation is largely unknown, but the degree of control is quite remarkable. Blood tests measure a large number of them and they tend to stay very constant over the years, even though other numbers, like glucose and triglycerides, are soaring and diving like an aerial circus act. Perhaps the fact that mineral regulation seldom seems to break accounts for the relative paucity of research.

Some of the minerals are controlled right at the intestine. If the body needs zinc, for instance, the cells of the intestine will express transporters that will grab it and yank it in.

Electrolytes are ionized versions of the trace minerals. These are tightly regulated as well.

ASSORTED FOOD TOPICS

Whole Grain

Whole grain is the most over-hyped dietary concept in decades, perhaps of all time, and given the swirl of hyperbole that seems part and parcel of the food industry, this is saying a lot. Whole grain simply means electing not to separate the indigestible cellulose grain husk (also known as fiber) from the digestible starch interior. Though the term is widely used, "whole grain" is not standardized and most industrial food that claims to be whole grain contains only about 50% of it.

Is whole grain healthier than refined grain? Yes, but only slightly. However, the cereal industry has directly poured enough money into research to firmly establish this slight benefit. Be that as it may, the colorful vegetables that we recommend have considerably more fiber than any industrial 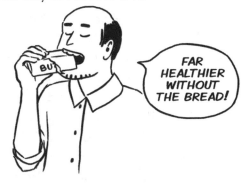 whole grain concoction. This is comparison you don't often see. The broccoli industry simply doesn't have the budget.

For those planning to eat bread or rice anyway, whole grain is obviously preferred. Our advice would be to eat something else. Eating starch, whole grain or otherwise, differs little from eating the equivalent (dry) weight of straight sugar. We should mention, though, that bread which is generously buttered results in a better food mix results and slows the glucose absorption.

Glycemic Index

At the end of the day, all carbohydrates that are eaten, including all the sugar, starch, and carbohydrate content of vegetables (but minus the fiber), end up as glucose. One way or another, the body has to find a home for all this glucose. Whether it is spread out in time, as is the case with low-glycemic-index foods, or arrives in a burst makes little difference to the overall energy picture.

However, if someone is hypoglycemic, their body will overreact to glucose, and choosing low-glycemic-index foods will clearly help. That said, following our dietary recommendations, while taking into account an individual's personal sugar tolerance, will prevent or control hypoglycemia.

Are There Foods We Are Missing?

The answer is surely yes, but the question is what? Our metabolism and health are optimized by a million years of the hunter-gatherer diet. Or, rather, diets. There was little homogeneity. The agricultural revolution—a seismic shift to a starch-based diet—is only 10,000 years old. This is but 1% of our evolutionary history. So what were they dining on that we are not? Here is some speculation:

- All their food was organic and grass-fed. It could have been diseased, though.
- They consumed the entire animal. In doing so, they took on a lot of parasites, and we doubt there is any benefit in that. However, they ate the brain, the gristle, the heart, the liver, and so on. These are different sorts of proteins with different properties. We eat the muscle and the fat. We are surely missing something here.
- Their diet varied seasonally and regionally. This might be good or bad. We have access to more geographic diversity, but they had their 200 local edible plants.

- They ate all sorts of animals, whatever they could catch. We restrict to a couple of mammals, a few birds, and perhaps a dozen fish. No mice, no raccoons, no snakes, no crows, no kangaroos.
- They ate bugs. Appalling? Few would disagree, but there is no clear winner in a beauty contest between a shrimp and a cricket. The Bay Area Bug Eating Society posts nutritional information on several bugs. Seems mainly a source of protein.

GRASSHOPPER BORDELAISE, BUT WITH THE ANTENNAE ON THE SIDE PLEASE.

Now of these five, we can adopt the more obvious ones. We already know to favor organic and grass-fed food. The rest of the animal—liver, brains, etc.—can be delicious, and is commonly consumed in most places outside the U.S.

Another missing piece in our diet is the collagen, the gristle, the tendons. Tough chewing, but a different amino acid profile. Should we be supplementing here?

Bugs? Maybe they are the future. Loaded with insectanoids, major antioxidant. We'll investigate. Any volunteers?

There never was a real "paleo diet." Hunter-gatherers ate whatever was available and they ate it all: muscle, fat, organs, intestines, etc. Few could afford to be picky. The most distinctive attribute of the paleo diet is what the hunter-gatherers did *not* eat: prepackaged industrial food was, of course, not on the menu, and sugar and starches were rare.

Fasting

Fasting used to be a part of Dr. Nichols's diet regime, but ultimately, it failed to produce the desired effects. Though fasting could, and frequently would, have an initial benefit, after a while the hypothalamus would somehow determine the fasting schedule and undermine it, putting the brakes on anabolism, and causing binge eating the night before. The numbers clearly showed the effect.

There may be some therapeutic use for extreme fasting, though this is in no way tested enough for any usable medical intervention at this point. In Dr. Nichols's training, he participated in an autopsy of a very sick man who had intentionally starved himself to death over a two-month period. The man had a very bad cancer and a very bad heart, and it was a toss-up as to which would get him first. Upon autopsy, Dr. Nichols discovered, to his and his colleague's astonishment, that the unfortunate man's heart was completely healed—clean, pink, like a baby's. While starvation has no place as a health procedure, this is quite a remarkable demonstration, if you will, of the incredible healing ability of the body.

Starving yourself might not be all that easy. In 1972 a 450-pound 27-year-old man walked into a Scottish hospital and asked to be put on a 30-day supervised fast. He took a daily multivitamin, water, coffee, and tea as desired. He did well, was discharged after two weeks, and continued the fast at home. When the month was up, he decided to keep fasting, visiting the hospital every couple of weeks. He continued this fast for a grand total of 382 days, well over a year. He was for all intents and purposes "normal" for this period of time, if not much of a dinner companion. His blood glucose dropped to as low as 30, which would usually be considered dangerous, but given some time, the hypothalamus will supplant it by turning on a process called ketosis. His final weight: 180 lbs. He kept it off too. Five years later he was 195. You can read about him in the medical literature or in the Guinness Book of World Records. Now fasting as a way of losing weight has a spotty record indeed, and we definitely recommend you don't try it, but this story certainly illustrates the body's capacity for storing energy.

Calorie Restriction

A Silicon Valley billboard proclaims: "The First Person to Live to 150 Is Alive Today." Prudential Life Insurance put up the sign, and it would certainly be a boon to their business were this to come true.

In pursuit of longevity, groups of people are practicing what is known as Calorie Restriction. These people take care to get sufficient nutrients and try to keep their caloric intake in the neighborhood of 2,000 calories per day. This is not in any sense starvation, but they would be considered thin, or on the thinner side of normal. This movement traces its roots to a long known fact: underfed lab mice live 40% longer. If such an increase would extend to humans as well, that first 150-year-old might well come from this crowd.

We can't really experiment on humans, nor are we mice, but how about something a bit closer on the evolutionary ladder? Twenty-something years ago, two separate calorie restriction experiments were started with rhesus monkeys. The results are in, and frankly, it doesn't look all that good for the calorie restrictors.

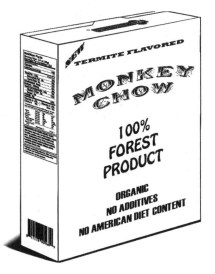

In the first experiment, some monkeys were fed all the Monkey Chow they wanted, and for the others, it was restricted. There was no difference in longevity for these two groups. In the second experiment, the calorie-restricted group was still fed restricted amounts of Monkey Chow, and that group did outlive the control group, but the control group wasn't fed Monkey Chow. The control group was fed a *simulated American diet*. Not exactly apples to apples here. What this mainly proves is that Monkey Chow is better for you than the American diet, but we probably already knew that. What's also proven, though, is that *calorie restriction didn't improve longevity for groups fed the same sort of food*, and this bodes poorly for the hopes of the calorie restrictors.

More to the point, recall that those with an "overweight" Body Mass Index had lower all-cause mortality than those with a "normal" BMI, a surprising result. There are also results for those with "thin" BMI and they do even worse.

The main objection we have to calorie restricting is that it places the body into catabolic mode way too much of the time, plus it isn't much fun.

Note that the human version of the "experiment" will eventually be completed. Many calorie restrictors will continue in spite of the monkey trial results and time will tell. We hope they prove us wrong, but that's not where the research is currently pointing.

Why did this work for mice and not for the monkeys? If you look at life expectancy versus weight for mammals, it's 2 years for a mouse and 25 years for a moose. That moose could weigh 400 pounds. This sort of "more weight means greater longevity" trend applies to all mammals with two exceptions: bats, in a class by themselves, and primates, which are all the monkeys, the apes, and ourselves (actually we are also apes, but that bothers some people). Specifically, our 10-pound rhesus monkeys will beat the 400-pound moose, living up to 30 years (depending on whether they get Monkey Chow or an American diet). A chimp, weighing in at around 100 pounds, might live 60 years. (Cheetah, from the '30s Tarzan films, only recently died, purportedly at age 80.)

We live longer still, 122 years being the current record. We are living a lot longer than the standard "mammal weight-longevity" trend. There are a lot of reasons for this and it is almost surely the case that we have already "evolved" whatever was needed to get that extra 40% the starving mice got. We humans are basically already there. We really don't know where that 150-year-old is going to come from.

The China Study

The China Study, by T. Colin Campbell, is the bible of veganism. It is a large book which covers a lot of ground and makes many valuable points. The name of the book comes from a series of observational studies done in 69 counties in China called the China-Oxford-Cornell Project. Dr. Campbell himself led two of these studies. From this project, he concludes that "plant-based foods are beneficial, and animal-based foods are not."

We found online data for the 1989 study and attempted to verify this conclusion. We looked at all-cause mortality versus dietary choices. There are several reasons for using all-cause mortality instead of specific diseases, such as cancer or heart disease. First, there is general agreement on the diagnosis, and second, a dietary item that decreases instance of one specific disease is of limited interest if it increases another.

We threw caution to the wind and looked first at red meat consumption. What a shock! Surprisingly, the study showed that people who consumed more red meat had lower mortality. Well, actually, this didn't surprise us.

The surprise is that data like this could somehow be used to advocate a vegan diet.

Ours was not an elaborate data analysis, the sort that might be subject to cherry picking or data mining. We did a simple scatter plot of red meat consumption versus all-cause medical mortality for the 67 counties in the study that reported this and observed the trend. Red meat was clearly beneficial. The more eaten, the lower the mortality. After this unexpected start, we tried a variety of other foodstuffs. The results are a pretty far cry from any sort of conclusion that animal product is bad and vegetable good. Here's a list of all the animal and plant categories found in the study:

Food	Mortality effect
Rice	Decreased
Wheat Flour	Increased
Other Cereal	Increased
Starchy Tubers	Increased
Legumes	Decreased
Light-Colored Vegetables	Increased
Green Vegetables	Decreased
Fruit	Decreased
Nuts	Decreased
Milk	Increased
Eggs	Decreased
Red Meat	Decreased
Poultry	Decreased
Fish	Decreased

What conclusion can be reached here? Here's the data. Is animal product harmful? Did it increase mortality? Are starches and cereals helpful? Did they decrease mortality? We don't want to be too picky, but the results strongly indicate that the ideal diet is a lot more like our own dietary guidelines than any vegan fare. We could even reasonably make a claim that the China-Oxford-Cornell Project "proves" our own diet is best.

The results for animal and plant product were amazingly consistent: more meat—less death. More grain or starch—less life.

We do not suppose these results actually "prove" meat is better than vegetables. Meat eaters probably had more money, and there were no doubt other factors. However, to claim this data proves animal product is bad for you is absurd. The raw data strongly and consistently contradicts any such notion.

In fact, *The China Study,* the book, that is, simply ignores most of the China study project data. People other than Campbell have used this data too, and have largely reached the same conclusions we reached. Oddly, Campbell's name appears on some of these papers. However, data is always a tricky business. In the hands of a skilled statistician, armed with a good stat package, most data will, under sufficient torture, confess to any result.

Our findings, though, are not very good news for vegans, and we would strongly suggest they consider the potential consequences of their diet and add lacto-ovo items. There seems to be a lot of attention paid these days to sustainable and humanely treated animal product. Perhaps a reasonable compromise could be reached.

Interestingly, the China-Oxford-Cornell Project counties with the highest blood cholesterol levels also had the lowest mortality.

The Omega-3 Omega-6 Controversy

Omega-6 and omega-3 are a couple of polyunsaturated fats the body can't make, or at least can't make enough of. These fats have kinks 6 or 3 carbons from the end (the omega). Generally, the body can easily manufacture the exact types of fats it needs, but for some reason, has a hard time installing the kink needed to produce these two, so these must be obtained from food. Omega-6 is abundant, but omega-3 is a bit rare, with fish being a good source. We need to get enough omega-3 as well. There is often talk of omega-6 to omega-3 ratio. Our hunter-gatherer ancestors probably got 1:1, but we are about 6:1. However, there is no real science supporting the value of the ratio, and the real issue seems to be omega-3 deficiency. Besides fish, eggs and grass-fed beef are good sources.

Who Is Making Nutritional Policy and Why?

Dietary advice is frequently filtered through lenses that may have little to do with nutrition. The National School Lunch Program was revised in 2012, following recommendations from the Institute of Medicine. The revision increased fruits, vegetables, and whole grain starch, and reduced saturated fat. In a nutshell, higher carb, lower fat. So what is the Institute of Medicine all about? It is a Non-Governmental Organization, but is 67% government funded. A lot of the Institute of Medicine's work seems to be about sustainability. Now sustainability is indeed a valid cause, and the Institute of Medicine's approach to this seems to be to eat more veggies and less meat.

However, the real issue at hand is the health and welfare of 32 million children being fed by the National School Lunch Program. Now there is certainly no universal agreement that a high-carb/low-fat diet is the best way to go, but the recommended revision is exactly that. We would hope the Institute of Medicine keep their goals clear, separated, and appropriate, though, in their school lunch recommendations, this does not seem to be the case.

Key Points

27 - Nutrition

- The body can metabolize fat, glucose, proteins, or ketones.
- The body can metabolize glucose by fermentation, and all four in the Krebs cycle.
- The brain runs on glucose, and the liver can manufacture it if it is not in the diet.
- The brain can also run on ketones, which the liver can generate as well.
- Fats gets to the cells bound up in VLDL or chylomicron particles.
- Glucose floats freely in the blood, but is not utilized by non-brain cells unless insulin is raised. This gives the brain first shot at it.
- Protein is broken down into constituent amino acids.
- The body will use amino acids in the diet, and will burn excess as fuel.
- Nine amino acids come only from food. The body can manufacture twelve.
- Vitamin supplementation has not proven to be a good idea with the exception of vitamin D and possibly B_{12}. Vitamin D is not a true vitamin, as the body can still make it.
- Phytochemicals, which give plants and fruits their colors, can fight cancer.
- Whole grain is slightly better than refined grain, but it is still starch. Avoiding grain altogether is the healthiest choice.
- The Glycemic Index is of little use. Glucose absorption depends heavily on the other food eaten, and whatever is eaten will eventually have to be metabolized.
- The China Study fails to prove that animal product is bad. In fact, it proves exactly the opposite.
- The National School Lunch Program may have been designed to support a different agenda than the health of school-age children.

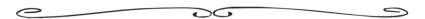

28 - EXERCISE

That exercise is healthy is well known, but less well known is that the type of exercise makes a tremendous difference. A little of the right kind can work wonders, whereas a lot of the wrong kind can be harmful.

WHY IS EXERCISE GOOD FOR US?

This is surprising really. Cars and machines don't behave this way; they wear out. We wear out too, but unlike cars and machines, we have a very elaborate built-in repair and maintenance system. But this system only operates if we are active, and (crucially) if the body's energy management system thinks it can spare the energy. We are a lot better off using our cells and replacing them, through activity, than attempting to conserve them.

What are people trying to accomplish at a gym? The three most common motives are losing weight, building muscle, and health. Of course our motivation for attempting to send people to a gym is the latter category, and here, in no particular order, are several of the broad benefits:

- Neurological—balance, coordination, foot speed, memory
- Posture
- Flexibility
- Range of motion and joint health
- Weight control—lose fat
- Increasing anabolic hormones
- Strengthening the bones
- Building muscle

Exercise is doing a lot more than building muscle. The right exercise maintains and improves all aspects of physical health, and this alone would be reason enough to engage in it. But there is yet a lot more.

Exercise will push back degenerative disease. It will jumpstart arterial wall cleaning, slow or reverse adult onset diabetes, and reduce cancer risk. If you were to enumerate the opposite of these benefits, you would have a good definition of aging. Are we claiming to be able to reverse aging? Yes! Well, sort of. A person who exercises will have the health attributes of a much younger person. Their "biological clock" will say they are much younger than their "chronological clock."

We think most people can do enough exercise to reap all these benefits in two 45-minute sessions a week. Two very intense 45-minute sessions to be sure, but still, that's only 90 minutes a week. This leaves a lot of time for everything else. Even better, add some time for stretching, balancing, general coordination work. Sessions could end with that.

Exercise should encompass these:

- Run the joints through their full range, with only modest weight.
- Stress the big bones in the legs and back.
- Run the heart up and down in bursts.
- Whole-body, explosive, concentric, multi-planar, closed-chain (WECMC) exercises.

These each have specific benefits. It is strongly recommended that all the exercise attributes be embodied in the WECMC exercises.

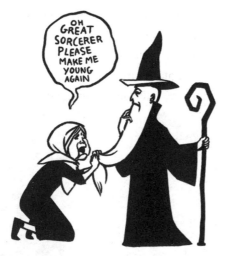
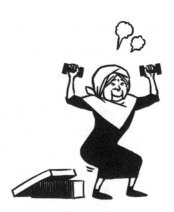

HEALTH EFFECTS OF THE EXERCISE TYPES

Joint Exercises - Maintaining Joint Health and Flexibility

Joint health is maintained if the joints are operated through their full range of motion, compressed and released. The critical joint surfaces, the articular cartilage, are comprised of cells that only get nourished via the joint's lubricating fluid. There is no blood supply, so it is vital to spread that nourishing lubricating fluid around with full-range motion, while applying pressure to force it into the cartilage.

These are easily accomplished by doing the WECMC exercises with full-range motion, reducing the weight, if necessary.

Stressing the Big Bones and Back - Resistance Exercise

Stressing the leg bones and the spine prevents and can reverse osteoporosis. The two best exercises for this are squats and deadlifts, which would usually be included in a WECMC program. For osteoporosis prevention, more weight should be added during the final set of squats and deadlifts, while making sure to maintain perfect form. Both men and women should do this.

Heart Rate Variability - Interval Exercise

Maintaining heart rate variability will slow atherosclerosis, slow calcium buildup, and contribute significantly to arterial health. The optimal exercise is intervals, the idea being to exercise briefly at your maximum level, a level that you cannot sustain for more than 20 or 30 seconds. Unless otherwise advised by a doctor, this is all-out effort. The 20 to 30-second surge should be repeated 5 times, with perhaps a 10 or 15-second rest in between.

This will cause blood pressure to temporarily soar. The arteries will contract, expand, and stretch with the pulses. The blood rushing by the arterial wall triggers all sorts of arterial repair processes. Mitochondrial number and efficiency are significantly increased.

Though intense, intervals are over with quickly. There have been many studies comparing interval training with aerobics, and the results are stunning. Interval exercise shows considerably more benefit, with far less time spent as well. It is, in fact, quite remarkable how much benefit is accrued in so little time.

Typical interval exercises would be:
- Hill runs. Running up a steep hill for 20 or 30 seconds, walking back down, repeated 2 to 4 times.
- Rowing. Most gyms have a couple of Concept 2 rowing machines. They can be programmed for 20 seconds of rowing, 10 seconds of rest.
- Other exercises could also serve as interval training. However, unless the legs and back are involved, the heart will probably not attain its maximum.

Whole-Body, Explosive, Concentric, Multi-Planar, Closed-Chain

The WECMC exercises are the key to peak health. They can be done in a fashion that incorporates the other desirable exercise attributes. Here is a description of each component:
- **Whole Body** means that several things are moving at once, as opposed to isolation exercises, where only one muscle is worked. This improves neural function and coordination.
- **Explosive** means pushing as hard and quickly as possible. The idea here is to place a rapidly increasing energy demand on the mitochondria. This sets in motion various processes that improve both mitochondrial efficiency and the mitochondrial population.
- **Concentric** means a muscle is contracting when it is doing the work. Consider a dumbbell curl. The exercise is concentric on the way up, and eccentric as the weight is let down. For both moves, the bicep is stressed, but on the way up, it is getting shorter, and vice versa on the way down. Why is this important? The hypothalamus, our energy manager, interprets concentric movement as hunting, and eccentric movement as migration. It has sensor nerves embedded in the muscles that can directly detect this. If we are "hunting," the hypothalamus thinks we will succeed and lets us burn energy, repair cells, and renew. If we are migrating, it thinks we are doing so to find

a new source of food. Sound a bit far-fetched? The nerves that measure concentric versus eccentric motion are there, and the hypothalamus responds to them in that way. That much is fact. The hunting vs. migration is supposition, but what else could explain it? Doesn't really matter anymore. It's the concentric exercise that turns on anabolism, and that's what we want.

- **Multi-planar** just means to not merely work in one plane, such as push/pull or extension/flexion. This improves balance, coordination, and neural function.
- **Closed-chain** means recruitment of the neurological chain: an exercise involving all the stabilizing small muscle movements. Tier One exercises, like squats and deadlifts, are examples of this. Most gym machines are not.

Good WECMC Exercises

There are several exercises that embody all of these. The concentric part should be explosive, done fast. The eccentric part, slow.

Squats are ideal, embodying all components. Plus squats are a very good exercise for osteoporosis prevention. Deadlifts are another osteoporosis-preventing exercise that also involves all the WECMC items. Others good examples are pull-ups, snatches, clean and jerk, power cleans, and kettlebell cross-body cleans. Squat-thrust-throw with a medicine ball would also be good, as are the 20/10 rowing intervals.

Most exercise machines found in a gym aren't of much use. It is difficult to do these exercises explosively, and usually only a single muscle is worked.

VO$_2$Max

VO$_2$Max correlates strongly with longevity and is a great measure of overall health and fitness, particularly mitochondrial health. Would improving it increase longevity? Given the effort needed to raise VO$_2$Max, we would reasonably assume so.

HURRY UP! PRESSURE'S RISING!!

There are a couple of ways to measure VO_2Max. The easy, but somewhat inaccurate method uses the Concept-2 rower. The concept2.com website will estimate a VO_2Max given a time for a two-kilometer row.

The preferred method is to find a facility that directly measures VO_2Max. They are a bit rare, but some are not too pricey, maybe around $150. Usually EKG and blood pressure are simultaneously measured. The test is normally done on a treadmill. This measurement represents extreme conditions, and a medical consultation beforehand is recommended.

VO_2Max is a direct measure of both mitochondrial number and efficiency. Increases in both are highly desirable.

HOW DO MUSCLE CELLS WORK?

We know that muscle cells contract, and we know this somehow runs on ATP, since everything else does. The details are interesting. Muscles are yet another amazing bodily invention. Cells typically stay put, and most mobile ones, like white cells, just ooze along like a snail.

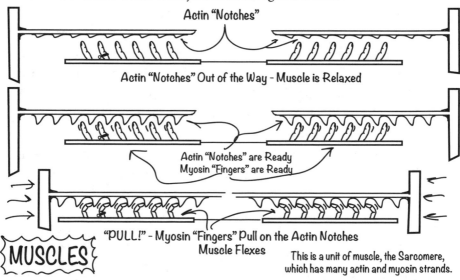

Imagine moving your finger in a "come-hither" sort of motion. Something like this is going on inside the muscle. The "finger" is attached to one sort of fiber called myosin. In fact, there are many fingers all along the length of this fiber. Of course, wiggling these fingers isn't going to accomplish anything unless they can pull on something. There is a different sort of fiber called actin lying alongside, which has notches the fingers can catch and pull. They don't just pull once. They pull, release, pull, release, and pull their way all the way down to the end of the notched actin. There are separate notched fibers attached to each end of a muscle. The myosin fibers with all the fingers sit in the middle and pull the notched actin fibers toward the center. This pulls the two ends of the unit closer together, giving us our contraction.

This "unit" of the myosin and actin fibers is called a sarcomere. It will have a bunch of actin-myosin pairs. Sarcomeres are the usual tiny size, but they are attached end-to-end, forming a long filament. The bicep might have 100,000 of these.

The entire 100,000-sarcomere-long filament is called "a" muscle cell. However, it has multiple nuclei. This is weird. So did 100,000 little cells fuse? If so, we would expect to see 100,000 nuclei, one per sarcomere. But that's not what we see. It's a much lower number. How many then? Oddly, this is unknown, but a lot less than 100,000.

It seems muscle is built from a progenitor cell called a myoblast. This cell has the standard-issue single nucleus. This cell morphs itself (differentiates) into several sarcomeres, each with bundles of actin and myosin fibers. This is called a myofibril, and by all rights, this ought to be called a cell. It started out as a cell and has a single nucleus as do all proper cells.

These myofibrils attach end-to-end to other myofibrils, as long as necessary, to form the muscle. It is this chain of fused myofibrils that is then called a single muscle cell or myocyte.

The extremely long myocyte is packed up in bundles of 10 to 100, and the bundles packed to form the final muscle, attached to the bones, and ready for action.

The actin fiber can cover its notches. This would be a muscle in a relaxed state. Here, the myosin and actin slide freely against one another. If you decide to flex the muscle, the brain sends a nerve signal to the long muscle cell. The signal travels the length of the muscle fiber electrically. The pulse goes to each of the individual sarcomeres, and opens the calcium channels. Calcium channels are transporters embedded in sarcomere cell walls. Calcium ions pour into the sarcomere and cause the actin notches to "expose" themselves. Now the fingers have something to pull on, and the sarcomeres all flex.

A single nerve will have multiple terminations into multiple nerve fibers. To get more muscle contraction, the nerve fires repeatedly.

It is interesting to note that the simplest multi-cellular creature known, a certain C. elegans, a tiny ancient worm with exactly 1,031 cells, has got muscle, and its workings are almost identical to ours, sarcomeres, myofibrils, the whole bit.

Sometimes people with high blood pressure are given Calcium Channel Blockers in order to slow down the heart. Sound foolhardy? So far, no mortality benefit has been reported, but numerous side effects have been. Given how fundamental the calcium step is in muscle contraction, this comes as no shock.

If someone goes from skin and bones to muscle-man, no new muscle cells were grown. Surprising, isn't it? Obviously the muscles are bigger, so something grew. When muscle needs to grow, the sarcomeres increase the number of myosin and actin fibers, and the number of mitochondria as well. Except in the case of injury, new muscle cells are not built.

Never? Well hardly ever. But almost forever, it was standard dogma that heart muscle never rebuilt, and now it is found to be doing so, and there is a grand debate on how much of this goes on, with estimates ranging from 1% to 7% per year.

Those following the QM program will probably have a pretty good idea of the speed at which new skeletal "muscle" is built. Of course we now know that it's just new myosin and actin fibers and mitochondria, and not new muscle at all.

GROWTH HORMONES

The right exercise triggers the release of growth hormones. We want this. Growth hormones trigger the repair and renewal of cells. Some of the repair is local, where it is needed—a sore muscle, for instance—and some of it is general. Repair and renewal are done from the fresh, pristine stem and progenitor cells. Repair and renewal keep the body young.

Not all exercise triggers these growth hormones. The hypothalamus will slow this system way down if it perceives an energy shortage. The hypothalamus's energy management notions are mired in our ancient past. Using the amount and type of our activity, it attempts to predict the future energy supply. Even though we have enough to eat today, if we aren't hunting or gathering, it concludes that energy (food) will soon run out. What cues are gotten from our activity level? Perhaps there is no activity. Conserve. Maybe we are snowed in, or waiting for a migrating herd that is late arriving.

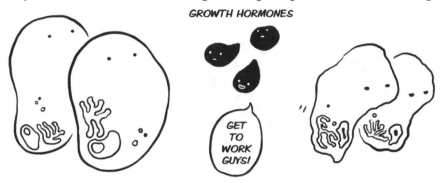

If the hypothalamus concludes that we are hunting and gathering, it will up-regulate circulating growth hormones. This is the anabolic state. Various local processes are enabled as well. At the local level, the tissue itself decides which cells are repaired or replaced. Stressed cells needing help will express receptors for the growth hormones.

Replacement and growth are enabled as well. Any new cells that may be needed come from stem or progenitor cells, which are usually protected from the day-to-day wear and tear. Because of this sequestering, the new cells are in far better shape than the old ones, and as such, they are less prone to cellular damage, more cancer resistant, more efficient, and so on. This system is as close to a Fountain of Youth as we are likely to attain.

The arteries likewise benefit. They have their own repair systems, and these are triggered by the variation in blood flow and the consequent direct stress on the artery walls.

Without exercise, none of this happens. The cells are powered down and sit and wait. Even if we could trick the hypothalamus into giving the green renewal light, things still would not work right. Underutilized cells would not request repair, the arteries would not be cleaned of plaque, and so on.

EXERCISE AS SEEN FROM AN ENDOTHELIAL CELL

Let's shrink the reader (you) down to the size of a cell and see what is going on in the endothelium. So far, it is pretty tranquil. Red and white cells are drifting by. They are about your size. However, the owner of this particular artery is about to plunge into high-intensity interval exercise. Get a real good grip on something, because this is going to be a wild ride.

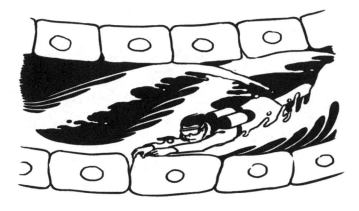

With every huge heartbeat, the whole artery expands, red and white cells along with the plasma rush by in a burst. The current tugs you and the endothelial wall as well. The blood pressure is almost double (210/150) our exerciser's normal value. (Blood pressure goes that high normally in intense exercise.) And the pounding. Three blasts a second. Hold on tight.

Fortunately, interval exercise doesn't last long. A couple of minutes later things are back to normal. Or are they? That 30 seconds of arterial chaos left an aftermath, and a very beneficial one.

The scene is transformed. The environment is pristine and clean. The shear force of the rushing, pulsing blood gave the endothelium a thorough scrubbing. The individual endothelial cells changed their alignment in response to the rushing blood. Several key endothelial cell functions were also triggered by the shear force, and, of course, blood will now flow more easily and uniformly.

The smooth muscle cells surrounding the endothelium got a workout as well. This improved their elasticity and responsiveness. Their mitochondria got their needed exercise, and this increased their health while reducing the amount of reactive oxygen species.

EXERCISE AS SEEN FROM MITOCHONDRIA

Mitochondria are largely self-regulating. If nothing is using any ATP, the internal processes, the Krebs cycle, will back up, and effectively, the mitochondria energy production plant will pause. Too much of this and the mitochondria will shut down entirely, may die, and might take out the cell as well.

Activity starts the mitochondrial engine up again. If demands are made, it will produce energy at its maximum rate, which tends to clear out any debris, making the mitochondria more efficient. In fact, in a pinch, the cells will burn some of that trash for energy.

The muscle uses ATP just like any other cell, but the demand can become huge in a hurry, so fuel supply is a big issue. The fuel burn rate, of course, depends on the exercise. Let's consider high-intensity and then aerobic.

In high-intensity exercise, the first burst of energy, good for about 20 to 30 seconds, uses up the available ATP in the muscle cells. Then fresh ATP is made from fermentation. This yields only 2 ATP per glucose molecule versus 38 for mitochondria, but fermentation is far faster than the Krebs cycle. The local free glucose and glucose stored in glycogen are rapidly burned through. After that, the interval exercise is over. This short but intense demand on the mitochondria has interesting consequences. First, the number of available mitochondria will be increased in anticipation of future demand, and second, the existing ones will operate more efficiently. This means healthier cells with more biological power. This is what we want.

Aerobic exercise is a different matter. In principle, aerobic exercise can continue for an hour or more. Again, the free ATP is burned first, but here the mitochondria *can* keep up with the lower energy demand. The glucose and glycogen are next, but in the aerobic case, these are processed by the mitochondria, not by fermentation. This lasts 15 or 20 minutes. After that, local and circulating fat is used. There is enough of this to run for hours. Since the mitochondria can keep up with the demand. there is no need to increase the mitochondrial supply or efficiency. This is not what we want.

Why Do Non-Muscular Areas Also Benefit?

Muscles and their arteries are not the sole beneficiaries of exercise. There is a general benefit, and two principal reasons for it. Blood flow is a managed resource. The arteries and veins can constrict to control this. The stomach can get more blood if it has a meal to digest. The muscles get the lion's share in a workout. However, this shuffling about of the blood supply is not total. If the heart is pumping furiously, the entire vascular system experiences it and benefits from it. Thus the arterial conditioning—the stretching, pulsing, and polishing—will occur in parts of the body not directly involved in the exercise.

The second reason is hormonal. The signal to renew and repair is local, regional, and global. The hypothalamus has its hand on the levers. If it concludes that energy conservation is not necessary, that the body can build and renew, it opens the growth-hormone gates. Specifically, IGF-1 and testosterone levels are increased. These can trigger renewal and repair wherever they are needed, not just the recently worked muscles. (That said, it is pretty likely that those muscles will need a bit of repair.)

WHY DO WE HATE EXERCISE? REVISITED

This was discussed in somewhat philosophical terms in chapter 10, STEP III - LIFESTYLE CHANGE GUIDELINES - EXERCISE. However, there may be "scientific" explanations as well. Or sort of. Consider this: The hypothalamus is always behaving like a stingy grump, and is forever trying to conserve resources and be efficient. So generally, it "permits" exercise only for hunting and self-defense (or offense).

Now then, suppose you think about exercising, and then come up with 101 reason not to do so. You know it's good for you, has benefits, as do we all. So who is supplying all this negativity? Most likely the hypothalamus, somehow. Procrastination hormones? The hypothalamus is famously well connected.

But why did it make this calculation? Most likely because the reward for the exercise wasn't immediate. The hypothalamus is thinking: "OK so you want to exercise. What's in it for me? Where's the food?" Hunting would have this payback, as would warfare. Food? OK. Survival? OK.

Place yourself in the hunter-gatherer's moccasins. You are sitting around the fire, playing games, spinning yarns, and suddenly a deer is spotted. There's no discussion of the relative benefits of exercise. The effect is immediate. To arms! The hunt is on! Feast tonight! The hypothalamus doesn't get in the way of this one. Warfare or defense would also receive the same hypothalamic OK. But lifting a heavy boulder 10 times, 3 sets, for no reason? No way.

Dr. Mike Case Study
Extreme Exercise Can Cause Problems

"Mr. Smith" was a 55-year-old ultra-runner. When I met him I had the only medical-grade gas exchange/stress machine on the West Coast and he was very curious about his VO$_2$Max. I was still building my research database so I only took patients for a complete work-up. He assured me—with almost a smirk of confidence—he was in such great shape there was no way he actually needed all of the testing I required, but out of curiosity he agreed to my full testing protocols.

Well, as it turned out he had osteoporosis and his coronary calcium score (CAC) was 939.8: above the 95th percentile. Bad, very bad coronary artery disease (CAD): not what he expected, nor I for that matter. His VO$_2$Max was very good; age adjusted he was in the top 5%.

Now there are lots of interesting numbers in his data but for this note I want to focus on his HDL. His first testing showed an HDL of 56 mg/dl. His total cholesterol was 165, LDL was 97 and his triglycerides were 61 mg/dl. How could this guy have CAD, you might ask? Surely he had high Lp(a) or homocysteine or CRP or something? Nope; all were OK. However, his activated HDL, HDL2b was only 17%. Could that be it or at least associated with his CAD?

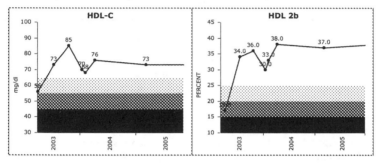

We decided to find out. He carefully followed all of my recommendations, mostly summarized in this book; in his case we cut his total weekly running mileage by about 50%, added in the weight training I advocate, and changed his diet to my basic diet also described elsewhere in this book. His HDL went up to 85mg/dl and his percent HDL 2b went up to 36%.

After two years his CAC went down to 884.7—normally this goes up, not down—and his bone mineral density went up 30%.

But, wait; there is more human detail to the story. Mr. Smith didn't make the changes I requested like a robot; he had opinions and a life too. After his first six months saw the improvements in HDL, he said he believed all of the improvements were from the diet change, and he wanted to go back to his old style of training. OK, let's see: his HDL went back down to 68 and HDL 2b down to 30%. This was a sequential change that we tracked, not just two random points. He conceded that perhaps the exercise change was the driver of his better numbers but missed his very long runs. We compromised, and thus with careful calibration he was able to up his mileage to about 65% of his old baseline with the weight training system still in place. Well his HDL went back up to 76 and his HDL 2b to an even better 38%. As you can see from the graphs, he "dialed this in" and maintained the training pattern and his BMD went up an additional 20% over the next year. Well done, "Mr. Smith."

We have to confess to a slight error in reasoning that the hypothalamus catches. We have claimed that exercise is anabolic. It will build you up. This is the net effect, but it is not the direct effect of exercise. Exercise itself is catabolic. Muscles are damaged, bones are stressed. The amazing thing is that the body not only repairs the damage in a day or so, but actually makes the bones and muscles better than they were.

However, the ever-skeptical hypothalamus may not be quite so sure. Suppose we exercised, a catabolic activity. Should the hypothalamus authorize repairs? It may not be sure we will have access to the energy needed to repair and improve, and indeed, if we don't get the food, the hypothalamus won't authorize those repairs. Now, we *know* we are going to get food and this is all going to work, but the hypothalamus, with its primordial ways of thinking, is not so sure. So it reasons: best not to exercise. And somehow it gets our conscious self thinking up excuses.

Could we meditate our way out of this conundrum? The hypothalamus needs to hear the other side of the story.

Key Points
28 - Exercise
- Exercise has benefits well beyond building muscle. Joint health is improved, bones are strengthened, coordination and neural circuitry are improved.
- Four goals of exercise: improve mitochondrial health, improve heart rate variability, improve joint health, and improve bone strength.
- All of these are simultaneously achieved by concentric, explosive, closed-chain, systemic exercise. Two good examples are squats and deadlifts.
- Squats and deadlifts will specifically improve large bone strength.
- Some exercises should be done full range with light weight for joint health.
- Some balance exercises should be done for coordination.
- Interval exercise improves mitochondrial health and is very "cost effective."
- Muscle is constructed from very long cells.
- The contraction is done by fibers that pull each other along.
- The number of muscle cells stays the same, but the number of pulling fibers will increase with exercise.
- The right sort of exercise triggers growth hormones at optimal levels.
- Exercise cleans and renews the artery wall: the endothelium.
- Because of the rise in blood pressure and heart rate, arterial areas not directly involved are also cleansed.

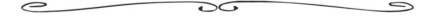

29 - SPIRITUAL DISCIPLINE

The three main modifiable components of a healthy lifestyle are:
- Sound nutrition
- Effective exercise
- Spiritual discipline

No one questions the importance of the first two, but spiritual discipline is a tough sell. Yet, it is very reasonably and arguably the most important of the three. Oddly, few want to hear this.

Any attempt at an honest evolutionary anthropology keeps bumping into the fact that all world-historical religions have a very distinctive "spiritual discipline," be that the yoga of the Hindus, or the Prayer of the Breath of the Eastern Orthodox Christians, or the rosary of Western Catholics, or the emptying meditation of Buddhists. Hasidic Jews praying at the Wailing Wall also know the ancient "secret" of spiritual discipline: rhythm, movement, breathing, and inner silence. As they rock back and forth on their feet they chant, in Hebrew, "Holy, Holy, Holy," to rhythmic breathing and speaking.

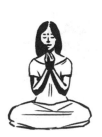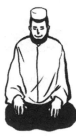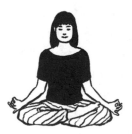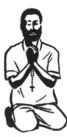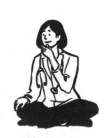

This universal sign of ancient man meant something—perhaps many things—but at least it meant deep biology, and almost anything that honors our deep, ancient biology helps us be healthier.

The chemistry and hormonal effects of spiritual discipline are scattered throughout the medical literature. Because medical science is, in principle at least, a secular enterprise, the findings are usually couched in oddly apologetic language; they are bashful about using the word "prayer" in the context of the *New England Journal of Medicine* or the *Journal of the American Medical Association*. Medical science seems finally to have become comfortable with the term "mindfulness-based meditation," and thus a body of literature is starting to grow up around this term. However, there is nothing magic about the referent of this term either. This synthetic Buddhist term still alludes to the basics: rhythm, movement, breathing, and inner silence.

The interior mental state attained with various spiritual disciplines is associated with less depression, anxiety, and addiction and fewer dysfunctional families. This list of maladies, when improved, are associated with a lower incidence of heart disease, sudden cardiac death, high blood pressure, suicide, cancer, obesity, dementia, and adult onset diabetes. Oh, and not incidentally, you will sleep better too.

Take this pill of spiritual discipline, and you will be happier and healthier, and, very likely—this is not as precise—more joyful.

From the rest of this book you will recognize the deleterious effects of prolonged elevated cortisol levels; you will recognize the anticancer, anti-atherosclerotic benefits of higher melatonin levels. You will recognize the calm of a happy hypothalamus more contentedly running your eating behavior. You will be less driven to non-productive over-work on obsessive-compulsive details of your work and family life. The lower cortisol levels encourage higher testosterone, which is one of the best antidepressants there is; natural testosterone, intra-testicular testosterone, not the kind you take as a pill, shot, or cream.

There is an enormous amount of "gee whiz" imaging and narrative accounts of neural patterning changes in those who meditate. We hope this book has set the table so that the benefits of metabolic transformation are clear and the roles of improving sleep and lowering the biochemistry of stress are freshly linked in your understanding, in such a way that we are beyond the "gee whiz" and down to the business of fundamental metabolic transformation.

HALLMARKS OF EFFECTIVE SPIRITUAL DISCIPLINE

All of the traditional disciplines share an emphasis on rhythmic breathing, some kind of repeated pattern of movement, even if it is the breathing itself, and the goal of interior silence.

Many health gurus who push calm, relaxation, breathing therapy, and the like seem to be advocating a particular discipline. This may make them more successful and may appeal, cult-like, to a strong following, but this may not be the best advice for most people. The benefits of spiritual discipline are found in biology more than in metaphysics.

Keep in mind, though, that while separating out the benefits from any specific religious affiliation, we do not mean to deny there are benefits there too, but merely assert that to properly benefit from Quantitative Medicine, that association need not be present.

You will need to find a discipline that is congenial to you. It can be as simple as an imaginary body scan. In this sense a body scan is lying down, closing your eyes, breathing slowly and rhythmically, casting your mind over your body in an orderly way, and thinking of each area in sequence, simultaneously intending the area of reflection and imagination to relax: first the toes, then the foot, and so on, head to toe or toe to head. Even something as simple as this, done with intention, in a quiet place, while breathing and relaxing can be profoundly relaxing and invigorating.

How much of this should be done to obtain the full benefit? The medical literature on this would indicate that to realize all the health benefits, any spiritual discipline needs at least an hour a week's attention: 20 minutes 3 times a week or 4-6 sessions of 10-15 minutes.

Ten minutes a day would be effective. There are many forms of spiritual discipline that incorporate the essential components of rhythm, movement, breathing, and inner silence; what recommends any of them is that you find them pleasurable, attractive, or effective. The list of choices is long, and for our purposes they are all fine, as long as they encourage you to the discipline part.

- Yoga
- Tai chi
- Qigong
- The rosary
- Via negativa Christian meditation
- Emptying meditation of Buddhism
- Contemplation in many forms

Choose one. The key is discipline. Those who finally make it and find their spiritual discipline "groove"—it is a hard slog adhering to a spiritual discipline—find that the rewards are deep, clear, and profound.

WELCOME TO THE SCHOOL OF SILENCE

One of the hallmarks of all spiritual disciplines, sometimes spelled out in various ways in various "sacred texts," is the call to a quiet mind. While speculation about what constitutes a just and peaceful society is a treatise well beyond our scope here, Pascal's dictum, "All of humanity's problems stem from man's inability to sit quietly in a room alone," captures the ancient understanding of the benefit of a calm mind.

The attention to breathing and rhythmic movement, as seen in the meditative martial art Taijiquan, for example, lead to and draw from a quiet mind. In the modern world, stilling the mind is one of the biggest challenges we face.

Different spiritual disciplines accomplish this in different ways. One of the most common draws on sitting still and attempting to not think about anything. This can be tough, but for those who can achieve this state, a simple clear path is provided to a quiet mind.

Another method is to attempt to hold before the "mind's eye" a simple, nearly abstract image like the horizon of a darkening sea. Another approach is to rehearse favorite or even "sacred" passages or images. The rosary is an example of this approach.

BREATHING AND THE HEART

One of the easiest connections between the elements of spiritual discipline and physiological effects is the focus on breathing. If we remember the role of the hypothalamus, the connection becomes clearer. The hypothalamus controls and integrates the sympathetic and parasympathetic autonomic systems. In simple terms, the sympathetic system is a rapidly activating system to give us that shot of adrenalin we sometimes need, you know, when that pesky saber-tooth tiger roams the neighborhood, while the parasympathetic system is there to help us relax and smell the roses.

THE GREAT CIRCLE OF VIPASSANA
(READ CLOCKWISE)

For the autonomic system to work properly, it needs to be supple; it needs to be rapidly compliant and responsive to change and need. In the same way that arteries become "hardened" as they age, the autonomic system can become rigid and unresponsive: it becomes stuck. This shows up in poor heart rate variability. Heart rate variability is of at least two kinds: the heartbeat-to-heartbeat variability at rest in response to very subtle changes in metabolic need, and the wildly dynamic heart rate response to exercise. Heart rate variability is a very important surrogate for measuring heart health, but what it reflects is the health or illness of the autonomic nervous system.

The hypothalamus has both incoming and outgoing nervous system information, which allows it to regulate virtually all organ system functions. Two of its most important functions are regulating the heart and breathing. For our purposes, we are now full circle; breathing and heart rate variability are very tightly connected and mediated through the hypothalamus. Just as heart rate variability is lost in an aging or unhealthy heart, so too, and for the same reasons, our breathing variability becomes suppressed or rigid. Well, conveniently enough, we can reestablish breathing variability, initially at least, consciously. We can provide afferent signals back to the brain and hypothalamus, signals that will coach variability and subtlety back into the hypothalamus and consequently the autonomic nervous system, just by consciously relearning to breathe, or at least to breathe freely and well.

The brain thrives or atrophies rather like a muscle, and without regular exercise, becomes flaccid, weak, and monotonic, but like a muscle, it can be retrained and invigorated. This isn't attained by playing chess or solving quadratic equations, but rather by helping it return to its ancient biological roots and wordless self-awareness. In the act of meditation, the conscious and noisy neocortex agrees to hand the reins back to the verbally shy hypothalamus and its efforts to maintain or restore a healthy balanced autonomic nervous system. Think of Michelangelo's "The Creation of Adam" in the Sistine Chapel—just so does the divine touch the fallen. Through spiritual discipline the hypothalamus and the neocortex sustain and enliven one another. And we become healthy

---

Key Points
29 - Physiology of Meditation
- Spiritual discipline can take many forms.
- Most medical literature calls it Mindful Meditation.
- A focus on breathing is a good starting point.

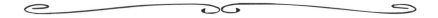

30 - SLEEP

The circadian rhythm is the 24-hour clock and is managed by the hypothalamus. It will maintain an approximate 24-hour cycle in the absence of light, but will synchronize to a the actual day-night cycle, if present. This synchronizing does not happen immediately, as any traveler knows.

The hypothalamus thinks we are still hunter-gatherers and that there is no artificial light other than the dim glow of a fire. For northerners, the winter night is long, and the summer day is long. For several hundred years or more, we have, in effect, departed from this ancient rhythm, likely to our detriment.

Of primary interest is sleep. Duration, timeliness, and quality are all important. Disturbed sleep cycles or onset times are associated with adult onset diabetes, cancer, and atherosclerosis.

For those involved in shift work, incidences of cancer, heart disease, and all-cause mortality are higher by up to 25% compared to day workers doing similar jobs.

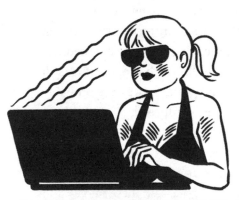

THE HYPOTHALAMUS MAY NOT BE ABLE TO INTERPRET ALL LIGHT SOURCES.

But even in the absence of something as disruptive as shift work, faulty sleep patterns cause a number of problems. Primarily, the body uses sleep as a massive repair time. This is essential. Lab rats prevented from sleeping soon die.

383

Melatonin

Melatonin is the sleep hormone. It starts to climb rapidly around 9 p.m. It is a simple and ancient hormone, found in plants as well as animals and triggered by darkness. Rather than controlling melatonin, the hypothalamus detects it and responds. Since the melatonin is circulating, any interested cell could express a receptor and take some action.

Circulating melatonin acts as an antioxidant, among other things. Because it is such a small molecule, it can easily get into cells and is able to cross the blood-brain barrier. Circulating melatonin also interacts with the immune system, apparently reducing inflammation. These are anti-cancer effects, and the disruption of the melatonin cycle by shift work is the probable cause of the higher cancer risk.

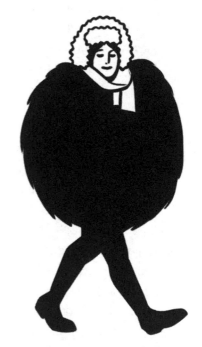

The seasonal variation in light causes a corresponding seasonal variation in melatonin, and apparently this triggers seasonal changes in some animals, change of fur color or thickness, or breeding behavior. We probably once responded to this as well. If this apparatus still functions within us, we have probably thoroughly confused it.

Melatonin is produced by the pineal gland, named for its resemblance to a pine cone. It reacts directly to retinal light-sensing nerves. These nerves also inform the hypothalamus.

LIKE OTHER ANIMALS, HUMANS ARE ALSO PRONE TO SEASONAL CHANGE.

Body Repaired While You Sleep

Soon after the onset of sleep, Growth Hormone (GH) shoots way up— maybe tenfold over daytime levels—and stays high for the first six hours of sleep. With this 10:1 ratio, one can immediately conclude that any benefit from GH occurs almost entirely during sleep. Insulin and glucose rise also, though not as dramatically. GH stimulates IGF-1 production, which gives any damaged cells needing to repair the green light to proceed. In the absence of IGF-1, non-urgent repairs, like sore muscles, will be postponed. Muscles aren't built at the gym, they are built during sleep. (Repair of a wound is a different matter entirely. It is locally controlled and obviously immediate.) Some sleeping pills suppress the growth hormone secretion, an undesirable side effect.

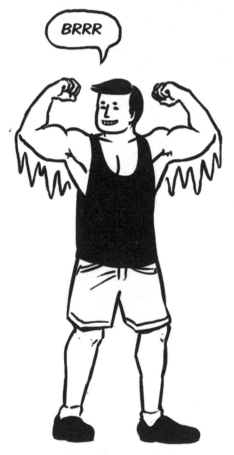

. . . **BUT IT IS OFTEN SECONDARY TO MATING BEHAVIOR.**

Testosterone, which functions as a body-wide "OK to rebuild" signal, also increases during sleep, as does thyroxin, another growth stimulator.

Sleep turns out to be a rather busy time. With so much activity going on all night, it's amazing we aren't exhausted when we wake up.

Around 4 a.m., cortisol starts to rise, peaking at 8 a.m. or so. The reason for this is unknown. Maybe it's to jar you awake.

REM Sleep—Memory Consolidation?

REM stands for Rapid Eye Movement. All parents have seen this in their sleeping baby. This is dreaming time. REM sleep may be necessary for the sorting and storing of recent memories. Results of research vary. If someone is deprived of REM sleep, it appears they will catch up at their next opportunity.

Almost all mammals and birds exhibit REM sleep, and many appear to dream.

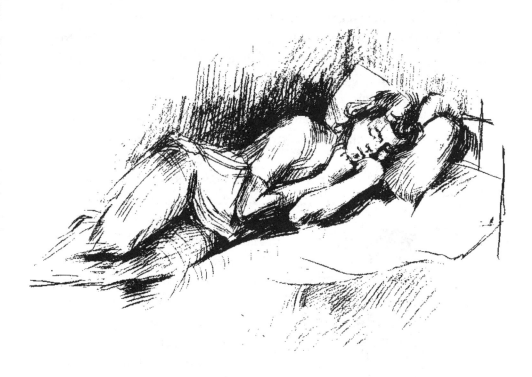

The Glymphatic System

This is new. Scoop your doctor. The body also uses sleep to drain the brain. Throughout the body, cellular junk is dumped into the lymph system. The notable exception is the brain—the lymph system doesn't extend there. So how do the neurons unload their waste?

For over a century, it was assumed that detritus from active neurons was somehow cleared by the cerebrospinal fluid. However, quite a few things didn't really add up. Apparently, there is not enough contact with the neurons to accomplish this.

The research that finally sorted this out will probably be worth a Nobel Prize. It is about two years old and quite amazing. It seems that all the blood vessels in the brain are surrounded by a second wall. So it's a tube within a tube. The inner tube performs its normal blood circulation function, but the space between the inner and outer tube carries the cellular junk away. The discoverers named this the glymphatic system, a combination of glia, the helper cells in the brain that build and maintain the structure, and the lymph system. The discoverer, Nedergaard, injected dye into a mouse and got a most amazing picture.

OK, nice to know the brain can drain, but what has this to do with sleep? It turns out this drainage system only works while you sleep. No sleep—no drainage. Poor sleep—poor drainage. So, for this reason, sound sleep is more crucial for proper brain function than previously imagined.

Does the brain drain during meditation? That might explain a thing or two. Hey Dr. Nedergaard . . .

Unihemispheric Sleep

Ever been half asleep? Some animals can literally do this. Whales are a good example. One half of the brain sleeps while the other half deals with periodically surfacing for a breath of air. It is thought that migrating birds may also use unihemispheric sleep, but this may be hard to observe.

Hibernation Isn't Sleep

Hibernation is a state of "torpor." The animal isn't asleep, but it isn't awake. In fact, hibernating animals come out of the torpor, "wake-up," and move about. Some then go to sleep, actual sleep, then wake up from that and return to hibernation. The obvious purpose of hibernation is to conserve energy, which is dramatically down-regulated. Northern bears will reduce their metabolism by 75%, and not eat or drink for months.

One might wonder why these animals don't just simply sleep.

Some recent research on meditation has suggested it is akin to hibernation.

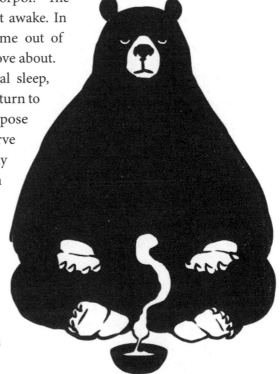

Napping Isn't Sleep—Or Is It?

At least some sleep-like functions go on during a nap. Memory consolidation is one. REM sleep sometimes occurs, but there is no melatonin spike. Some hormones are elevated.

Many cultures regularly nap—the siesta—and sleep less at night. These cultures do not appear to be more or less healthy than those that do not nap, so one could conclude that a nap plus less sleep is equivalent.

Key Points
30 - Circadian Rhythm and Sleep

- The hypothalamus regulates sleep, and will keep the cycle in the absence of light.
- Darkness triggers the melatonin cycle. This is independent of the hypothalamus.
- Melatonin acts as an antioxidant and may have anti-cancer properties.
- The body is repaired during sleep. Growth hormone increases considerably while sleeping, and this triggers a rise in other growth hormones.
- The brain has an drainage system called the glymphatic system. However, it only operates during sleep.
- Some animals, whales for instance, and possibly migrating birds, can sleep one-half of their brain at a time.
- Hibernation is not sleep, and may be a state akin to meditation.
- Napping plus a shorter night's sleep appears to be equivalent to a full nights sleep.

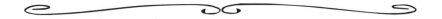

31 - BLUE SKIES

The history of medicine is replete with foolish ideas. From leeches to beta-blockers, institutional medicine has advocated treatments that have all too frequently caused more harm than good. The process that leads to such errors is hubris. Pride. And to be fair, some of the motivation has also been desperation. Who could blame a mother for fearing demons in the vapors of a damp night when that was the wisdom of the time and her son was sick?

Thus desperation, foolishness, and greed have killed millions, and this calculation is easily made, especially in modern times when we know how many die from hospital-acquired infections, medication reactions, side effects, and, after the fact, calculations of the harmful effects of the aforementioned beta-blockers and other widely prescribed medications.

Hope for the magic pill springs eternal. The latest goes by the name of "big data." It is imagined that all of the interconnectedness of centralized medical data will generate astounding new avenues of therapy and diagnosis. Just crunch enough numbers and the answers will magically appear in the numerical tea leaves.

Sadly this is not true and harkens back the same hubris that gave us leeches and beta-blockers. The root problem is that we are all incalculably complex, and the combination of genetics and environment that defines ourselves and our health means we need to each be our own specific experiment.

In this book we have offered a narrative of our biological past as a way to see the layered complexity of systems as they accreted in our genome and cultures and are finally reflected in how our bodies respond to disease and are programmed to heal and be restored when the right conditions are provided. We have attempted to give you a line of thought, cause and effect, so that you can see how basically simple choices could encourage or defeat the intrinsic systems as they attempt to restore us to health.

While we have listed only a few surrogate markers of health, like resting and peak heart rates, fasting insulin, morning cortisol, and glycation markers like A1C, there are potentially thousands that matter. The rich enough array of markers brought into our graphing environment and tracked through the simple application of the scientific method outlined here mean that you and I and institutional medicine can be truly healed. The future of QM with your help—help yourself—is as nearly boundless as the universe itself.

Quantitative Medicine is a thoroughly different approach to degenerative disease management and prevention. Medicine at its best helps the body stay well. Consider vaccines. They don't kill pathogens. They only tell our body how to identify them. It's up to our body to do the rest. And it can. And it does. Degenerative disease follows the same model. If you "inoculate" yourself by driving your numbers to known healthy regions, your body will do the rest. It will prevent degenerative disease.

Start graphing things and measure the markers we discuss: they have been well chosen. There are others—help us find more and add your own—and join the game of life in earnest. Your body wants to heal; your body wants to be vibrant. It waits for you to care and then to measure and change.

HEALING

The agency of the will makes us sick or well. The argument over the roles of biological determinism (hormones made me do it) and free will (if I can do it, then something is wrong with those who can't) plays out continually.

So many people fail at being or becoming well that something more is needed. That people fail to choose to be well is indisputable. It is further true that they could choose to be well but don't. But why? This failure is from not giving biology its due. It is simply that one cannot progress without knowledge of the biology and genetics driving the healing process, and we are simply no longer tuned into these vital forces. In effect, it means we don't honor our ancient ancestry. We can no longer see the long, tortured, and elegant chain of life and struggle that is buried in behavior and genetics. The cultural reminders no longer even exist.

Humans survived the evolutionary pageant, the epics of our struggle to become the dominant predator of biological life on earth as clans, as tribes, as social beings. We hunted in packs, we ate as families and clans and tribes. The will of our ancestors ranged freely over many choices: hunt alone, hunt together, eat alone, eat together. Our ancestors were every bit as intelligent as we are and were great scientists of the possible and the actual that worked so that they might live another day; to thrive or die in the death-haunted beauty of the world. This success story became embedded in our facial-recognition-coded genetics; in our auditory lie detectors; again genetically encoded in our sensory world as the desire for the touch of another's skin. Simply put, our genetics, the bountiful fruit of millions of years of perfect honing, play a powerful role in how and what we *can* choose. Our cortex, our "higher mind," sees the incoming waves, but our biology remains as a riptide to wash us out again into the deep waters of genetic history: the deep ocean of clan, tribe, and cultural behavior.

Our genes *didn't* make us do it. We reject biological determinism. But if we don't adequately take into account the riptide of the genetic signals, we cannot stand informed by our intelligence and liberated as agents of free will to make the right choices, to choose to be healthy. The genetics pulls as biological determinism, the moral imagination pulls into an unseen but imagined better future; but in this day, this very day, we are balanced between the dreary abyss of our mortality and the eternal longing of our family, clan, and tribe: we must survive, work too late, eat too poorly. We succeeded, we lived another day. "I" failed because I died too soon, became unhappy, weak, and sad. I chose what my genetics foretold. The problem is that our genetics are lost in this place in time and space. Our clan is lost in this time and space. We must construct a clan deferential to our ancient ancestry, the anthropology of our biology, and informed by the higher mind, the neocortex, but empowered by our very free, very human will.

Strange indeed that all our civilization and technology leave us so disconnected and so vulnerable, and that all our abundance and ease should cause horrible diseases and shorten our lives. We have left this in the hands of the doctors, and their response has been to find cleverer and cleverer ways to repair the damage and prolong things. What else could they do? They are no more connected than we are. Besides, they are indeed very good at this. They do pay some attention to preventive strategies, but it is mostly *pro forma*. There appears to be little knowledge or conviction that behavior changes can completely prevent all these seemingly inevitable horrors. Or perhaps they believe that people will not make those changes. Possibly they are right, but then, possibly people don't know that profound differences are achievable. The evidence for this is compelling in many ways. Many highly studied drugs and interventions have but slight benefit—15% reductions in this disease or that, and the like. Yet if one drives ones health with the correct life choices, the reduction is more like 100%, or at least can be if begun early enough.

This ability is at hand. Quantitative Medicine brings this ability to all. Anyone can take it up and do it. Amazingly, culture pushes us strongly away from this. We are bombarded with suggestions to eat things that would not even be recognized as food by a hunter-gatherer. We can be as sedentary as we desire, though this seems to be changing for the better. But changing for the worse is the 24/7 assault on our senses that all the modern connectivity and gadgetry provide.

So if you can chop your way through the cultural forest and find, in your own personal fashion, the ways and paths that lead to a long disease-free life, you will have triumphed not only for your own benefit, but for those around you, who will take similar cues and steps.

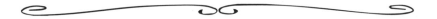

APPENDICES

APPENDIX 1 - MEDICAL RESEARCH

WHERE TO FIND MEDICAL RESEARCH

Virtually all medical research is available on the Internet, but a fair amount of it is behind a paywall. Policy varies from organization to organization. All the papers listed in APPENDIX-2 are available on the Internet, and are not paywalled. If you are interested, the same appendix (or, more likely, an updated one) is repeated at QuantitativeMedicine.net, with links to the various papers. Search for "bibliography."

Generally there are two places to start: Google Scholar (scholar.google.com) and PubMed (www.ncbi.nlm.nih.gov/pubmed). Most documents will be found on both these sites, but there is a major advantage to Google Scholar: if a document is available in a non-paywalled version, Google Scholar will list it in the right margin.

If diving into a new topic, search first for review articles. They are generally better written, less technical, and provide the "big picture."

HOW TO READ MEDICAL RESEARCH

In our opinion, doctors write better than physicists. Nonetheless, the readability of the papers runs the gamut from lucid to incomprehensible. However, unlike physics, statistics tends to pervade all the papers, which can be confusing, sometimes deliberately.

The jargon can be a bit imposing at first, but here is a short guide:

- Cohort - A group of people.
- Epidemiology - A data set of a large group of people—health and lifestyle records typically.
- Epidemiological Study - Analysis of an epidemiology.
- Efficacy - effectiveness, ability to produce desired result
- Prospective study - These studies follow the development of disease in groups of people and attempt to determine the effect of factors such as lifestyle.
- Retrospective study - A retrospective study is similar to a prospective study, but looks at people that have already contracted a disease and attempts to associate the disease with some possibly causative factors.
- Cross-sectional study - Cross-sectional studies are one-shot events typically. A group of people could be asked to fill out a medical history and current eating and drinking habits to attempt to determine causes of lung cancer.
- Case-control studies - Here the outcomes are gathered, and the histories examined for possible causes. Dr. Nichols could divide his cohort into a high-triglyceride group (the "Cases") and a normal-triglyceride group (the "Controls"), and explore what prior lifestyle choices had been made.
- Hazard ratio (HR), Relative risk (RR) - Odds of an event. If the experimental group got 15% less cancer than the control group, the HR would be 0.85. Technically these are slightly different, HR being instantaneous and RR the average over the experiment.
- Confidence interval - A confidence interval, 95% for instance, will be stated with a pair of numbers representing the interval. It means that 95% of the results fell within the interval. Sometimes the interval is absurdly wide.
- Confounding factors - Other things that could affect the results. Heavy smokers are probably heavy drinkers. When they say "controlling for confounding factors," it means they took such things into account.

- Controlled for age - When comparing disease between two different groups, results may be skewed because one group is younger. Controlling for age adjusts this.
- Quintiles - Splitting a cohort into five groups based on some attribute, perhaps smoking. The lowest quintile would include the non-smokers and the highest quintile would cover the chain smokers. They would then likely compare something else in the quintiles, like lung cancer.
- Pre-prandial and post-prandial - Before and after a meal.
- Fasting glucose (or other circulating marker) - The level 12 hours after the most recent meal.

Here are a few more tips:

- If the cohort is small, say under a couple of hundred, the paper will probably not talk in statistical terms, though it might.
- Beware of papers that just talk about a single item without addressing side effects. These are numerous. Frequently the possible side effects will often be mentioned, but summarily dismissed. It is best to select papers that examine all-cause mortality, as this tends to catch all relevant side effects.
- Many researchers are not statisticians and may simply plug numbers into an available stat program. This can be hazardous.
- We are not mice. If a drug works on mice, it isn't necessarily going to work on us. Resveratrol would be a good example of this. If a trial drug doesn't even work on mice, it won't likely see the light of day.
- In vitro versus in vivo. This is cute talk for cultures in a petri dish versus a living animal. Again, just because something kills cancer in a lab cell-culture doesn't mean it would work in humans. It is a lot harder for a drug to get into a cell somewhere in our body than to get into a cell in a petri dish.
- Look for obvious conflicts of interest, such as employment by a pharmaceutical or packaged food company, or by funding by any of these.

- If there is a lot of money involved, look very hard indeed.
- If results are strong, you don't need 10,000 cases. If 24 of 25 people responded to some therapy, that is a strong result.
- If the benefit is more or less a toss-up, you will see studies involving tens of thousands. Conversely, if a study involves tens of thousands, expect a toss-up. Vitamins would be a good example of this.

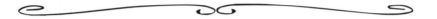

APPENDIX 2 - ANNOTATED BIBLIOGRAPHY

Most medical research listed below has to do with the effect of lifestyle on various degenerative diseases, so typically, some experiment will be described where a lifestyle element was varied and its effect on a degenerative disease measured.

On the Internet, you can find research supporting any view you like. This research below obviously supports our own point of view, but we also believe we have chosen research that was well done. Much of the research flew strongly in the face of conventional wisdom at the time of its publication, so the collection represents some studies in courage as well.

One pervasive theme throughout is the glacial pace at which the medical profession revises its thinking. A quicker reaction to the dangers of trans fat could have saved hundreds of thousands. When we look at the possible implications of the high-carb diet, the number affected is considerably greater.

In defense of policy makers, it must be noted that it is not easy to promulgate policy when there may be conflicting interests at stake, and any policy needs to be sufficiently simple to avoid erroneous interpretation.

All these papers were found somewhere on the Internet non-paywalled. If you are interested, the same appendix is repeated at QuantitativeMedicine. net, with live links to the various papers. Search for "bibliography."

NEJM=*New England Journal of Medicine,*

JAMA=*Journal of the American Medical Association,*

BMJ=*British Medical Journal.*

One or more papers are available on these topics . . .

CAUSES OF DISEASE - EXCESS GLUCOSE
  Glycation, Insulin, and Sugar
CAUSES OF DISEASE - CANCER
  Cancer Screening
  Prostate Cancer
  Cancer and Glucose Levels
  Cancer and High-Protein Diets
  Cancer Progression
  Cancer and Sun Exposure
  Cancer and HDL
  Cancer and Inflammation
CAUSES OF DISEASE - HEART DISEASE
  Heart Disease and Lifestyle
  Inflammation
  The Endothelium
  Heart Rate
  Predicting of Heart Attacks
  Lipoprotein(a)
CAUSES OF DISEASE - DEMENTIA
  Dementia and Lifestyle
CAUSES OF DISEASE - OSTEOPOROSIS
  Osteoporosis
CAUSES OF DISEASE - AGING
  Mitochondria

CAUSES OF DISEASE - ADULT ONSET DIABETES
  Insulin and Glucose
  Adult Onset Diabetes and Low-carb Diet
  Adult Onset Diabetes and Insulin
  Adult Onset Diabetes and Exercise
  Adult Onset Diabetes and Glycation
EFFECTS OF LIFESTYLE
  Cancer and Lifestyle
EATING
  Gluttony
  Low-carb Diets
  The Omega66 - Omega-3 Controversy
  Nuts
  Trans Fat
  Fructose
EXERCISE
  Interval Versus Aerobic Exercise
  Your Wate and Fate
SLEEP AND MEDITATION
EVERYTHING ELSE
  Hunter-Gatherer Health and Lifestyle
  Pathogens and the Immune System
  Stem Cells
  Statins

CAUSES OF DISEASE - EXCESS GLUCOSE

Glycation, Insulin, and Sugar

Glucose, especially in excess, has a tendency to "stick" to other molecules, which are then said to be glycated. This is usually deleterious. The more the glucose, the more the glycation. Glucose that sticks to (glycates) hemoglobin in red blood cells is measured in a standard blood test, as Hemoglobin A1C or simply A1C. This measure is used as a surrogate for average blood glucose level. If this is high, excess glycation is occurring somewhere. Glycation in the brain causes dementia. If in the arteries, atherosclerosis. Adult onset diabetics have elevated blood sugar, and hence are prone to the various problems of excess glycation. These problems include cancer, heart disease, and dementia. Thus glycation would appear to be a major bad actor in most degenerative disease.

The A1C measurement is in percent and indicates the portion of your hemoglobin that is sugar coated. The ideal number for A1C is 5% or less. Listing A1C as a percentage is confusing, and a change from say, 7% to 5% would be a huge improvement, but doesn't sound like much.

This paper rather clearly explains A1C and finds that adult onset diabetics with an A1C greater than 7% have 2½-fold increased all-cause mortality rate and an even higher risk of heart disease.

K. Khaw et al. "Glycated haemoglobin, diabetes, and mortality in men in Norfolk cohort of European Prospective Investigation of Cancer and Nutrition (EPIC-Norfolk)." BMJ VOLUME 322 6 JANUARY 2001

Glycation causes inflammation. The progression of Advanced Glycation End products (with AGE as its acronym) is discussed in this paper:

R. Ramasamy et al., "Advanced glycation end products and RAGE: a common thread in aging, diabetes, neurodegeneration, and inflammation," Glycobiology vol. 15 no. 7 pp. 16R–28R, 2005

Glycation is further reviewed here:

R. Singh, A. Barden, T. Mori, L. Beilin., "Advanced glycation end-products: a review," Diabetologia ⏹2001) 44: 129±146

Glycation is tied to cancer in this paper:

Louis J Sparvero et al., "RAGE (Receptor for Advanced Glycation Endproducts), RAGE Ligands, and their role in Cancer and Inflammation," Journal of Translational Medicine 2009, 7:17

Here, glycation's role in dementia is discussed:

Enzo Emanuele et al., "Circulating Levels of Soluble Receptor for Advanced Glycation End Products in Alzheimer," Disease and Vascular Dementia." ARCH NEUROL / VOL 62, NOV 2005

CAUSES OF DISEASE - CANCER

Cancer Screening

Is early screening for colon cancer beneficial? Although something suspicious was found in over 20% of those screened, these doctors conclude that screening for colon cancer for those under 50 is not "cost effective." They have evidently already decided what we are worth.

T. Imperiale, D. Wagner, C. Lin, G. Larkin, J. Rogge, and D. Ransohoff, "Results Of Screening Colonoscopy Among Persons 40 To 49 Years Of Age," N Engl J Med, Vol. 346, No. 23 · June 6, 2002

This prompted a well-deserved scolding in a later issue:

J. Romagnuolo. "Correspondence: Screening Colonoscopy Among Persons 40 To 49 Years Of Age." N Engl J Med, Vol. 347, No. 15 · October 10, 2002

Here can be found the survival rate for early versus late detection of colon cancer:

J. O'Connell, M. Maggard, and C. Ko, "Colon Cancer Survival Rates With the New American Joint Committee on Cancer Sixth Edition Staging," Journal of the National Cancer Institute, Vol. 96, No. 19, October 6, 2004

Prostate Cancer

The progression of prostate cancer has been dramatically slowed by drinking pomegranate juice and taking other supplements. Here are three papers presenting results:

Allan J. Pantuck et al., "Phase II Study of Pomegranate Juice for Men with Rising Prostate-Specific Antigen following Surgery or Radiation for Prostate Cancer," Clin Cancer Res 2006;12(13) July 1, 2006

Pantuck et al., "Long Term Follow Up Of Phase 2 Study Of Pomegranate Juice For Men With Prostate Cancer Shows Durable Prolongation Of PSA Doubling Time," The Journal Of Urology Vol. 181, No. 4, Supplement, Monday, April 27, 2009

R Thomas et al., "A double-blind, placebo-controlled randomised trial evaluating the effect of a polyphenol-rich whole food supplement on PSA progression in men with prostate cancer—the UK NCRN Pomi-T study," Prostate Cancer and Prostatic Disease (2014), 1–7

This is an excellent paper comparing the outcomes of a variety of prostate cancer treatments:

P. Grimm et al., "Comparative analysis of prostate-specific antigen free survival outcomes for patients with low, intermediate and high risk prostate cancer treatment by radical therapy.," BJU INTERNATIONAL © 2012 BJU INTERNATIONAL | 109, SUPPLEMENT 1, 22–29

Cancer and Glucose Levels

Saydah et al. find that people who fail glucose testing have an 87% higher risk of cancer:

S. Saydah, C. Loria, M. Eberhardt, and F. Brancati, "Abnormal Glucose Tolerance and the Risk of Cancer Death in the United States," Am J Epidemiology 2003;157:1092–1100

This study finds a strong relationship between high sugar levels and certain cancers, particularly liver cancer:

K.Rapp et al., "Fasting blood glucose and cancer risk in a cohort of more than 140,000 adults in Austria," Diabetologia (2006) 49

This group finds a more than doubling of breast cancer risk for women with high blood glucose:

P. Muti, T. Quattrin, B. Grant, et al. "Fasting Glucose Is a Risk Factor For Breast Cancer: A Prospective Study," Cancer Epidemiol Biomarkers Prev 2002;11:1361-1368.

Near doubling of pancreatic risk in the presence of high glucose:

S. Jee et al, "Fasting Serum Glucose Level and Cancer Risk in Korean Men and Women," JAMA, January 12, 2005—Vol 293, No. 2

Here is an article from the *New York Times* about a doctor who was on the right track in 1887. Look how he was treated:

SUGAR AND CANCER.

The theories of Dr. Freund of Vienna concerning the cause of the cancer in the German Crown Prince's throat are generally discredited by New-York medical men. According to recent dispatches Dr. Freund's theory is that the blood of patients suffering from cancer contains an abnormal quantity of sugar, and that cancerous growths may be destroyed by a reduction of the amount of sugar.

Dr. George F. Shrady, editor of the *Medical Record*, was inclined to be conservative on this subject yesterday. He did not care to speak against a new theory just because it was new, for new theories had frequently developed into something practical. In this case, however, it was different. Dr. Freund, who is unknown as an authority, has advanced a theory wholly inconsistent with the results of years of scientific research. In the first place sugar is present normally 'in the blood in small quantities. Various diseased conditions of the system occasionally produce an excessive quantity of sugar in the blood, the direct cause of diabetes mellitus, which is most difficult to cure. There is no relation whatever between cancer and sugar in the blood as cause and effect, either active or retroactive. A patient may have diabetes and cancer both at the same time, and the treatment of one would have no effect upon the other. Dr. Shrady did not think that Dr. Mackenzie and the other eminent physicians associated with him would experiment upon the Crown Prince with a new theory. They have always been accustomed to using their own opinions, and independent of outside influence.

Specific lifestyle changes that affect cancer are broadly examined in this paper:

P. Anand et al., "Cancer is a Preventable Disease that Requires Major Lifestyle changes," Pharmaceutical Research, Vol. 25, No. 9, September 2008 (# 2008) DOI: 10.1007/s11095-008-9661-9

The Warburg effect, which is that cancers need sugar to thrive and have lost much of their mitochondrial function, is discussed here:

Jung-whan Kim1 and Chi V. Dang, "Cancer's Molecular Sweet Tooth and the Warburg Effect," Cancer Res 2006; 66: (18). September 15, 2006

More on the sugar connection and the Warburg Effect can be found here:

Patrick Quillin, "Cancer's Sweet Tooth," Nutrition Science News, April 2000

More on the Warburg effect and mitochondria:

M. Boland, A. Chourasia1, and K Macleod, "Mitochondrial Dysfunction in Cancer," Frontiers in Oncology, 02 December 2013

This paper describes the Warburg effect in breast cancer:

D Ciavardelli, "Breast cancer stem cells rely on fermentative glycolysis and are sensitive to 2-deoxyglucose treatment," Cell Death and Disease (2014) 5, e1336

Alcohol greatly increases the risk of esophageal cancer; even a single drink a day raises the risk 33%:

Paolo Boffetta, Mia Hashibe, "Alcohol and cancer," Lancet Oncol 2006; 7: 149–56

Cancer and High-Protein Diets

Despite a steady and shrill stream of warnings from the vegan crowd that high protein kills, we have this:

Victor W. Ho et al., "A Low Carbohydrate, High Protein Diet Slows Tumor Growth and Prevents Cancer Initiation," Cancer Res; 71(13) July 1, 2011

Cancer Progression

Michor et al. go through the various steps of cancer progression:

F. Michor, Y. Iwasa, And M. Nowak, "Dynamics Of Cancer Progression," Nature Reviews | Cancer, Volume 4, 2004

Cancer and Sun Exposure

It is commonly believed that exposure to the sun is associated with malignant melanoma, but this only appears to be the case if there are repeated instances of sunburn. Magnus examines this and finds more malignant melanoma in parts of the body which have the least exposure toward skin.

Knut Magnus, "Habits of Sun Exposure and Risk of Malignant Melanoma," Cancer 48:2329-2335, 1981.

Cancer and HDL

This key paper identifies the amazing protective effect of increased HDL. A 10 mg/dl increase in HDL was associated with a 36% reduction in cancer, a very powerful result:

H. Jafri et al., "Baseline and On-Treatment High-Density Lipoprotein Cholesterol and the Risk of Cancer in Randomized Controlled Trials of Lipid-Altering Therapy," Journal of the American College of Cardiology, Vol. 55, No. 25, 2010

Another paper on HDL's tumor-fighting properties:

Feng Su et al., "HDL Mimetics Inhibit Tumor Development in Both Induced and Spontaneous Mouse Models of Colon Cancer," Mol Cancer Ther; 11(6) June 2012

Cancer and Inflammation

This paper examines the relationship between cancer and inflammation, particularly the specific mechanisms involved:

Seth Rakoff-Nahoum, "Why Cancer and Inflammation?" Yale Journal Of Biology And Medicine 79 (2006), pp.123-130.

CAUSES OF DISEASE - HEART DISEASE

Heart Disease and Lifestyle

Tuzcu et al. examined hearts from relatively young people and found a surprising amount of heart disease. Perhaps atherosclerosis should be considered a childhood disease:

E. Murat Tuzcu et al, "High Prevalence of Coronary Atherosclerosis in Asymptomatic Teenagers and Young Adults," Circulation June 5, 2001

A macrophage is a large white cell that "eats" bad stuff. These are handy to have around. How do they know what to eat? They have receptors on their surface that detect various debris. The macrophages described below have receptors that look for damaged LDL (oxidized, glycated, etc.) The paper is a bit technical, but includes a description of the various receptors in the cell's receptor kit: bad LDL, staph bacteria, hepatitis, pneumonia, and so on. There seems no end to the body's gadget collection

David R. Greaves1 and Siamon Gordon, "The macrophage scavenger receptor at 30 years of age: current knowledge and future challenges," Journal of Lipid Research April Supplement, 2009

Inflammation

In 2002, inflammation was beginning to appear on the scene as the new bad guy:

Peter Libby, Paul M. Ridker, Attilio Maseri, "Inflammation and Atherosclerosis," Circulation. 2002;105:1135-1143.

One of HDL's tricks in inflammation reduction:

Marcus D. Saemann et al., "The versatility of HDL: a crucial anti-inflammatory Regulator," European Journal of Clinical Investigation Vol 40.

The Endothelium

For decades, the endothelium was thought to be merely a blood vessel lining and of little importance. It is now viewed as essential to arterial health. Here is a good survey paper from 2005:

Lerman and Zeiher, "Endothelial Function Cardiac Events," Circulation. 2005;111;363-368.

One important endothelial function is nitric oxide synthesis. Low nitric oxide is a cause of high blood pressure.

Forstermann and Sessa, "Nitric oxide synthases: regulation and function," European Heart Journal (2012) 33, 829–837

"You are only as old as your arteries" is respun here in medicalese:

Zoltan Ungvari et al., "Mechanisms of Vascular Aging: New Perspectives," J Gerontol A Biol Sci Med Sci. 2010 October;65A(10):1028–1041

Most atherosclerosis forms in places where the endothelium is frequently replaced. Here, a researcher determines that LDL (and everything else) leaks through during replacement, and replacement happens frequently in areas of low or no blood flow.,

L. Cancel and J. Tarbell, "The role of mitosis in LDL transport through cultured endothelial cell monolayers," Am J Physiol Heart Circ Physiol 300: H769–H776, 2011

HDL, on the other hand, is welcome behind the artery wall, and the endothelial cells will escort it right through. This paper reviews this amazing process:

R. Frank, "Caveolae and transcytosis in endothelial cells: role in atherosclerosis," Cell Tissue Res (2009) 335:41–47 DOI 10.1007/s00441-008-0659-8

Heart Rate

Resting heart rate, maximum heart rate during exercise, and heart rate recovery after peak exercise all provide substantial information about heart attack risk. (Again, don't attempt extreme exercise without your doctor's blessing.) Resting heart rate should be taken before you get out of bed in the morning. There is considerably more detail in the paper, but here is a quick summary. Those with a resting heart rate over 75 bpm (beats per minute) had a fourfold higher risk than those 60 or less. For peak heart rate, those whose peak was less than 90 bpm higher than their resting heart rate also had a four-fold higher risk than those whose peak rate exceeded their resting rate by more than 113. Finally, for recovery after peak exercise, those whose heart rate dropped more than 25 bpm one minute after peak exercise had more then a twofold risk increase over those whose rate declined by more than 40. If you have a watch that will monitor heart rate, you can track your progress.

X. Jouven et al., "Heart-Rate Profile during Exercise as a Predictor of Sudden Death," NEJM 352;19 May 12, 2005

Predicting Heart Attacks

Coronary calcium directly measures plaque load. One would think a "direct view" of the problem would be a no-brainer, yet this test remains an outlier. Insurance won't pay for it and so on. This paper is a bit obfuscated by statistical analysis, but, in fact, the rate of heart attacks between the highest to lowest heart calcium groups was a whopping 20:1. Are you at risk? Forget cholesterol—get a heart scan. This paper is 10 years old, yet a heart scan is still not a standard procedure for determining cardiac risk. (An interesting aside: statins have no effect on heart calcium.)

Michael J. LaMonte et al., "Coronary Artery Calcium Score and Coronary Heart Disease Events in a Large Cohort of Asymptomatic Men and Women," Am J Epidemiol 2005;162:421–429

On the other hand, here we have a paper trying to predict heart attacks from cholesterol, triglycerides, and the other typical measurements. Instead of getting results like 20 times more likely, we get results for high LDL or high triglycerides of 0.3 times more likely. This is a weak predictor at best. Yet this is the standard procedure for determining heart risk. Go figure.

A.R. Sharrett et al., "Coronary Heart Disease Prediction From Lipoprotein Cholesterol Levels, Triglycerides, Lipoprotein(a), Apolipoproteins A-I and B, and HDL Density Subfractions: The Atherosclerosis Risk in Communities (ARIC) Study," Circulation. 2001;104:1108-1113

CAUSES OF DISEASE - DEMENTIA

Dementia and Lifestyle

Here cortisol level is shown to have an adverse effect on the hippocampus.

S. Lupien et al., "Cortisol levels during human aging predict hippocampal atrophy and memory deficits," Nature Neuroscience volume 1 no. 1 may 1998

This paper is a survey of factors affecting Alzheimer's. It discusses low cholesterol and low fat intake as possible contributing causes:

Barry Groves, "Alzheimer's and Parkinson's Diseases," Second Opinions, 1 Aug 2008

A ketogenic diet (little or no carbs) has shown some effectiveness against Alzheimer's:

Robert Krikorian et al., "Dietary ketosis enhances memory in mild cognitive impairment," Neurobiol Aging. 2012 February

The following review article discusses the causes of Alzheimer's. He notes that exercise and "cognitive stimulation" may reduce the risk:

Mark P. Mattson. "Pathways towards and away from Alzheimer's disease," Nature vol 430 |5 AUG 2004

Alzheimer's is significantly reduced by a mediterranean Diet and by exercise:

Nikolaos Scarmeas et al., "Physical Activity, Diet, and Risk of Alzheimer Disease," JAMA, August 12, 2009—Vol 302, No. 6

The ketogenic diet is again examined here. The author posits, "While the mechanisms through which the ketogenic diet works remain unclear, there is now compelling evidence that its efficacy is likely related to the normalization of aberrant energy metabolism." Let's hear it for "normalization of aberrant energy metabolism," the most oblique reference to "eating right" on record.

Carl E. Stafstrom and Jong M. Rho, "The ketogenic diet as a treatment paradigm for diverse neurological disorders," Frontiers in Pharmacology | Neuropharmacology,April 2012 | Volume 3 | Article 59 | 2

The higher the total cholesterol, the better the cognition, in this paper from 2005. This is, by the way, the same cholesterol the medical profession has spent the last two decades trying to lower at all costs. Since statins lower cholesterol, the interesting experiment would be the effect of statins on cognition. Any volunteers?

Penelope k. Elias et al, "Serum Cholesterol and Cognitive Performance in the Framingham Heart Study," Psychosomatic Medicine 67:24–30 2005

In this review article, the author suggests that Alzheimer's should be called type 3 diabetes, as sugar/insulin is way out of regulation:

Suzanne M. de la Monte and Jack R. Wands, "Alzheimer's Disease Is Type 3 Diabetes—Evidence Reviewed," Journal of Diabetes Science and Technology IEW ARTICLE Volume 2, Issue 6, November 2008

These researchers also see Alzheimer's as a metabolic disorder:

Sergio T. Ferreira et al., "Inflammation, defective insulin signaling, and neuronal dysfunction in Alzheimer's disease," Alzheimer's & Dementia 10 (2014) S76–S83

McNay is also supporting the metabolic syndrome hypothesis of Alzheimer's:

Ewan McNay, "Your Brain on Insulin: From Heresy to Dogma," Perspectives on Psychological Science 2014, Vol 9(1) 88–90

More research indicating glucose and insulin are at the root of the Alzheimer's epidemic:

Enrique Blázquez et al., "Insulin in the brain: its pathophysiological implications for states related with central insulin resistance, type 2 diabetes and Alzheimer's disease," Frontiers of Endocrinology, October 2014 | Volume 5 | Article 161 | 1

Lipoprotein(a)

Also known as Lp(a), this variant form of the LDL lipoprotein particle significantly increases the risk of heart disease and clotting. The variation consists of the attachment of a protein string called apo(a). Lp(a)'s evolutionary benefit is unknown, but it may confer some resistance to cancer and adult onset diabetes. This review paper is an excellent overview. A molecular biology section that is a bit difficult follows the introduction. Then follows a very interesting review of known benefits and treatments.

JWu, "Lipoprotein(a) in Vascular Disease, Cancer and Longevity," Chang Gung Med J Vol. 34 No. 6 November-December 2011

Anti-sense therapy is proposed for high Lp(a). In this therapy, a molecule is introduced that binds to the specific RNA that initiates the Lp(a) apo(a) string. However, such drugs often bind to similar molecules and end up showing no benefit or even harm. Here are two recent papers:

F. Stroes and F. van der Valk, "A sense of excitement for a specific Lp(a)-lowering therapy," www.thelancet.com Vol386 October10,2015

S. Tsimikas, "Antisense therapy targeting apolipoprotein(a): a randomised, double-blind, placebo-controlled phase 1 study," www.thelancet.com Vol386 October10,201

Details of the attached apo(a) protein string are discussed here. The string comes in various lengths (isoforms), and the longer ones are significantly less harmful.

Erqou et al., "Apolipoprotein(a) Isoforms and the Risk of Vascular Disease," JACC Vol. 55, No. 19, 2010 May 11, 2010:2160–7

L. Stefania et al., "Lipoprotein(a) levels, apo(a) isoform size, and coronary heart disease risk in the Framingham Offspring Study," J Lipid Res. 2011 Jun; 52(6): 1181–1187. PMCID: PMC3090239 doi: 10.1194/jlr.M012526

CAUSES OF DISEASE - ADULT ONSET DIABETES

Insulin and Glucose

This paper is a transcript of a talk given in 1999. Though not at all kind to the medical establishment, it has a very broad range, and establishes the crucial importance of managing insulin:

Rosedale, Ron, "Insulin and Its Metabolic Effects," Presented at Designs for Health Institute's BoulderFest, August 1999 Seminar

Insulin resistance is a hallmark of type 2 (adult onset) diabetes. It is a syndrome wherein insulin is unable to clear blood glucose effectively. (The body becomes "resistant.") One interpretation is that the various cells already have all the glucose that they want. This paper describes insulin resistance at the cellular level in some detail:

S. Schenk, M. Saberi, and J. Olefsky, "Insulin sensitivity: modulation by nutrients and inflammation," J. Clin. Invest. 118:2992–3002 2008

This paper ties insulin resistance to inflammation:

Jerrold M. Olefsky and Christopher K. Glass, "Macrophages, Inflammation, and Insulin Resistance," Annu. Rev. Physiol. 2010. 72:219–46

Is whole grain better for you? This paper looks at glucose and insulin after consumption of either whole or refined grain and finds no difference:

Katri S Juntunen et al., "Postprandial glucose, insulin, and incretin responses to grain products in healthy subjects," Am J Clin Nutr 2002;75:254–62

Here is an important paper wherein adult onset diabetics were treated with insulin, rather than the standard, metformin. The insulin caused a significant increase of various cancers. Three conclusions here: 1) Thousands were treated with insulin. Where were the vaunted safety measures? This protocol went very wrong. 2) There is no logic here. If there is no demand for the excess glucose, the solution is to reduce the supply, not "force" an increased demand. 3) High insulin causes cancer.

C. J. Currie, C. D. Poole, and E. A. M. Gale, "The influence of glucose-lowering therapies on cancer risk in type 2 diabetes," Diabetologia (2009) 52:1766–1777 DOI 10.1007/s00125-009-1440-6

Adult Onset Diabetes and Low-carb Diet

A cohort of 28 diabetics undertook a low-carb diet, with very impressive results. Seven were able to stop taking their meds.

William S Yancy Jr. et al., "A Low-carbohydrate, Ketogenic Diet To Treat Type 2 Diabetes," Nutrition & Metabolism 2005, 2:34

Adult Onset Diabetes and Insulin

Insulin use in type 2 diabetics is associated with significant increase in cancer risk. It's double the risk in this paper.

Samantha I. Bowker et al., "Increased Cancer-Related Mortality for Patients With Type 2 Diabetes Who Use Sulfonylureas or Insulin," Diabetes Care, Volume 29, Number 2, February 2006

Adult Onset Diabetes and Exercise

Interval training was associated with significant glucose improvement in a group of adult onset diabetics.

Jonathan P. Little et al., "Low-volume high-intensity interval training reduces hyperglycemia and increases muscle mitochondrial capacity in patients with type 2 diabetes," J Appl Physiol 111: 1554–1560, 2011.

Adult Onset Diabetes and Glycation

Glycation is the attachment of a sugar molecule to some other molecule. The can be quite detrimental and is a factor in Alzheimer's, atherosclerosis, and other diseases. Here glycated hemoglobin is identified in diabetes.

Kay-Tee Khaw et al.m "Glycated haemoglobin, diabetes, and mortality in men in Norfolk cohort of European Prospective Investigation of Cancer and Nutrition (EPIC-Norfolk)," BMJ Volume 322 6 January 2001

CAUSES OF DISEASE - OSTEOPOROSIS

Osteoporosis

This is an important paper. Those calcium supplements, which are almost universally recommended to treat osteoporosis, appear to increase the occurrence of heart attacks 25%, while having little effect on osteoporosis.

Mark J Bolland, "Calcium supplements with or without vitamin D and risk of cardiovascular events: reanalysis of the Women's Health Initiative limited access dataset and meta-analysis," BMJ 2011;342:d2040

Here is a paper showing the mild effect on bone from calcium/ vitamin D supplementation. Basically calcium/vitamin D can only slow things down a bit.

B. Dawson-Hughes et al., "Effect Of Calcium And Vitamin D Supplementation On Bone Density In Men And Women 65 Years Of Age Or Older," NEJM, September 4, 1997

And here is the cure. Note the date. The benefit of resistance exercise on osteoporosis is not a new story, yet it still is not mainstream medicine.

Vincent, K. R., and R. W. Braith, "Resistance Exercise And Bone Turnover In Elderly Men And Women," Med. Sci. Sports Exerc.,Vol. 34, No. 1, 2002, pp. 17–23.

CAUSES OF DISEASE - AGING

Free radicals were the new bad boy 15 years ago, launching an antioxidant industry featuring all sorts of supplements designed to gobble them up. Things are a bit more settled now. Like everything else, free radicals have a purpose and are regulated. This paper broadly reviews research on the free radical theory of aging. Nothing definite can be concluded.

Kenneth B. Beckman And Bruce N. Ames, "The Free Radical Theory of Aging Matures," Physiological Reviews Vol. 78, No. 2, April 1998.

Mitochondria

The mitochondrial theory of aging holds that mitochondrial DNA, which indeed hasn't the precision of repair and maintenance of our regular cellular DNA, degrades with time, causing the mitochondria to perform less efficiently, thus contributing to accelerated aging and degenerative disease. This is somewhat controversial, though it undoubtedly is a significant factor, perhaps the most significant factor. This entire book is available online, is very well written, and gives a great overview.

Aubrey D.N.J. de Grey, "The Mitochondrial Free Radical Theory of Aging," 1999 R.G. Landes Company (ENTIRE BOOK)

Numerous aspects of the mitochondria theory have been examined since de Grey's publication. Some have survived and others have not. The following paper gives a good overview of this 14 years later.

Gustavo Barja, "Updating the Mitochondrial Free Radical Theory of Aging: An Integrated View, Key Aspects, and Confounding Concepts," Antioxidants & Redox Signaling. October 20, 2013, 19(12): 1420-1445

The cause of insulin resistance is somewhat controversial. It is known that the muscles either won't or can't take up the glucose. This paper argues that excess fat in the cell interferes with insulin signaling and that is the cause. This could be interpreted as "the cell is full and doesn't want any more stuff."

Timothy R. Koves et al., "Mitochondrial Overload and Incomplete Fatty Acid Oxidation Contribute to Skeletal Muscle Insulin Resistance," Cell Metabolism 7, 45–56, January 2008

EFFECTS OF LIFESTYLE

Cancer and Lifestyle

The number of people in this study was a bit small, but the results were quite stunning. Around 200 people with high blood pressure (around 140 mm Hg) either meditated or received "standard" health instruction. They were followed for some years. The meditators had a 23% decrease in all-cause mortality, a 30% decrease in mortality from heart disease, and a huge 50% decrease in cancer mortality.

R. Schneider, et al., "Long-Term Effects of Stress Reduction on Mortality in Persons ≥55 Years of Age With Systemic Hypertension," Am J Cardiol. 2005 May 1

This paper represents the other side of the coin: depression, which could likely be alleviated by meditation. Chronic depression increased cancer risk 88%.

Brenda W. J. H. Penninx, et al., "Chronically Depressed Mood and Cancer Risk in Older Persons," Journal of the National Cancer Institute, Vol. 90, No. 24, December 16, 1998

These papers examines the incidence of cancer in night and shift workers. Megdal et al. find a 50% increase in breast cancer.

P. Bhatti, D. Mirick, S. Davis, "Invited Commentary: Shift Work and Cancer.," Am J Epidemiol. 2012;

S. Megdal et al., "Night work and breast cancer risk: A systematic review and meta-analysis," European Journal of Cancer 41 (2005)

Cancer incidence in the Nurses' Health Study is computed for many lifestyle choices, including smoking, drinking, and nut consumption.

H. Baer et al., "Risk Factors for Mortality in the Nurses' Health Study: A Competing Risks Analysis," Am J Epidemiology 2011

EATING

Gluttony

In an experiment likely to never be repeated, we have two charmingly titled papers wherein subjects consumed enormous amounts of fat, some as much as 6,000 calories/day. To the astonishment of the researchers, they essentially did not gain weight. There were hot and sweaty all the time. If you want proof positive that fat doesn't make you fat, here it is.

D. Miller and P. Mumford, "Gluttony 1. An Experimental Study of Overeating Low or High Protein Diets," The American Journal of Clinical Nutrition, Vol. 20, No. 11, November 1967.

D. Miller and P. Mumford, "Gluttony 2. Thermogenesis in Overeating Man," The American Journal of Clinical Nutrition, Vol. 20, No. 11, November 1967.

Another "gluttony" experiment. These people either took excess olive oil (they gained some weight) or corn oil (they lost weight).

H Kasper, H Thiel, M Ehl, "Response of body weight to a low carbohydrate, high-fat diet in normal and obese subjects," The American journal of clinical Nutririon, 1973 - Am Soc Nutrition

Low-carb Diets

Here's a marvelous paper from Stanford where a group was given a very high-fat diet for several weeks, then a high-carbohydrate diet for several more. As we would expect in light of today's knowledge, cholesterol and triglycerides were stable on the high-fat diet, but soared on the high-carb one. What's remarkable is the date of the study—1966—after which followed 50 years of high-carb, low-fat diet recommendations, with endless wonderment all the while as to why everyone was getting so fat.

J. Farquhar, A. Frank, R. Gross, and G. Reaven, "Glucose, Insulin, and Triglyceride Responses to High and Low Carbohydrate Diets in Man," Journal of Clinical Investigation Vol. 45, No. 10, 1966

The following papers discuss low-carb diets, such as the Atkins Diet. Invariably, LDL, HDL, and triglycerides show marked improvement.

Richard J. Wood et al., "Carbohydrate Restriction Alters Lipoprotein Metabolism by Modifying VLDL, LDL, and HDL Subfraction Distribution and Size in Overweight Men," J. Nutr. February 2006 vol. 136 no. 2 384-389

This review article examines the very strong association of high carbohydrate consumption and high triglycerides. Its conclusion is that "the American public has increased its consumption of carbohydrate, either through the consumption of more food per day or through replacement of fats with carbohydrates. At the same time, the incidence of obesity in this country is rising. Whether these 2 trends are linked is unknown." Aren't we ignoring an elephant in the room here?

Elizabeth J Parks and Marc K Hellerstein, "Carbohydrate-Induced Hypertriacylglycerolemia: Historical Perspective And Review Of Biological Mechanisms," Am J Clin Nutr February 2000 vol. 71 no. 2 412-433

Here is a paper astonishing for its prescience in 2004. Specifically we have this: "In postmenopausal women with relatively low total fat intake, a greater saturated fat intake is associated with less progression of coronary atherosclerosis, whereas carbohydrate intake is associated with a greater progression." Translation: "saturated fat good—carbs bad." Ten years later, the medical world has grasped about half of this: carbs are bad. Saturated fat is still in nutritional limbo.

D. Mozaffarian, E. Rimm, and D. Herrington, "Dietary fats, carbohydrate, and progression of coronary atherosclerosis in postmenopausal women," Am J Clin Nutr 2004;80:1175–84

A survey paper summarizing the huge shift in attitude concerning saturated fat.

Arne Astrup, "A Changing View On SFAs and Dairy: From Enemy To Friend," Am J Clin Nutr doi: 10.3945/ajcn.114.099986.

Yet another paper indicating that high-carb diets cause heart disease. This one dates from 1997.

Jeppesen J et al., "Effects of low-fat, high-carbohydrate diets on risk factors for ischemic heart disease in postmenopausal women," Am J Clin Nutr. 1997 Apr;65(4):1027-33.

This huge meta-analysis concludes there is no association of saturated fat with heart disease. These were highest to lowest quintile comparisons, which would mean that one group that consumed a lot of saturated fat was compared to another that consumed very little. Saturated fat was mildly protective for heart attack, and neutral for strokes and atherosclerosis.

P. Siri-Tarino, Q. Sun, F. Hu, and R. Krauss, "Meta-analysis of prospective cohort studies evaluating the association of saturated fat with cardiovascular disease," Am J Clin Nutr 2010;91:535–46.

The Mediterranean diet shows a 30% reduction in heart disease.

Ramón Estruch et al., "Primary Prevention of Cardiovascular Disease with a Mediterranean Diet," n engl j med 368;14

The Omega-6 - Omega-3 Controversy

There is abundant popular literature suggesting that we reduce omega-6 oils or maintain some ration of omega-6 to omega-3. This paper dives into that controversy and finds that omega-6 oil is beneficial, particularly for reduction of heart disease risk, and further that excess omega-6 is not harmful and may have additional benefit.

William S. Harris et al., "Omega-6 Fatty Acids and Risk for Cardiovascular Disease," Circulation. 2009;119:902-907.

Nuts

Here heart disease is reduced around 30% for people who eat nuts five times a week or more. Ischemic heart disease is cut in half and all-cause mortality is also reduced around 30%.

Joan Sabaté, "Nut consumption, vegetarian diets, ischemic heart disease risk, and all-cause mortality: evidence from epidemiologic studies," Am J Clin Nutr 1999;70(suppl):500S–3S

Also see this one for nuts versus cancer.

H. Baer, et al., "Risk Factors for Mortality in the Nurses' Health Study: A Competing Risks Analysis," Am. J. Epidemiol. (2011) 173 (3): 319-329.

Trans fat

By the mid-'90s, trans fat had been nailed as a really bad actor. Ascherio and Willett conclude that it caused 30,000 premature deaths annually in the United States alone. Sixteen years later, the FDA decided to start looking at it, and is currently (2016) considering measures to further reduce it. If you are wondering why there wasn't an outright ban two decades ago, you are not alone.

A Ascherio, WC Willett, "Health effects of trans fatty acids," Am J Clin Nutr October 1997vol. 66 no. 4 1006S-1010S

Fructose

We do not appear to be well adapted to deal with the unnaturally large amounts of fructose present in the Western diet. The effects are summarized in this short editorial. Apparently curtailing fructose in processed food has a deleterious effect on profits, as there is significant industry pushback. Will the FDA ban added fructose anytime soon? Perhaps they should be encouraged to require the industry to prove s high-fructose corn syrup is good for you before they allow its use—as they do with drugs.

George A Bray. "How bad is fructose?" Am J Clin Nutr 2007;86:895–6.

EXERCISE

Interval Versus Aerobic Exercise

This is about as close as you can come to a free lunch or magic pill. Here one group cycled at 65% maximum heart rate for 4 ½ hours per week, and another group did high-intensity exercise for 10 minutes per week. That's 10 minutes spent doing the actual exercises, which typically involve a 30-second all-out effort and a 30-second rest. So the actual time involved may be 20 minutes. In spite of spending less than a tenth of the time as the bikers, the interval people had significantly greater improvement in VO_2Max and also in a measure of mitochondrial function.

M. Gibala, J. Little, M. MacDonald and J. Hawley, "Physiological adaptations to low-volume, high-intensity interval training in health and disease," Physiol 590.5 (2012) pp 1077–1084

Here the same experiment was done, except this time both groups had heart issues. Again, the interval group did better.

Darren E.R. Warburton et al., "Effectiveness of High-Intensity Interval Training for the Rehabilitation of Patients With Coronary Artery Disease," The American Journal of Cardiology Vol. 95 May 1, 2005

Finally, here is a broad review of results of interval training. There seems to be no downside to interval training.

Paul B. Laursen and David G. Jenkins, "The Scientific Basis for High-Intensity Interval Training," Sports Med 2002; 32 (1)

Your Wate and Fate

Here's one of the articles that identifies the healthiest body mass index as "overweight."

K. Flegal, B. Kit, H. Orpana, B. Graubard, "Association of All-Cause Mortality With Overweight and Obesity Using Standard Body Mass Index Categories: A Systematic Review and Meta-analysis," JAMA. 2013;309(1):71-82.

Here's the paper about the 450-pound Scotsman who fasted for over a year.

A Ascherio, WC Willett, "Health effects of trans fatty acids," ;2DW. K. Stewart, Laura W. Fleming, "Features of a successful therapeutic fast of 382 days' duration," Postgrad Med J 1973;49:203-209

How would you measure jollity? Find out here.

A H Crisp and B McGuiness, "Jolly fat: relation between obesity and psychoneurosis in general population," Br Med J. Jan 3, 1976; 1(6000): 7–9.

SLEEP AND MEDITATION

There is little research on meditation, but in all cases where it was measured, meditation caused a significant reduction in cortisol. As cortisol is a launch pad for both cancer and adult onset diabetes, keeping it under control merits attention.

There is far more research on sleep. Poor sleep patterns are so strongly associated with cancer that it could be said to be causative. Shift work and irregular sleep derail the melatonin cycle, which sets off a whole series of subsequent problems.

Sleep and low stress are far more important than generally recognized. This 50-year-old article established that Human Growth Hormone only comes out at night, effectively being zero during the day. This hormone triggers a number of renew and repair hormones, including IGF-1:

Y. Takahashi, et al., "Growth Hormone Secretion during Sleep," The Journal of Clinical Investigation Volume 47 1968

Young and Taylor argue that meditation has survival roots, and was a form of hibernation.

John Ding-E Young and Eugene Taylor, "Meditation as a Voluntary Hypometabolic State of Biological Estivation," News Physiol. Sci. Volume 13 June 1998

A course of transcendental meditation lowers cortisol.

Christopher R. K. et al., "Effects Of The Transcendental Meditation Program On Adaptive Mechanisms: Changes In Hormone Levels And Responses To Stress After 4 Months Of Practice," Psychoneuroendocrinology, Vol. 22, No. 4, pp. 277-295, 1997

In this meta-analysis, night work, primarily airline work, led to a 50% higher risk of breast cancer.

Sarah P. Megdal et al., "Night work and breast cancer risk: A systematic review and meta-analysis," European Journal of Cancer 41 (2005) 2023–2032

This paper tends to close the loop on the preceding one. Melatonin is substantially disrupted if sleep is disturbed. Here it is shown to have direct breast-cancer-fighting properties.

E. J. Sánchez-Barceló et al., "Melatonin: An Endogenous Antiestrogen with Oncostatic Properties," Melatonin: From Molecules to Therapy- Chapter XV

These researchers find that poor sleep patterns in the elderly are strongly associated with all-cause mortality. Of course, terminal diseases are likely to cause poor sleep. These researchers studied healthy people and found that poor sleep doubled the risk of death.

Mary Amanda Dew et al., "Healthy Older Adults' Sleep Predicts All-Cause Mortality at 4 to 19 Years of Follow-Up," Psychosomatic Medicine 65:63–73 (2003) (ABSTRACT ONLY)

Kreuger and Friedman did a large meta-analysis and concluded that the average amount of sleep in the U.S. is between seven and eight hours, and that those sleeping seven hours had the lowest mortality.

Patrick M. Krueger and Elliot M. Friedman, "Sleep Duration in the United States: A Cross-sectional Population-based Study," 1052 Am J Epidemiol 2009;169:1052–1063

These researchers found essentially the same result.

Kripke er al., "Mortality Associated With Sleep Duration and Insomnia," Arch Gen Psychiatriatry Vol 50, Feb 2002

EVERYTHING ELSE

Hunter-Gatherer Health and Lifestyle

This article, dating from 1937, identifies cancer among various societies. It does not indicate the cause for the cancer.

C. Bonne, "Cancer and Human Races," Am J Cancer 1937;30:435-454.

Gurven and Kaplan study mortality patterns of 14 different hunter-gatherer tribes—very thorough and analytical. They develop expected longevity given current age and have various other analyses. Pertinent to our endeavor are causes of death. For the elderly, degenerative disease appears to cause it 20% to 25% of the time.

M. Gurven and H. Kaplan, "Longevity Among Hunter-Gatherers: A Cross-Cultural Examination," Population and Development Review 33(2): 321–365 (June 2007)

Milton offers interesting comments on the diversity of hunter-gatherer diets.

Katharine Milton, "Hunter-gatherer diets—a different perspective," Am J Clin Nutr 2000;71:665–7.

Here's a cure to degenerative disease that appears to work. O'Dea follows 10 middle-aged Australian aboriginal hunter-gatherers who returned to the bush after attempting to acclimate to city life, noting: "In conclusion, the major metabolic abnormalities of type 2 diabetes were either greatly improved or completely normalized in this group of Aborigines by relatively short reversal of the urbanization process." Blood test measurements were done before the reintroduction and seven weeks later. The group's sugar numbers improved dramatically in these seven weeks.

Kerin O'Dea, "Marked Improvement in Carbohydrate and Lipid Metabolism in Diabetic Australian Aborigines After Temporary Reversion to Traditional Lifestyle," Diabetes, vol. 33, June 1984

Weston Price was a dentist as well as a university anthropologist who traveled worldwide in the 1920s and 1930s examining the health of various isolated people, particularly their dental health. This is reinforced with numerous dental photos. There is detailed information on diet. Weston-Price attributes the near absence of dental problems among isolated people and hunter-gatherers to their traditional diet.

Weston A. Price, "Nutrition and Physical Degeneration: A Comparison of Primitive and Modern Diets and Their Effects," Harper & Brothers New York London, 1939 (ENTIRE BOOK)

A variety of health observations of various hunter-gatherers can be found here.

Zac Goldsmith, "Cancer: A Disease of Industrialization," Pharmaceutical Research, Vol. 25, No. 9, September 2008

The wide variety of Paleolithic fare is quite thoroughly described.

S. Eaton, M. Konner, "Paleolithic Nutrition: A consideration of it Nature and Current Implications," NEJM, Jan 31, 1985

The authors of the previous paper re-examine the Discordance Hypothesis. Oddly, they rehash paleo dietary items in the context of conventional wisdom (saturated fat and cholesterol are bad), almost as though setting out to "prove" this by hunter-gatherer behavior. They then conclude that hunter-gatherers ate little saturated fat, but a lot of cholesterol, and then conclude that the lesser amount of saturated fat counteracts the excess cholesterol. Quite a lot of logical gymnastics to go through to protect the party line. Then they start in on salt.

Melvin Konner, and S. Boyd Eaton, "Paleolithic Nutrition Twenty-Five Years Later," Nutrition in Clinical Practice Vol. 25, No. 6, December 2010

Again the same authors with a general discussion of degenerative disease.

S. Eaton, M. Konner, M. Shostak, "Stone agers in the fast lane: chronic degenerative diseases in evolutionary perspective," The American Journal of Medicine Volume 84, 1988

These people conclude that hunter-gatherer societies will eat meat when they can and 73% get over half their energy from meat.

L. Cordain, J. Miller, S., N. Mann, S. Holt, and J. Speth, "Plant-animal subsistence ratios and macronutrient energy estimations in worldwide hunter-gatherer diets," Am J Clin Nutr 2000;71:682–92

These hunter-gatherers in India appear to frequently live to 100, and easily outlive the people in the surrounding areas.

R.K. Anuradha et al., "Cultural and Nutritional Perspective of Indian Hunter-Gatherers (Kurichia Tribe)," American Medical Journal 3 (1): 1-7, 2012

Here, a 1974 paper concluding that beyond a certain age, hunter-gatherers outlive others.

Alexander R. P. Walker, "Survival rate at middle age in developing and Western populations," Postgraduate Medical Journal (January 1974) 50, 29-32.

An excellent book on hunter-gatherer lifestyles would be:

McMichael, AJ, "Human Frontiers, Environments and Disease: Past Patterns, Uncertain Futures," 250–282 (Cambridge Univ. Press, Cambridge, 2001) (BOOK-VARIOUS PARTS AVAILABLE ONLINE)

Pathogens and the Immune System

Here is a fascinating paper describing the various tricks bacteria and viruses use to fool the immune system.

Leigh A. Knodler, Jean Celli And B. Brett Finlay, "Pathogenic Trickery: Deception Of Host Cell Processes," Nature Reviews | Molecular Cell Biology Volume 2 | August 2001

Stem Cells

Here is a very readable paper on intestinal stem cells.

Barker, Wetering, and Clevers, "The intestinal stem cell," Genes & Development 22:1856–1864 2008

More on stem cells.

Petersen and Polyak, "Stem Cells in the Human Breast," Cold Spring Harbor Perspect Biol 2010;2:a003160

Statins

The title of this paper says it all. ENHANCE was a trial that tested statins used alone or in combination with another drug, ezetimibe, which also lowered cholesterol. The trial was a flop. People taking both the drugs got worse even though their cholesterol was further reduced. Now statins do, in fact, lower cholesterol, but they are also anti-inflammatory, like aspirin, and may suppress the immune system. The ENHANCE result would tend to indicate that cholesterol reduction is not doing the heavy lifting.

B. Greg Brown, M.D., Ph.D., and Allen J. Taylor, "Does ENHANCE Diminish Confidence in Lowering LDL or in Ezetimibe?" NEJM 358;14, April 3, 2008

This is a bizarre paper of the relation between ezetimibe and cancer. In the abstract, results are stated as "Assignment to ezetimibe was associated with an increase in any new onset of cancer (101 patients in the active-treatment group vs. 65 in the control group) from several cancer sites." and "Among patients assigned to ezetimibe, there were more, albeit not significantly more, deaths from cancer." Yet the conclusion was, "The available results from these three trials do not provide credible evidence of any adverse effect of ezetimibe on rates of cancer." What—50% more cancer is not credible? Go reread your abstract, docs.

Richard Peto et al., "Analyses of Cancer Data from Three Ezetimibe Trials," NEJM 359;13 September 25, 2008

This is a 10-year-old result on the benefits of statins on women of all ages. With no heart disease, statins had no effect on heart disease mortality (and a negative effect otherwise). For women with heart disease, statins did reduce heart disease mortality, but not overall mortality. Conclusion: no women get any benefit from statins. This 10-year-old result is from the prestigious *Journal of the American Medical Association* (JAMA), and you would think this would not be taken lightly. Do you suppose statin prescriptions are still being written to women 10 years later? Remember the takeaway: Statins+Women=no benefit. How did this ever get to be a blockbuster drug?

Judith M. E. Walsh, Michael Pignone, "Drug Treatment of Hyperlipidemia in Women," JAMA, May 12, 2004—Vol 291, No. 18

A study to determine if statins reduce heart calcium. They didn't.

Y. Arad, L. Spadaro, M. Roth, D. Newstein, A. Guerci, "Treatment of Asymptomatic Adults With Elevated Coronary Calcium Scores With Atorvastatin, Vitamin C, and Vitamin E," Journal of the American College of Cardiology, Vol. 46, No. 1, 2005 ISSN 0735-1097/05/$30.00 doi:10.1016/j.jacc.2005.02.089

The statin results reported here were for people over 55 with moderate heart disease risk. Statins did not lower all-cause mortality or cardiac heart disease in this group.

The ALLHAT Officers and Coordinators for the ALLHAT Collaborative Research Group, "Major Outcomes in Moderately Hypercholesterolemic, Hypertensive Patients Randomized to Pravastatin vs Usual Care," JAMA, December 18, 2002—Vol 288, No. 23

This paper is a meta-study, which concluded statins showed no all-cause mortality benefit even with a high-risk group. The study covers 244,000 person-years.

Ray, et al., "Statins and All-Cause Mortality in High-Risk Primary Prevention," ARCH INTERN MED/VOL 170 (NO. 12), JUNE 28, 2010

For those at low risk, this paper finds that statins increase all-cause mortality with no benefit for heart disease:

Jackson, P., "Statins for primary prevention: at what coronary risk is safety assured?" Br J Clin Pharmacol, 52, 439±446

What is amazing is that this was even still being discussed in 2013.

J. Abramson lecturer, H. Rosenberg, N. Jewell, and J. Wright, "Should people at low risk of cardiovascular disease take a statin?" BMJ 2013;347:f6123

This almost completely covers it. So far, the only data we don't have is the effect on men under 55 who are neither low risk nor high risk. Will this group rescue statins from the jaws of complete uselessness? These men are the last hope: if they fail to cooperate and get some sort of overall benefit from statins, it will mean that the only benefit of the drug is to the pharmaceutical industry bottom line.

So what do statins do? Besides providing no overall benefit, they do at least three things we definitely do not want. First, they lower LDL particle size. This would tend to *increase* atherosclerosis. Here is this onerous result:

Choi, C., "Statins Do Not Decrease Small, Dense Low-Density Lipoprotein," Texas Heart Institute Journal Volume 37, Number 4, 2010

Statins increase the risk of adult onset diabetes almost 50% according to this paper:

Cederberg, H., "Increased risk of diabetes with statin treatment is associated with impaired insulin sensitivity and insulin secretion," Diabetologia (2015) 58:1109-1117"

Finally, it seems statins lower the efficacy of the immune system, the last thing we want:

Izadpanah, R., "The impact of statins on biological characteristics of stem cells provides anovel explanation for their pleiotropic beneficial and adverse clinical effects," Am J Physiol Cell Physiol 309: C522–C531, 2015

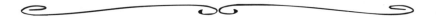

APPENDIX 3 - MEDICAL GADGETRY

We have evaluated several devices which could be useful for purposes of health monitoring. We do not explicitly endorse any of these devices nor are we in any way associated with any of the companies producing them. The remarks simply express our findings.

Heart Rate Monitor

This one is important for exercise. Specifically, it is important to know maximum heart rate, resting heart rate, and how much the heart rate goes down one minute after peak exercise. The "leader" in heart rate monitors is Polar. The monitors are a bit pricey and not awfully user-friendly.

The Polar system involves a chest strap, which some find uncomfortable. The chest strap transmits heart rate information to a watch, which displays it. You can have the simple display model for around $50, or one that can download general data to a PC for around $70. You can get one that will record every heartbeat for around $250. The software is Windows only.

Ideally, every heartbeat of an exercise session should be recorded. This can reveal any heart abnormalities that occur under stress. It seems that only the Polar model can do this.

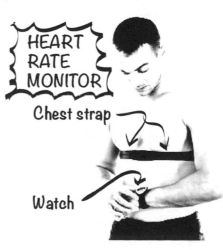

425

However, besides being pricey, this high-end model a bit cranky, and has a tendency to eat batteries. A better solution would be welcome.

There are other watches that measure heart rate without the strap. These are significantly cheaper. You have to touch the watch and wait five seconds or so. This isn't really adequate and can be inconvenient.

There are now Bluetooth chest straps that connect directly to smartphones. How well this works is unknown. Perhaps this is the way to go. Any readers who know about this, please chime in.

Glucose Level

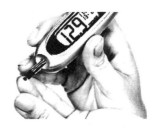

These are not very accurate. Two that were tested had a spread of around 20 mg/dl. This degree of accuracy may be fine for a diabetic's use, but it is rather useless for determining glucose to the accuracy we would want.

Cuff Blood Pressure

This device consists of a doctor's-office-like cuff that goes around the upper arm, and a machine that inflates it and makes the measurements. It measures systolic and diastolic blood pressure as well as pulse rate. The official name for this device is sphygmomanometer. The leader appears to be Omron, so we bought one. The cuff has to be positioned just so, but the machine will warn you if you don't have it right. It seems to be quite accurate and consistent. You see these same machines in doctors' offices. Street price: $65.

Keto-Sticks

If you are doing a very low-carb diet, you might be interested in knowing if you are in "ketosis." There is nothing wrong or dangerous about ketosis. If the liver cannot make enough glucose for the brain, it will make ketones as a backup supply. This is ketosis. The brain functions perfectly well on ketones. It may, in fact, function better, as very low-carb diets are sometimes recommended for people with Alzheimer's. Cost is around 10¢ per strip.

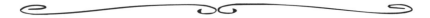

INDEX

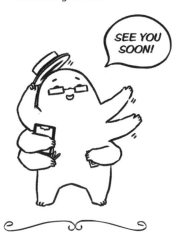

SEE YOU SOON!